Endoscopic Ear Surgery

Editors

MANUELA X. FINA
JUSTIN S. GOLUB
DANIEL J. LEE

OTOLARYNGOLOGIC CLINICS OF NORTH AMERICA

www.oto.theclinics.com

Consulting Editor
SUJANA S. CHANDRASEKHAR

February 2021 • Volume 54 • Number 1

ELSEVIER

1600 John F. Kennedy Boulevard ● Suite 1800 ● Philadelphia, Pennsylvania, 19103-2899

http://www.oto.theclinics.com

OTOLARYNGOLOGIC CLINICS OF NORTH AMERICA Volume 54, Number 1
February 2021 ISSN 0030-6665, ISBN-13: 978-0-323-75700-3

Editor: Stacy Eastman
Developmental Editor: Julia McKenzie

Otolaryngologic Clinics of North America (ISSN 0030-6665) is published bimonthly by Elsevier, Inc., 360 Park Avenue South, New York, NY 10010-1710. Months of issue are February, April, June, August, October, and December. Business and Editorial Offices: 1600 John F. Kennedy Blvd., Suite 1800, Philadelphia, PA 19103-2899. Customer Service Office: 6277 Sea Harbor Drive, Orlando, FL 32887-4800. Periodicals postage paid at New York, NY and additional mailing offices. Subscription prices are $437.00 per year (US individuals), $1278.00 per year (US institutions), $100.00 per year (US & Canadian student/resident), $559.00 per year (Canadian individuals), $1348.00 per year (Canadian institutions), $610.00 per year (international individuals), $1348.00 per year (international institutions), $270.00 per year (international student/resident). Foreign air speed delivery is included in all *Clinics*' subscription prices. All prices are subject to change without notice. POSTMASTER: Send address changes to *Otolaryngologic Clinics of North America*, Elsevier Health Sciences Division, Subscription Customer Service, 3251 Riverport Lane, Maryland Heights, MO 63043. **Telephone: 1-800-654-2452 (U.S. and Canada); 314-447-8871 (outside U.S. and Canada). Fax: 314-447-8029. E-mail: journalscustomerservice-usa@elsevier.com (for print support); journalsonlinesupport-usa@elsevier.com (for online support).**

Reprints. For copies of 100 or more of articles in this publication, please contact the Commercial Reprints Department, Elsevier Inc., 360 Park Avenue South, New York, NY 10010-1710. Tel.: 212-633-3874; Fax: 212-633-3820; E-mail: reprints@elsevier.com.

Otolaryngologic Clinics of North America is also published in Spanish by McGraw-Hill Interamericana Editores S.A., P.O. Box 5-237, 06500 Mexico D.F., Mexico.

Otolaryngologic Clinics of North America is covered in *MEDLINE/PubMed (Index Medicus), Current Contents/Clinical Medicine, Excerpta Medica, BIOSIS, Science Citation Index,* and *ISI/BIOMED.*

Contributors

CONSULTING EDITOR

SUJANA S. CHANDRASEKHAR, MD, FACS, FAAOHNS
Past President, American Academy of Otolaryngology–Head and Neck Surgery,
Secretary-Treasurer, American Otological Society, Partner, ENT & Allergy Associates,
LLP, Clinical Professor, Department of Otolaryngology–Head and Neck Surgery, Donald
and Barbara Zucker School of Medicine at Hofstra-Northwell, Hempstead, New York,
USA; Clinical Associate Professor, Department of Otolaryngology–Head and Neck
Surgery, Icahn School of Medicine at Mount Sinai, New York, New York, USA

EDITORS

MANUELA X. FINA, MD
Assistant Professor, Department of Otolaryngology–Head and Neck Surgery, University of
Minnesota, Minneapolis, Minnesota, USA

JUSTIN S. GOLUB, MD, MS
Associate Professor, Otology, Neurotology, and Skull Base Surgery, Department of
Otolaryngology–Head and Neck Surgery, Vagelos College of Physicians and Surgeons,
NewYork-Presbyterian/Columbia University Irving Medical Center, New York, New York,
USA

DANIEL J. LEE, MD, FACS
Associate Professor of Otolaryngology–Head and Neck Surgery, Harvard Medical School,
Director, Pediatric Otology and Neurotology, Director, Fellowship in Neurotology, Director,
Wilson Auditory Brainstem Implant (ABI) Program, Department of Otolaryngology,
Massachusetts Eye and Ear, Boston, Massachusetts, USA

JENNIFER A. VILLWOCK, MD, FAAOA
Department of Otolaryngology–Head and Neck Surgery, University of Kansas Medical
Center, Kansas City, Kansas, USA

AUTHORS

ZAINAB ARSIWALA, MD
Department of Otolaryngology, American Hospital Dubai, Dubai, United Arab Emirates

SAMUEL R. BARBER, MD
Resident Physician, Department of Otolaryngology–Head and Neck Surgery, University of
Arizona College of Medicine, Tucson, Arizona, USA

LUCA BIANCONI, MD
ENT Department, University Hospital of Verona, Verona, Italy

TICIANA CABRAL DA COSTA, MD
Cepto – Otos, Fortaleza, Brazil

SUJANA S. CHANDRASEKHAR, MD, FACS, FAAOHNS
Past President, American Academy of Otolaryngology–Head and Neck Surgery,
Secretary-Treasurer, American Otological Society, Partner, ENT & Allergy Associates,
LLP, Clinical Professor, Department of Otolaryngology–Head and Neck Surgery, Donald
and Barbara Zucker School of Medicine at Hofstra-Northwell, Hempstead, New York,
USA; Clinical Associate Professor, Department of Otolaryngology–Head and Neck
Surgery, Icahn School of Medicine at Mount Sinai, New York, New York, USA

DIVYA A. CHARI, MD
Department of Otolaryngology–Head and Neck Surgery, Massachusetts Eye and Ear,
Harvard Medical School, Boston, Massachusetts, USA

ALEXANDER CHERN, MD
Department of Otolaryngology–Head and Neck Surgery, Vagelos College of Physicians
and Surgeons, NewYork-Presbyterian/Columbia University Irving Medical Center,
Columbia University, New York, New York, USA

WHITNEY CHIAO, MD
Resident, Department of Otolaryngology, University of Minnesota, Minneapolis,
Minnesota, USA

DOUG CHIEFFE, MD
Resident, Department of Otolaryngology, University of Minnesota, Minneapolis,
Minnesota, USA

MICHAEL S. COHEN, MD
Assistant Professor, Department of Otolaryngology, Massachusetts Eye and Ear, Harvard
Medical School, Boston, Massachusetts, USA

MAURA K. COSETTI, MD
Associate Professor, Department of Otolaryngology–Head and Neck Surgery, Icahn
School of Medicine at Mount Sinai, Department of Otolaryngology–Head and Neck
Surgery, New York Eye and Ear Infirmary of Mount Sinai, New York, New York, USA

RAQUEL DE SOUSA LOBO FERREIRA QUERIDO, MD
Postdoctoral Research Scientist, Columbia University, Department of Otolaryngology–
Head and Neck Surgery, New York, New York, USA

MANUELA X. FINA, MD
Assistant Professor, Department of Otolaryngology–Head and Neck Surgery, University
of Minnesota, Minneapolis, Minnesota, USA

CANDACE A. FLAGG, MD
Department of Otolaryngology–Head and Neck Surgery, San Antonio Uniformed Services
Health Education Consortium, Ft. Sam Houston, Texas, USA

JUSTIN S. GOLUB, MD, MS
Associate Professor, Otology, Neurotology, and Skull Base Surgery, Department of
Otolaryngology–Head and Neck Surgery, Vagelos College of Physicians and Surgeons,
NewYork-Presbyterian/Columbia University Irving Medical Center, New York, New York,
USA

JANAINA GONÇALVES DA SILVA LEITE, MD, MS
Surgery Post-Graduation, Professor, Federal University of Ceará, Fortaleza, Brazil

SCOTT HARRISON, PhD
Director of Liberal Studies and Associate Vice President of Academic Affairs, Boston Architectural College, Boston, Massachusetts, USA

SANDRA HO, MD
Otolaryngologist, TJH Medical Services, P.C., Jamaica, New York, USA

JOHN W. HOUSE, MD
President, House Ear Institute, Clinical Professor of Otolaryngology, Geffen-UCLA Medical Center, Los Angeles, California, USA

BRANDON ISAACSON, MD, FACS
Professor and Co-Director of the Comprehensive Skull Base Program, Department of Otolaryngology, UT Southwestern Medical Center, Dallas, Texas, USA

NICHOLAS JUFAS, DISCIPLINE OF SURGERY, MBBS (Hons), BSc (Med), FRACS, MS
Clinical Associate Professor, Department of Otolaryngology–Head and Neck Surgery, Royal North Shore Hospital, Macquarie University, University of Sydney, Sydney Endoscopic Ear Surgery Research Group, Sydney, Australia

JUDITH S. KEMPFLE, MD
Resident, Senior Research Associate, Department of Otolaryngology, Massachusetts Eye and Ear, Harvard Medical School, Boston, Massachusetts, USA

DANIEL E. KILLEEN, MD
Neurotology Fellow, Department of Otolaryngology, UT Southwestern Medical Center, Dallas, Texas, USA

JONATHAN H.K. KONG, DISCIPLINE OF SURGERY, MBBS, FRACS, FRCS, MS
Clinical Associate Professor, Department of Otolaryngology–Head and Neck Surgery, Royal Prince Alfred Hospital, Macquarie University, University of Sydney, Sydney Endoscopic Ear Surgery Research Group, Sydney, Australia

ELLIOTT D. KOZIN, MD
Department of Otolaryngology, Massachusetts Eye and Ear Infirmary, Harvard Medical School, Boston, Massachusetts, USA

BARRY KRIEGSMAN, BS
University of Massachusetts Medical School, Worcester, Massachusetts, USA

DANIEL J. LEE, MD, FACS
Associate Professor of Otolaryngology–Head and Neck Surgery, Harvard Medical School, Director, Pediatric Otology and Neurotology, Director, Fellowship in Neurotology, Director, Wilson Auditory Brainstem Implant (ABI) Program, Department of Otolaryngology, Massachusetts Eye and Ear, Boston, Massachusetts, USA

MICHELLE F. LIU, MD, MPH, FAAOA
Department of Otolaryngology–Head and Neck Surgery, Walter Reed Military Medical Center, Bethesda, Maryland, USA

NAUMAN F. MANZOOR, MD
Department of Otolaryngology–Head and Neck Surgery, Case Western Reserve University, University Hospitals Cleveland Medical Center, Cleveland, Ohio, USA

DANIELE MARCHIONI, MD
Department of Otolaryngology–Head and Neck Surgery, Professor and Chair of the ENT Department, Azienda Ospedaliera Universitaria Integrata Verona, Verona, Italy
RACHEL McCABE, MD
Department of Otolaryngology, University of Minnesota, Minneapolis, Minnesota, USA

ALLISON NEWEY, DISCIPLINE OF RADIOLOGY, MBBS (hons), FRANZCR
Department of Radiology, Royal North Shore Hospital, University of Sydney, Sydney, Australia

JOAO FLAVIO NOGUEIRA, MD
Medicine Faculty, State University of Ceará, Fortaleza, Brazil

NIRMAL P. PATEL, DISCIPLINE OF SURGERY, MBBS (Hons), FRACS, MS
Clinical Associate Professor, Department of Otolaryngology–Head and Neck Surgery, Royal North Shore Hospital, Macquarie University, University of Sydney, Sydney Endoscopic Ear Surgery Research Group, Sydney, Australia

ALEXANDER G. PITMAN, DISCIPLINE OF RADIOLOGY, MBBS, B.Med.Sc, M. Med, FRACR
Clinical Associate Professor, Department of Radiology, Northern Beaches Hospital, University of Sydney, Sydney, Australia

NATASHA POLLAK, MD
Department of Otolaryngology–Head and Neck Surgery, Lewis Katz School of Medicine, Philadelphia, Pennsylvania, USA

MICHAL PREIS, MD
Department of Otolaryngology, Maimonides Medical Center, State University of New York Downstate, Brooklyn, New York, USA

ALICIA M. QUESNEL, MD
Department of Otolaryngology–Head and Neck Surgery, Massachusetts Eye and Ear, Harvard Medical School, Boston, Massachusetts, USA

SARAH E. RIDGE, BA
Department of Otolaryngology, Massachusetts Eye and Ear Infirmary, Harvard Medical School, Boston, Massachusetts, USA

ALEJANDRO RIVAS, MD
Department of Otolaryngology–Head and Neck Surgery, Case Western Reserve University, University Hospitals Cleveland Medical Center, Cleveland, Ohio, USA

EVETTE RONNER, BA
MD Degree Candidate, Dartmouth Geisel School of Medicine, Hanover, New Hampshire, USA

ALESSIA RUBINI, MD
Department of Otolaryngology–Head and Neck Surgery, Azienda Ospedaliera Universitaria Integrata Verona, Verona, Italy

ALEXANDER J. SAXBY, DISCIPLINE OF SURGERY, MB BChir, MA (Cantab.), FRACS
Clinical Associate Professor, Department of Otolaryngology–Head and Neck Surgery, Royal Prince Alfred Hospital, University of Sydney, Sydney Endoscopic Ear Surgery Research Group, Sydney, Australia

ZACHARY G. SCHWAM, MD
Resident Physician, Department of Otolaryngology–Head and Neck Surgery, Icahn School of Medicine at Mount Sinai, New York, New York, USA; Department of Otolaryngology–Head and Neck Surgery, New York Eye and Ear Infirmary of Mount Sinai, New York, New York, USA

RAHUL K. SHARMA, BS
Department of Otolaryngology–Head and Neck Surgery, Vagelos College of Physicians and Surgeons, NewYork-Presbyterian/Columbia University Irving Medical Center, Columbia University, New York, New York, USA

KUNAL R. SHETTY, MD
Department of Otolaryngology, Massachusetts Eye and Ear Infirmary, Harvard Medical School, Boston, Massachusetts, USA

LINDSAY SOBIN, MD
Division Director of Pediatric Otolaryngology and Assistant Professor, Department of Otolaryngology, University of Massachusetts Medical School, Worcester, Massachusetts, USA

DAVIDE SOLOPERTO, MD, PhD
Department of Otolaryngology–Head and Neck Surgery, Azienda Ospedaliera Universitaria Integrata Verona, Verona, Italy

SAGIT STERN SHAVIT, MD
Department of Otolaryngology–Head and Neck Surgery, Vagelos College of Physicians and Surgeons, NewYork-Presbyterian/Columbia University Irving Medical Center, Columbia University, New York, New York, USA

MUAAZ TARABICHI, MD
Tarabichi Stammberger Ear and Sinus Institute, Dubai, United Arab Emirates

KRISTEN L. YANCEY, MD
Department of Otolaryngology–Head and Neck Surgery, The Bill Wilkerson Center for Otolaryngology & Communication Sciences, South, Nashville, Tennessee, USA

Contents

> The introduction of the microscope to ear surgery by Wullstein has been a transformative event in ear surgery. The ability to visualize disease and anatomy has resulted in more effective surgery and better functional outcomes. Many surgical disciplines have adapted the endoscope as the instrument of choice to access and correct internal pathology without disruption of overlying tissue. Multiple discussions and attempts at using the endoscope in ear surgery over the years have culminated in the development of transcanal endoscopic ear surgery. This article discusses the integration of the endoscope into the practice of otologic surgery.

> A new era of surgical visualization and magnification is poised to disrupt the field of otology and neurotology. The once revolutionary benefits of the binocular microscope now are shared with rigid endoscopes and exoscopes. These 2 modalities are complementary. The endoscope improves visualization of the hidden recesses through the external auditory canal or canal-up mastoidectomy. The exoscope provides an immersive visual experience and superior ergonomics compared with binocular microscopy. Endoscopes and exoscopes are poised to disrupt the standard of care for surgical visualization and magnification in otology and neurotology.

> Middle ear anatomy and physiology is highly complex, yet familiarity is important to perform middle ear surgery and understand surgically relevant ventilation pathways of the ear compartments. The middle ear is divided into five subspaces: the mesotympanum, the retrotympanum posteriorly, the epitympanum superiorly, the protympanum anteriorly, and the hypotympanum inferiorly. The Eustachian tube plays a crucial role in maintaining middle ear aeration and atmospheric pressure. There are two independent aeration routes of the epitympanum. Thanks to the advent of the endoscope, this anatomic and physiologic knowledge has allowed one to

understand the pathophysiology of ear diseases, improving surgical concepts.

Endoscopic technology has matured over the past several decades. Ear surgeons have increasingly used endoscopy to address some of the limitations of operative microscopy. The wide field of view and high-resolution images provided by endoscopes allow for improved visualization of the tympanic cavity using minimally invasive surgical portals compared with the standard operative binocular microscope. The endoscope is becoming an essential tool in the otologist's armamentarium. In this article, the authors discuss rationale for endoscopic ear surgery, terminology and classification, surgical indications, essential equipment, surgical ergonomics, and practical steps to incorporate endoscopic ear surgery into practice.

Since its introduction into the field of otology in 1967 endoscopes are gaining acceptance in evaluation and treatment of middle ear disease. Endoscopes offer a wide field view enabling looking "around the corner" with reduced need for soft tissue and bone removal. Outcomes of middle ear surgery for cholesteatoma and need for second-look procedures are improving because of the addition of endoscopic evaluation. Trainee education using the endoscope improves knowledge of middle ear anatomy. The portability of the endoscopic unit allows performing ear surgery in remote locations.

Endoscopic ear surgery (EES) has become an integral part of otologic surgery. Training in EES involves learning fundamental techniques for endoscopic visualization, becoming proficient at one-handed dissection, mastering use of instruments designed for endoscopic ear surgery, and learning to optimize the operating room setup specifically for EES. Despite the steep learning curve, EES offers several advantages over the microscope for otologic procedures. With the rise in the demand for minimally invasive approaches, EES has a clear role in the future of otologic surgery. Identifying strategies to improve the training process of EES for the novice and experienced otolaryngologist is paramount.

Herein we provide a broad overview of the literature as it applies to endoscopic myringoplasty and type I tympanoplasty. Advantages and disadvantages of the endoscopic approach are reviewed for both the adult and pediatric populations and are compared with conventional microscopic techniques.

Endoscopic ear surgery is increasingly accepted as a primary modality for cholesteatoma surgery. A major advantage is the enhanced visualization of the middle ear in traditionally poorly accessible locations by the microscope. We discuss novel techniques for selective mastoid obliteration when a canal wall down mastoidectomy is necessary. Postoperatively, indications for non-echo planar diffusion-weighted imaging MRI versus second-look surgery are discussed. Finally, outcome data for endoscopic versus microscopic ear surgery are reviewed, which show equivalent outcomes regarding residual and recurrent disease, similar rates of complications, decreased pain, and shorter healing time.

 Video content accompanies this article at http://www.oto.theclinics.com.

The endoscopic approach to stapes surgery affords unique advantages but is not without its specific challenges. The following reviews the equipment and surgical steps required to perform endoscopic stapes surgery safely and effectively, highlighting tips and potential points of failure through a series of case examples.

Pathology of the lateral skull base poses a unique challenge for the surgeon. An intimate knowledge of the anatomy and the various approaches used for accessing pathology of the lateral skull base is critical. Three novel, minimally invasive, transcanal approaches for the management of lateral skull base pathology are described herein along with their respective indications, advantages, and disadvantages.

Image-guided navigation is well established for surgery of the brain and anterior skull base. Although navigation workstations have been used widely by neurosurgeons and rhinologists for decades, utilization in the lateral skull base (LSB) has been less due to stricter requirements for overall accuracy less than 1 mm in this region. Endoscopic approaches to the LSB facilitate minimally invasive surgeries with less morbidity, yet there are risks of injury to critical structures. With improvements in technology over the years, image-guided navigation for endoscopic LSB surgery can reduce operative time, optimize exposure for surgical corridors, and increase safety in difficult cases.

Sensorineural hearing loss is caused by irreversible loss of auditory hair cells and/or neurons and is increasing in prevalence. Hair cells and neurons do not regenerate after damage, but novel regeneration therapies based on small molecule drugs, gene therapy, and cell replacement strategies offer promising therapeutic options. Endogenous and exogenous regeneration techniques are discussed in context of their feasibility for hair cell and neuron regeneration. Gene therapy and treatment of synaptopathy represent promising future therapies. Minimally invasive endoscopic ear surgery offers a viable approach to aid in delivery of pharmacologic compounds, cells, or viral vectors to the inner ear for all of these techniques.

Endoscopic ear surgery (EES) has become increasingly popular due to numerous visualization benefits, including angled optics that enable the surgeon to see and dissect around corners. These advantages help the surgeon overcome the visualization limitations of microscopic ear surgery, reducing the need for a post-auricular incision and bone removal. This chapter discusses useful pearls and pitfalls of EES, technical tips and ergonomic strategies, so the learner can understand and solve common obstacles faced when learning EES and incorporate it into his or her practice.

Microscopic ear surgery (MES) has been used since the 1950s whereas endoscopic ear surgery (EES) was introduced in the mid-1990s. The advantages of MES should not be forgotten as surgeons turn their attention to new technology. These include depth perception, wide angle view, and the ability to operate with 2 hands. EES affords the ability to look around corners but needs a pristine field and is limited to single-handed surgery in a narrow field. Trainees should be taught both, and technique used should reflect the experience and abilities of the surgeon and the nature of the disease in the particular patient.

Endoscopic ear surgery has gained popularity in recent years, becoming standard practice in otology centers around the world as an adjunct to conventional microscopic surgery and as a sole tool for limited disease. During the last years, technical improvements and growing expertise in the handling of the endoscope allowed introducing an exclusive endoscopic approach to the middle ear, lateral skull base, middle cranial fossa, and posterior fossa/cerebellopontine angle pathologies. Endoscopic instrumentation, techniques, and knowledge have improved during the last few years, and in the future, endoscopic surgical techniques will gain even more importance in otologic surgery.

Special Article Series: Intentionally Shaping the Future of Otolaryngology

Over the course of the last century, otolaryngology–head and neck surgery has made significant medical and surgical advancements. Several of these efforts are credited to women and minorities despite their having faced systemic barriers to entering medical schools and the medical professions. This article highlights some of these pioneering doctors and their contributions to the field. Additionally, the current representation of women and minorities in otolaryngology residency programs and the gender and racial disparities in academic positions are reviewed. The need for mentorship during undergraduate medical education to improve diversity and inclusion within this surgical subspecialty is reinforced.

The medical community is no exception when it comes to structural racism and implicit bias, often present in dangerously subtle ways. To enter a residency program in which one is the only black person seems odd, especially considering the decades-long calls to action for increasing diversity. Unless the societal majority removes the blinders and steps out of their realm of privilege to address personal and systemic racist and biased views, progress will not be made. Sponsorship and inclusion of those Underrepresented in Medicine also lead to a stronger, more diverse academic community, and ultimately better health care.

OTOLARYNGOLOGIC CLINICS OF NORTH AMERICA

SERIES OF RELATED INTEREST

Facial Plastic Surgery Clinics
Available at: https://www.facialplastic.theclinics.com/

THE CLINICS ARE AVAILABLE ONLINE!
Access your subscription at:
www.theclinics.com

Foreword

Big Ear Surgeons Don't Need to Make Such Big Incisions

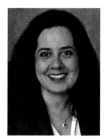

Sujana S. Chandrasekhar, MD, FACS, FAAOHNS
Consulting Editor

Physicians have always been trying to peer into places that are difficult to access. The first described endoscope was the *lichtleiter*, which used concave mirrors to reflect candlelight through an open tube into the esophagus, bladder, or rectum. It was created in 1806 by urologist Phillip Bozzini (**Fig. 1**). The first useable cystoscope was created in 1877 by urologist Maximilian Carl-Friedrich Nitze, using a series of lenses to increase magnification. He was also the first to place light inside the organ of interest to aid visualization. That system was modified into the first gastroscope by Johann von Mikulicz in 1880. Modern endoscopy was born with the introduction of the fiberoptic endoscope in the late 1950s.[1] During the 1960s and 1970s, gynecologists took the lead in the development of endoscopic surgery, while most of the surgical community continued to ignore the possibilities of the new technique. This was due in part to the introduction of ever more sophisticated drugs, the impressive results of intensive care medicine, and advances in anesthesia, which led to the development of more radical and extensive operations, or "major surgery."

I was told repeatedly during my training that, "Big surgeons make big incisions." This was for general surgery cases as well as in the head and neck. The idea that large problems require large incisions so deeply dominated surgical thinking that there was essentially no respect for surgeons attempting "key-hole" surgery. Working against this current, some general surgeons took up the challenge. In 1976, the Surgical Study Group on Endoscopy and Ultrasound was formed in Hamburg. Five years later, in the United States, the Society of American Gastrointestinal Endoscopic Surgeons was formed. The year 1987 saw the first issue of the journal *Surgical Endoscopy*, and in 1988, the First World Congress on Surgical Endoscopy took place in Berlin. The sweeping success of the "laparoscopic revolution" (1989–1990) marked the end of traditional open surgery and encouraged surgeons to consider new perspectives.

Otolaryngol Clin N Am 54 (2021) xvii–xix
https://doi.org/10.1016/j.otc.2020.10.002
0030-6665/21/© 2020 Published by Elsevier Inc.

By the 1990s, the breakthrough had been accomplished and endoscopy was incorporated into surgical thinking.[2]

In Otolaryngology, the adoption of functional endoscopic sinus surgery (FESS) was seen as a necessity, due to poor visualization and outcomes of current techniques. While the first attempt at nasal endoscopy is credited to Alfred Hirschman in 1901, and the term "sinuscopy" was introduced in 1925 by Maxwell Maltz, the creation of the Hopkins rod system in the 1960s was the major turning point in the field of sinonasal endoscopy. This new telescope design resulted in markedly enhanced light delivery and superior optical quality. In 1978, Walter Messerklinger wrote a landmark book on diagnostic endoscopy of the nose.[3] FESS was introduced into the United States in 1985, with avid adoption and simultaneous enhancements in computed tomography allowing the salient anatomical details to be understood.[4]

Dennis Poe introduced the concept of endoscope-assisted ear surgery in 1995.[5] The number of publications on the use of endoscopes in ear surgery increased from 6 in 1990 to an accumulated total of 451 in 2018, with an additional 132 articles on this subject published between January of 2019 and September of 2020. This technique can be used as an adjunct to microsurgery or as a stand-alone approach. With the burgeoning body of experience and literature, this is the right time for an entire issue of *Otolaryngologic Clinics of North America* to be devoted to this subject. Guest Editors Drs Manuela Fina, Justin Golub, and Daniel Lee have drawn from their varied experiences to assemble an outstanding collection of articles that detail to the reader how to start using endoscopes, where they are indicated and where one might take caution, and what the future might hold for this technology and for our patients. The articles are written generously, and the reader who takes in all of this information

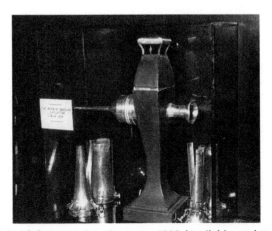

Fig. 1. The Bozzini Lichtleiter, Mainz, Germany, 1806 (Available at: https://www.facs.org/about-acs/archives/pasthighlights/bozzinihighlight. Accessed November 4, 2020)

will find themself well equipped to embark on the "big surgeons make small incisions" endoscopic ear surgery journey.

Sujana S. Chandrasekhar, MD, FACS, FAAOHNS
Consulting Editor
Otolaryngologic Clinics of North America
Past President
American Academy of Otolaryngology–
Head and Neck Surgery
Secretary-Treasurer
American Otological Society
Partner, ENT & Allergy Associates LLP
18 East 48th Street, 2nd Floor
New York, NY 10017, USA

Clinical Professor
Department of Otolaryngology–
Head and Neck Surgery
Zucker School of Medicine at Hofstra-Northwell
Hempstead, NY, USA

Clinical Associate Professor
Department of Otolaryngology–
Head and Neck Surgery
Icahn School of Medicine at Mount Sinai
New York, NY, USA

E-mail address:
ssc@nyotology.com

Website:
http://www.ears.nyc

REFERENCES

1. Morgenthal CB, Richards WO, Dunkin BJ, et al, SAGES Flexible Endoscopy Committee. The role of the surgeon in the evolution of flexible endoscopy. Surg Endosc 2007;21(6):838–53.
2. Litynski GS. Endoscopic surgery: the history, the pioneers. World J Surg 1999; 23(8):745–53.
3. Tajudeen BA, Kennedy DW. Thirty years of endoscopic sinus surgery: what have we learned? World J Otorhinolaryngol Head Neck Surg 2017;3(2):115–21.
4. Cashman EC, Macmahon PJ, Smyth D. Computed tomography scans of paranasal sinuses before functional endoscopic sinus surgery. World J Radiol 2011;3(8): 199–204.
5. Bollrill ID, Poe DS. Endoscopic ear surgery, ANS Papers. Am J Otol 1995;(16): 158–63.

Preface

A New Window to the Ear

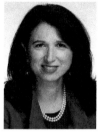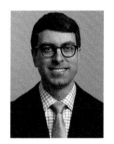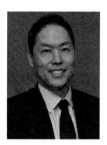

Manuela X. Fina, MD   Justin S. Golub, MD, MS   Daniel J. Lee, MD

Editors

Visualization is the key feature of safe and effective surgery. Until the introduction of the operative microscope in the mid 1900s, middle ear surgery was a crude endeavor, and ossicular reconstruction was merely an idea. Once the tympanic cavity could be illuminated and magnified, a new golden era of otologic surgery emerged.

For more than half a century, the operative microscope remained the near-exclusive visualization tool for otologists and neurotologists. However, fundamental limitations to microscope technology have hampered certain facets of middle ear surgery. The microscope optics remain outside the body at a distance to the target tissue. This means that the field of view, or how wide one can see, is defined by the narrowest part of the external auditory canal. A wide, panoramic view is unattainable. Attempting to compensate for this limitation demands extensive soft tissue or bone removal approaches. Certain parts of the middle ear, such as the sinus tympani, remain nearly impossible to see, except on the pages of anatomy textbooks.

The endoscope, long used in other subspecialties of otolaryngology, allows the optic to bypass the narrow waist of the ear canal and visualize the middle ear contents from only a couple centimeters away. The experience of using an endoscope is akin to stepping inside a room and moving freely with a magnifying glass, instead of standing at the door with binoculars.

In the past decade, interest in endoscopic ear surgery has grown tremendously. Procedures that previously required a postauricular approach can now be safely and efficiency performed transcanal with an endoscope. Hidden recesses have simply become recesses. For those at teaching centers, the magnificent anatomy of the middle ear can be optimally enjoyed by all in the operating room, not just the surgeon.

This issue of *Otolaryngologic Clinics of North America*, authored by the worldwide pioneers of endoscopic ear surgery, covers the full breadth of this exciting and growing field. Topics span from history to the future, from myringoplasty to skull base surgery, and from pearls to pitfalls. We hope that learning about this new technique will inspire

Otolaryngol Clin N Am 54 (2021) xxi–xxii
https://doi.org/10.1016/j.otc.2020.10.001
0030-6665/21/© 2020 Published by Elsevier Inc.

oto.theclinics.com

you to incorporate and master it in your own otologic practice. Like any surgical technology, the endoscope is just a tool. But put into the right hands, and the hands of many, we believe that the care of patients with otologic and neurotologic disease can be advanced.

Manuela X. Fina, MD
420 Delaware Street SE, MMC 396
Minneapolis, MN 55455, USA

Justin S. Golub, MD, MS
180 Fort Washington Avenue, HP8
New York, NY 10032, USA

Daniel J. Lee, MD
243 Charles Street
Boston, MA 02114, USA

E-mail addresses:
finax003@umn.edu (M.X. Fina)
justin.golub@columbia.edu (J.S. Golub)
daniel_lee@meei.harvard.edu (D.J. Lee)

History of Endoscopic Ear Surgery

Muaaz Tarabichi, MD[a],*, Zainab Arsiwala, MD[b]

KEYWORDS

- Otoendoscopy • Endoscopic ear surgery • History • Chronic ear surgery
- Endoscopy • Cholesteatoma

KEY POINTS

- The ability to visualize disease and anatomy has resulted in more effective surgery and better functional outcomes.
- Many surgical disciplines have adapted the endoscope as the instrument of choice to access and correct internal pathology without disruption of overlying tissue.
- Multiple discussions and attempts at using the endoscope in ear surgery over the years have culminated in the development of transcanal endoscopic ear surgery (TEES).

HISTORY OF ENDOSCOPIC EAR SURGERY

It is hard to separate the history of endoscopic ear surgery (EES) from the three-decade-long timeline of the process of integrating the endoscope into ear surgery. What constitutes EES is sometimes difficult to define in clinical practice. Throughout the early years of advocating EES to the otologic community, I was always faced with the argument that "we too are using the endoscope." The concept of EES as understood and practiced by the International Working Group On Endoscopic Ear Surgery (IWGEES) goes far beyond the simple idea of integrating the endoscope to selective tasks of operative otology. An attempt to define this issue was made by Cohen and colleagues[1] when they introduced a classification system to define EES:

1. The diagnostic and documentation aspect of the endoscope (Cohen class 1) initially had the most widely recognized role. Transtympanic middle ear endoscopy was initially reported by Nomura[2] and Takahashi and colleagues.[3] Poe and Bottrill[4] used transtympanic endoscopy for the confirmation of perilymphatic fistula and the identification of other middle ear pathologic conditions. Kakehata and

Financial Disclosures: None.
[a] Tarabichi Stammberger Ear and Sinus Institute, PO Box 73101, 143 Umm Suqiem Road, Dubai, United Arab Emirates; [b] Department of Otolaryngology, American Hospital Dubai, PO Box 5566, Oud Metha, Dubai, United Arab Emirates
* Corresponding author.
E-mail address: mtarabichi@ahdubai.com

Otolaryngol Clin N Am 54 (2021) 1–9
https://doi.org/10.1016/j.otc.2020.09.002
0030-6665/21/© 2020 Elsevier Inc. All rights reserved.

coworkers[5–7] used microendoscopy and transtympanic endoscopy for evaluation of conductive hearing loss and inspection of retraction pockets.

2. The second phase (Cohen class 2a) involved the use of the endoscope to assist in removal of disease, as an adjunct to the main workhorse, the microscope. Thomassin and colleagues[8] reported on operative ear endoscopy for mastoid cavities and designed an instrument set to be used for that purpose. Badr-el-Dine and coworkers[9] and El-Meselaty and coworkers[10] reported on the value of endoscopy as an adjunct in cholesteatoma surgery and documented a reduced risk of recurrence when the endoscope was used. The reduction in residual disease was further confirmed by Yung[11] and Ayache and coworkers.[12] Abdel Baki and coworkers[13] reported on using endoscopic technique to evaluate disease within the sinus tympani. Mattox[14] reported on endoscopy-assisted surgery of the petrous apex. Magnan and Sanna,[15] Bader-el-Dine and El-Garem,[16–18] and Rosenberg and colleagues[19] reviewed the role of the endoscope in neurotologic procedures. McKennan[20] described the second-look endoscopic inspection of mastoid cavities that was achieved through a small postauricular incision.

3. The third wave involved the advent of transcanal EES (TEES), using the endoscope as the main workhorse in ear surgery and the ear canal as the main access point (Cohen class 2B and 3). The author adopted this approach in his clinical practice in 1992 and published an initial report in 1997 on his experience with endoscopic cholesteatoma surgery,[21] then tympanoplasty, and stapes surgery.[22] Before that, there was one earlier report in 1992 of endoscopic myringoplasty from El-Guindy.[23] In 2007, Stephane Ayache (France) proposed "the creation of an international society of otoendoscopy" (later to be named IWGEES) to advocate and collaborate for further development of this approach to ear surgery. The founding members included Muaaz Tarabichi (UAE), Daniele Marchioni (Italy), Livio Presutti (Italy), Dave Pothier (Canada), Mohamed Badr-el-Dine (Egypt), and Seiji Kakehata (Japan). The IWGEES has grown to a substantial membership representing almost all countries and has been instrumental in standardizing, teaching, and spreading of the technique.

We believe that the previously mentioned patterns of use of the endoscope represent the process of integrating the endoscope into ear surgery rather than different approaches or techniques. Kapadiya and Tarabichi[24] performed a comprehensive literature search to identify abstracts that reported on the use of the endoscope in otology. They showed that TEES seems to be the area emerging with most of the research interest and the interest in the ancillary use of endoscope as adjunct to routinely performed microscopic procedures seems to have peaked (**Fig. 1**). Questionnaire data reported in the same paper from US-based otologists and performed 8 years apart confirm these findings and document the decreased interest in the use of the endoscope as an ancillary instrument to the microscope and increased recognition of TEES as viable option (**Fig. 2**).

The arguments for and against the endoscope have been diverse and heated. There is an emerging concept that basic advantages of the endoscope are better alignment of surgical access with underlying anatomy, disease process, and ventilation.

ALIGNING SURGICAL ACCESS WITH UNDERLYING ANATOMY AND DISEASE PROCESS

Acquired cholesteatoma is usually a manifestation of advanced retraction of the tympanic membrane that occurs when the sac advances into the tympanic cavity

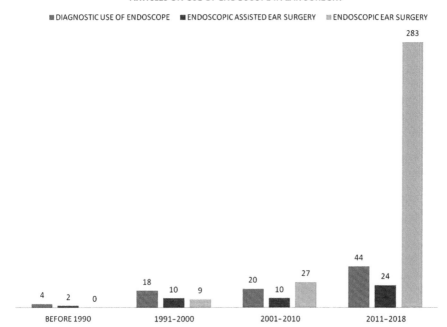

Fig. 1. Number of publications over the past four decades categorized by the pattern of endoscope use in ear surgery. (*From* Kapadiya M, Tarabichi M. An overview of endoscopic ear surgery in 2018. Laryngoscope Investig Otolaryngol. 2019 May 24;4(3):365-373.)

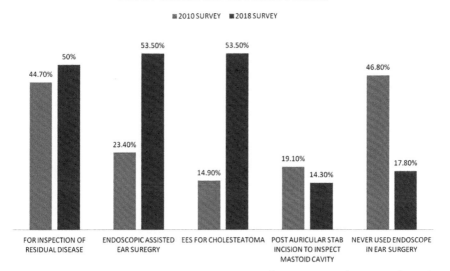

Fig. 2. Survey results in 2010 versus 2018 in response to the question "When using the endoscope, which technique do you apply?" There is a trend toward more endoscopic experience, particularly for dissection. (*From* Kapadiya M, Tarabichi M. An overview of endoscopic ear surgery in 2018. Laryngoscope Investig Otolaryngol. 2019 May 24;4(3):365-373.)

proper and then into its extensions, such as the sinus tympani, the facial recess, the hypotympanum, and the attic.[25] Only in advanced cases does a cholesteatoma progress further to reach the mastoid cavity proper. Most surgical failures associated with a postauricular approach seem to occur within the tympanic cavity and its hard-to-reach extensions rather than in the mastoid.[26,27] Therefore, the most logical approach to the excision of a cholesteatoma involves transcanal access to the tympanic membrane and tympanic cavity and the subsequent step-by-step pursuit of the sac as it passes through the middle ear. Mainstream ear surgery has usually involved the mastoid and the postauricular approaches because operating with the microscope through the external auditory canal allows for limited surgical field. The view during microscopic surgery is defined and limited by the narrowest segment of the ear canal (**Fig. 3**). This basic limitation has forced surgeons to create a parallel port through the mastoid to gain access to the attic, the facial recess, and the hypotympanum (**Fig. 4**). In contrast, transcanal operative endoscopy bypasses the narrow segment of the ear canal and provides a wide view that enables surgeons to look "around the corner." Even with a zero-degree endoscope, a structure like the facial recess becomes widely accessible for inspection and removal of disease (**Fig. 5**). Rediscovering the ear canal as the access port to the tympanic cavity is the main story and the main advantage of EES. **Fig. 6** shows a transcanal endoscopic view of the tympanic cavity with the center of endoscopic field aligning with the cochleariform process,

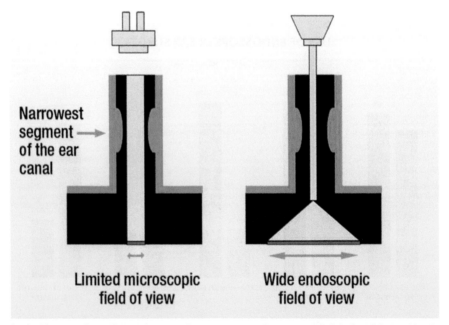

Narrowest segment of the ear canal

Limited microscopic field of view

Wide endoscopic field of view

Fig. 3. The view from the microscope during transcanal surgery is defined and limited by the narrowest segment of the ear canal. In contrast, the endoscope bypasses this narrow segment and provides a very wide view that allows the surgeon to "look around corners," even when the zero-degree scope is used.

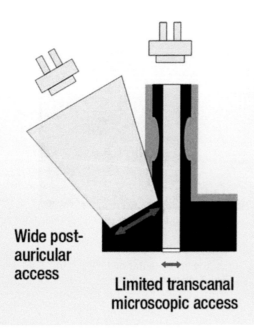

Fig. 4. The limited view provided by the microscope during transcanal procedures has forced surgeons to perform postauricular mastoidectomy, in which a port parallel to the attic is created after a considerable amount of healthy bone has been removed to enable anterior keyhole access to the attic and access to facial recess and posterior mesotympanum.

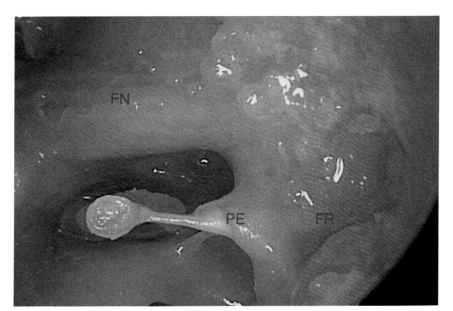

Fig. 5. Left ear. Transcanal endoscopic view after minor removal of bone; the facial recess (FR) is shallow and more of a flat depression, located at about the same level as the pyramidal eminence (PE) and the vertical segment of facial nerve (FN).

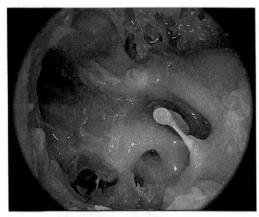

Fig. 6. Transcanal wide view of the tympanic cavity with the cochleariform process at the center of the visual field.

a structure that usually marks the most anterior limit of the field during micro-scopic transcanal surgery. **Fig. 7** shows multiplanar images of a normal middle ear cleft with the cochleariform process being the anatomic center of the tym-panic cavity. Therefore, transcanal endoscopic access aligns surgical access

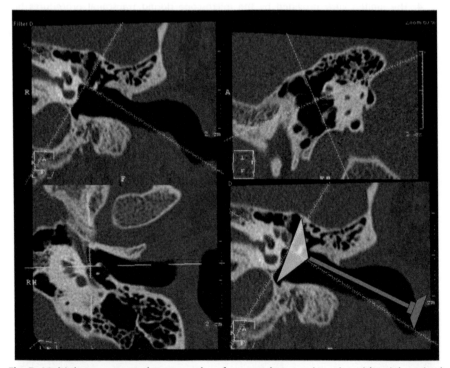

Fig. 7. Multiplanar computed tomography of a normal tympanic cavity with axial, sagittal, and coronal views demonstrating that the cochleariform process (intersection of *green lines*) is the anatomic center of the cavity, which is aligned with what is seen endoscopically in **Fig. 6**.

with anatomic reality and allows wide access to the tympanic cavity, the birth-place of chronic ear disease.

ALIGNING SURGICAL ACCESS WITH VENTILATION

Microscopic access through the mastoid is focused on the most posterior part of the air cell system, and therefore, the most downstream in terms of ventilation. The upstream parts of the ventilation system, the Eustachian tube isthmus, pro-tympanum, anterior mesotympanum, and the tympanic isthmus are barely visual-ized with the posterior, mastoid-based, microscopic approach. The endoscope allows access to be oriented toward the anterior upstream areas of the ventilation system, therefore aligning ventilation with surgical access as demonstrated in **Fig. 8**.

Chronic ear surgery has always revolved around removing disease and regaining function without much attention to the pathophysiologic process underlying the dis-ease. Because much of the obstruction sites lie anteriorly, out of reach of traditional instruments, it is always assumed that time and age have resolved any obstruction.[28] Failures in chronic ear surgery have been shown to correlate to persistent ventilation failure and Eustachian tube dysfunction.[29] The more anterior approach of EES has provided access to the "twin isthmus" of the temporal bone air cell system: the tym-panic isthmus and the Eustachian tube isthmus as a possible source of ventilation failure.

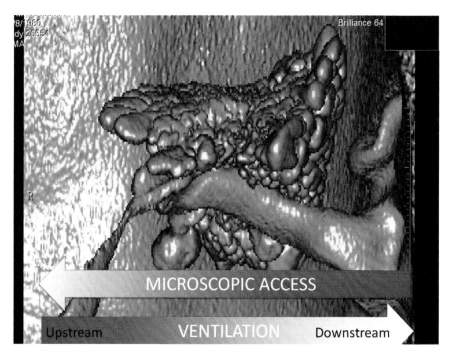

Fig. 8. Three-dimensional reconstruction of the air spaces within the temporal bone derived from a Valsalva computed tomography of a normal temporal bone. Note that microscopic access is misaligned with the most important areas of ventilation, the upstream part of the air cell system.

SUMMARY

TEES has transformed certain aspects of chronic ear surgery. The ability to better match the surgical access with the disease process should provide more room for improving the care of the chronic ear patient. The field is attracting the interest of young clinical investigators and industry and we should see further developments in the future.

CLINICS CARE POINTS

- Attempts at incorporating endoscopy in clinical practice have been ongoing for the last 40 years.
- Endoscopic Ear Surgery is increasingly the subject for research and publication in Otolarygology.
- Endoscopic transcanal access to many areas of the middle ear is far superior to existing microscopic means.

CONFLICT OF INTEREST

None. This research did not receive any specific grant from funding agencies in the public, commercial, or not-for-profit sectors.

REFERENCES

1. Cohen MS, Basonbul RA, Barber SR, et al. Development and validation of an endoscopic ear surgery classification system. Laryngoscope 2018;128(4):967-70.
2. Nomura Y. Effective photography in otolaryngology-head and neck surgery: endoscopic photography of the middle ear. Otolaryngol Head Neck Surg 1982;90:395-8.
3. Takahashi H, Honjo I, Fujita A, et al. Transtympanic endoscopic findings in patients with otitis media with effusion. Arch Otolaryngol Head Neck Surg 1990;116:1186-9.
4. Poe DS, Bottrill ID. Comparison of endoscopic and surgical explorations for perilymphatic fistulas. Am J Otol 1994;15:735-8.
5. Kakehata S, Futai K, Sasaki A, et al. Endoscopic transtympanic tympanoplasty in the treatment of conductive hearing loss: early results. Otol Neurotol 2006;27(1):14-9.
6. Kakehata S, Hozawa K, Futai K, et al. Evaluation of attic retraction pockets by microendoscopy. Otol Neurotol 2005;26(5):834-7.
7. Kakehata S, Futai K, Kuroda R, et al. Office-based endoscopic procedure for diagnosis in conductive hearing loss cases using OtoScan Laser-Assisted Myringotomy. Laryngoscope 2004;114(7):1285-9.
8. Thomassin JM, Korchia D, Doris JM. Endoscopic-guided otosurgery in the prevention of residual cholesteatomas. Laryngoscope 1993;103:939-43.
9. Badr-el-Dine M. Value of ear endoscopy in cholesteatoma surgery. Otol Neurotol 2002;23:631-5.
10. El-Meselaty K, Badr-El-Dine M, Mandour M, et al. Endoscope affects decision making in cholesteatoma surgery. Otolaryngol Head Neck Surg 2003;129:490-6.
11. Yung MW. The use of middle ear endoscopy: has residual cholesteatoma been eliminated? J Laryngol Otol 2001;115:958-61.
12. Ayache S, Tramier B, Strunski V. Otoendoscopy in cholesteatoma surgery of the middle ear. What benefits can be expected? Otol Neurotol 2008;29(8):1085-90.

13. Abdel Baki F, Badr-El-Dine M, El Saiid I, et al. Sinus tympani endoscopic anatomy. Otolaryngol Head Neck Surg 2002;127:158–62.
14. Mattox DE. Endoscopy-assisted surgery of the petrous apex. Otolaryngol Head Neck Surg 2004;130:229–41.
15. Magnan J, Sanna M. Endoscopy in neuro-otology. Stuttgart (Germany): Georg Thieme Verlag; 2003.
16. Badr-El-Dine M, El-Garem HF, Talaat AM, et al. Endoscopically assisted minimally invasive microvascular decompression of hemifacial spasm. Otol Neurotol 2002; 23:122–8.
17. El-Garem HF, Badr-El-Dine M, Talaat AM, et al. Endoscopy as a tool in minimally invasive trigeminal neuralgia surgery. Otol Neurotol 2002;23:132–5.
18. Badr-El-Dine M, El-Garem HF, El-Ashram Y, et al. Endoscope assisted minimal invasive microvascular decompression of hemifacial spasm. Abstracts of the 9th International Facial Nerve Symposium. Otol Neurotol Suppl 2002;23(3):68–72.
19. Rosenberg SI, Silverstein H, Willcox TO, et al. Endoscopy in otology and neuro-tology. Am J Otol 1994;15:168–72.
20. McKennan KX. Endoscopic 'second look' mastoidoscopy to rule out residual epi-tympanic/mastoid cholesteatoma. Laryngoscope 1993;103:810–4.
21. Tarabichi M. Endoscopic management of acquired cholesteatoma. Am J Otol 1997;18(5):544–9.
22. Tarabichi M. Endoscopic middle ear surgery. Ann Otol Rhinol Laryngol 1999; 108(1):39–46.
23. El-Guindy A. Endoscopic transcanal myringoplasty. J Laryngol Otol 1992;106(6): 493–5.
24. Kapadiya M, Tarabichi M. An overview of endoscopic ear surgery in 2018. Laryn-goscope Investig Otolaryngol 2019;4(3):365–73.
25. Tos M. Modification of combined-approach tympanoplasty in attic cholesteatoma. Arch Otolaryngol 1982;108:772–8.
26. Sheehy JL, Brackmann DE, Graham MD. Cholesteatoma surgery: residual and recurrent disease. A review of 1,024 cases. Ann Otol Rhinol Laryngol 1977;86: 451–62.
27. Glasscock ME, Miller GW. Intact canal wall tympanoplasty in the management of cholesteatoma. Laryngoscope 1976;86:1639–57.
28. Linstrom CJ, Carol AS, Arie R, et al. Eustachian tube endoscopy in patients with chronic ear disease. Laryngoscope 2000;110:1884–9.
29. Sato H, Hajime N, Iwao H, et al. Eustachian tube function in tympanoplasty. Acta Otolaryngol 1990;110:9–12.

Heads-up Surgery

Endoscopes and Exoscopes for Otology and Neurotology in the Era of the COVID-19 Pandemic

Sarah E. Ridge, BA, Kunal R. Shetty, MD, Daniel J. Lee, MD*

KEYWORDS

- Endoscopic ear surgery • Exoscopic ear surgery • Microscope • Ergonomics
- Minimally-invasive • Mastoidectomy • PPE • Aerosol generating procedure

KEY POINTS

- Traditional binocular microscopy provides excellent image quality, magnification, and illumination and 2-handed dissection.
- Binocular microscopy offer a heads-down approach that results in compromised ergonomics and a narrow field of view when operating in a small corridor.
- Endoscopes offers superior ergonomics with a heads-up approach that enhances visual access through the external auditory canal and decreases the need for mastoidectomy.
- Exoscopes also offer a heads-up approach and complement the endoscope. Exoscopes are a viable alternative to binocular microscopy to deliver comparable image quality, an immersive visual experience, and two handed dissection.
- Full eye-covering personal protection equipment, such as face shields and powered air-purifying respirator hoods, can be used with endoscopes and exoscopes to offer risk mitigation during the coronavirus disease pandemic without compromising visualization.

INTRODUCTION

The field of otology and neurotology requires dissection at high magnification to ensure successful management of middle ear and mastoid disease and preservation of anatomic structures. The ideal method of visualization should provide an unobstructed wide field of view and excellent ergonomics **Box 1**. Although the binocular microscope remains the cornerstone of surgical illumination and magnification, advances in video technology have enabled the use of heads-up techniques offered by endoscopes and exoscopes (**Fig. 1**). The endoscope is ideal when utilizing small surgical corridors to access the hidden recesses of the middle ear. The digital

Department of Otolaryngology, Massachusetts Eye and Ear Infirmary, Harvard Medical School, 243 Charles Street, Boston, MA 02114, USA
* Corresponding author.
E-mail address: daniel_lee@meei.harvard.edu

Otolaryngol Clin N Am 54 (2021) 11–23
https://doi.org/10.1016/j.otc.2020.09.024
0030-6665/21/© 2020 Elsevier Inc. All rights reserved.

Box 1
Timeline—A brief history of endoscopes in otolaryngology

1960s: Walter Messerklinger in Austria performed endoscopic sinus surgery using a modified cystoscope under local anesthesia.

1967: Bruce Mer described middle ear anatomy using otoendoscopy in cadavers, animal models, and living patients.[53]

1982: Yasuya Nomura used a needle otoscope to explore the middle ear using myringotomy in living patients.[54]

1985 to 1987: Rhinologist David Kennedy and radiologist Simion Zinreich developed computed tomography parameters for sinus imaging and originated functional endoscopic sinus surgery at Johns Hopkins University.[5,6,55–57]

1990s: Jean-Marc Thomassin, Dennis Poe, and Muaaz Tarabichi described new otologic applications of endoscopy, including management of cholesteatomas and perilymphatic fistulas.[58–67]

1995: First workshop on otoendoscopy in the United States, at Saint Louis university (directed by Eric Sargent, featuring Dennis Poe and Robert Jackler)[68]

2008: International Working Group on Endoscopic Ear Surgery established

2010: First EES course in Europe, Malta (featuring Schembri Mismayer, Livio Presutti, Daniele Marchioni, and Stephane Ayache)

2012: First workshop on EES in the United States, Saint Louis University (chairs: Anthony Mikulec and Daniel Lee)

2015: 1st World Congress on Endoscopic Ear Surgery, Dubai, UAE (chair: Muaaz Tarabichi)

2017: 2nd World Congress on Endoscopic Ear Surgery, Bologna, Italy (chairs: Livio Presutti and Daniele Marchioni)

2019: 3rd World Congress on Endoscopic Ear Surgery, Boston, Massachusetts (chairs: Michael Cohen, Daniel Lee, Alicia Quesnel)

2022: 4th World Congress on Endoscopic Ear Surgery will be held in Kyoto, Japan (chair: Seiji Kakehata)

---

extracorporeal scope, or exoscope, is complementary to the endoscope and was designed to replace the operating microscope. The exoscope can be used for transcanal, transmastoid, and craniotomy procedures requiring two handed dissection. When compared with the microscope, these two heads-up modalities provide an immersive surgical view, greater depth of field, improved ergonomics, and enhanced compatibility with personal protective equipment (PPE).

DISCUSSION
Limitations of the Operating Microscope

The traditional binocular microscope greatly advanced the field of otology and neurotology by providing a stable, illuminated, magnified, and 3-dimensional (3-D) view of ear and skull base anatomy. The ability to perform two handed dissection under high magnification facilitated more accurate manipulation of delicate ear structures, leading to the refinement of procedures, such as the tympanoplasty and stapedectomy.[1]

The surgical microscope consists of a binocular head with two adjustable eyepieces, an objective lens, and an illuminator (see **Fig. 1**). This system is attached to a suspension arm and a stand, making the system bulky. Improvements in microscopic technology also have taken a toll on the stack height of the binocular head, compromising ergonomics for the user (**Fig. 2**A). The stack obstructs the view of

	Microscope	2-D ENDOSCOPE	3-D EXOSCOPE
3-D Image	✓		✓
Focal distance	20–50 cm	1–3 cm	20–50 cm
Visualization	Line of Sight	HD/4K Video	HD/4K Video + 3-D Glasses

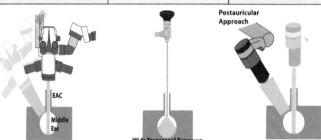

Fig. 1. General specifications for binocular microscope, 2-D Hopkins rod telescope, and 3-D exoscope. The microscope and exoscope are used with a line of sight approach, with similar focal distances and true depth perception, allowing the user to operate with both hands. In contrast, the 2-D endoscope has a much shorter focal distance but can be used in small corridors to provide a high contrast wide-angle view with enhanced depth of field. EAC, external auditory canal. (*Adapted from* Smith S, Kozin ED, Kanumuri V V., et al. Initial Experience with 3-Dimensional Exoscope-Assisted Transmastoid and Lateral Skull Base Surgery. Otolaryngol - Head Neck Surg (United States). 2019; with permission.)

the surgical field for operating room (OR) personnel and requires a static posture with the neck flexed and arms stretched forward (**see Fig. 2**A). The optical system also is far from the surgical field, and magnification and illumination are needed to maximize image quality. Field of view and depth of field, however, decrease as magnification

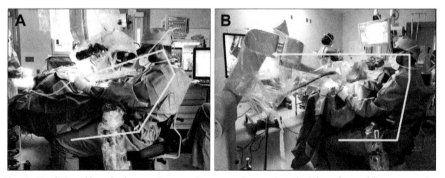

Fig. 2. Traditional heads-down microscopic surgery is associated with unfavorable ergonomics. Arrows illustrate the posture of the surgeon and the corresponding line of sight when using each device. (*A*) Binocular microscopy, even with armrests, Trendelenburg positioning, and 250-mm focal length places strain on the neck, shoulders and back during prolonged dissection. The stack height of the microscope increases the distance between the end of the oculars to the ear, requiring outstretched arms. (*B*) Heads-up exoscopic surgery results in a relaxed posture and enhanced body mechanics. (*Adapted from* Smith S, Kozin ED, Kanumuri V V., et al. Initial Experience with 3-Dimensional Exoscope-Assisted Transmastoid and Lateral Skull Base Surgery. Otolaryngol - Head Neck Surg (United States). 2019; with permission.)

increases, and anatomic boundaries can obstruct light transmission. Consequently, the microscope has a shallow depth of field and narrow field of view, necessitating soft tissue and bony dissection to overcome these limitations. These constraints necessitate frequent adjustments intraoperatively. A 2015 study found that neurosurgeons used the microscope handgrip controls to change focal length, zoom, or position an average of once every 114 seconds, which accounted for 8% of the total case time. Remarkably, surgeons modified several behaviors in order to prevent loss of alignment and further need for microscopic readjustment, such as avoiding looking away from the oculars during handoffs, maintaining unergonomic body postures, and even operating using a nonfocused view or at the edge of the field of view.[2]

Endoscopes

The endoscope has become an essential tool in many otolaryngologic disciplines, including rhinology. In otology and neurotology, endoscopes have advanced from an observational instrument (otoendoscopy) to an operative one (endoscopic ear surgery [EES]) at a growing number of centers. Although there has been a rapid increase in the adoption of EES within the past decade,[3] the endoscope continues to generate debate among surgeons as a primary modality for performing middle ear surgery. Many of the arguments raised against EES match those made by rhinologists when the Hopkins rod telescope was introduced for sinus surgery.[4–6]

The most common endoscope used in EES is the Hopkins rod telescope (see **Fig. 1**). The endoscope can be used with the naked eye or coupled to a standard definition, high-definition, or 4K video camera. A flexible fiberoptic cable is attached to the endoscope to provide radiant energy from a halogen, xenon, or light-emitting diode (LED) light source. The system integrates with proprietary components that enable transmission of a live video feed to a monitor (mounted on a tower or surgical boom) as well as recording of imaging data for documentation.[7] This feature allows all participants to (1) share an operative view with the surgeon, improving both teaching and coordination with OR personnel, and (2) allows the surgeon to sit comfortably in an ergonomic heads-up posture.

Endoscopes have a short focal length and deliver light through small openings, bypassing visual obstructions (see **Fig. 1**). These features make the endoscope an ideal choice for transcanal dissection, especially in patients with small or tortuous canals. Additionally, the wide-angle view, angled optics, and high-contrast light source allow surgeons to look around corners,[8] gaining visual access to hidden recesses (**Fig. 3**). Importantly, this reduces the need for soft tissue retraction and bony dissection.[3] Finally, mastoidectomy is an aerosol-generating procedure (AGP),[9,10] and surgical aerosols can carry viral pathogens.[11] Endoscopes play an important role in risk mitigation during the era of the coronavirus disease (COVID-19) pandemic, reducing the need for mastoidectomy.

Transcanal EES (TEES) is an ideal approach for the management of cholesteatoma, because the pathology can be followed along the anatomic growth pattern from the tympanic membrane to the tympanic cavity and hidden recesses.[3] A scope holder is not recommended because motion parallax creates a sense of depth perception when using a 2-D video camera system. TEES diminishes the need for a canal wall–up mastoidectomy in some cases[12] and facilitates en bloc removal of cholesteatoma, with an improved chance of ossicular preservation[13] and decreased rates of residual and recurrent disease.[14] In studies comparing TEES to microscopic surgery for cholesteatoma, results have shown comparable or improved rates of control,[15] improved quality of life, decreased surgical morbidity, shorter healing time, and less postoperative pain due to avoidance of postauricular incisions.[16] TEES for tympanoplasty

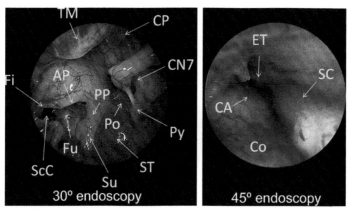

Fig. 3. Transcanal endoscopic tympanotomy, left ear. Endoscopes provide a wide-angle view and greater depth of field with minimal soft tissue and bony dissection compared with binocular microscopy. (*Left panel*) A 30° endoscopic view of the left ear mesotympanum and retrotympanum. (*Right panel*) A 45° endoscopic view of the protympanum. AP, anterior pillar; CA, carotid artery; CN7, facial nerve; Co, cochlea; CP, cochleariform process; ET, eEustachian tube; Fi, finiculus; Fu, fustis; Po, ponticulus; PP, posterior pillar; Py, pyramidal process. SC, semicanal; ScC, subcochlear canaliculus; ST, sinus tympani; Su, subiculum; TM, tympanic membrane.

results in similar outcomes compared with microscopic approaches.[17,18] Endoscopic-assisted stapedectomy in some series was associated with decreased chorda tympani injury and postoperative pain along with comparable audiological outcomes and operative times.[17]

In cases where a postauricular approach cannot be avoided, an endoscopic-assisted transmastoid approach can be used (**Fig. 4**). Transmastoid EES (TMEES) requires a smaller mastoidectomy compared with a traditional microscopic transmastoid approach. In the treatment of extensive cholesteatoma extending to the antrum, the use of TMEES has been shown to decrease the need for a canal wall–down mastoidectomy.[15]

The endoscope is an invaluable tool for the management of neurotology patients. Underwater endoscopic-assisted dissection can be used with a transmastoid approach for the management of superior canal dehiscence.[19] Angled endoscopes aid in the identification of subtle superior canal defects located along a down-sloping tegmen following middle fossa craniotomy that otherwise escape detection when using the microscope.[20] Fully endoscopic resection of vestibular schwannomas has been reported to be a safe and effective means for hearing preservation and requires a smaller cranial opening and less manipulation of the cerebellum and other structures.[21] Finally, the endoscope can be utilized to visualize the posterior fossa using a transmastoid craniotomy (**Fig. 5** for labyrinth-sparing resection of endolymphatic sac tumor) or dissection of the lateral recess of the fourth ventricle through a retrolabyrinthine craniotomy for auditory brainstem implant surgery (**Fig. 6**).

Disadvantages of endoscopic surgery include lack of true depth perception (some systems now are available with 4K 3-D), one handed dissection, steep learning curve, and fewer opportunities for training (especially during residency and fellowship) compared with the microscope.[8] Special consideration for safe EES include conservative use of antifog solution (shown to be ototoxic in animal models) and avoidance of thermal injury. Excess antifog solution can be prevented from entering the middle

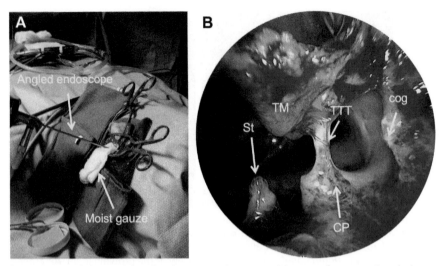

Fig. 4. TMEES, left ear. (*A*) Following a canal-up mastoidectomy for extensive cholesteatoma, a 30° or 45° endoscope (stabilized with a gauze sponge) is introduced into the aditus ad antrum to visualize residual disease. (*B*) Angled endoscopy directed anteroinferiorly reveals the posterosuperior surfaces of relevant anatomy that can be difficult to visualize transcanal. CP, cochleariform process. St, stapes; TM, tympanic membrane; TTT, tensor tympani tendon.

ear by wiping the endoscope with saline after application.[22] Endoscopes have the potential to cause thermal damage to middle ear structures,[23] but injury can be avoided by maintaining light intensity at 50%, using suction and irrigation for rapid cooling, keeping the endoscope tip at least 8 mm away from tissues, and removing the endoscope frequently.[24–26]

Exoscopes

The extracorporeal video microscope or exoscope is a recent addition to the microsurgical armamentarium and was designed to replace the operative microscope.[27] Most of the initial experiences with exoscopes are documented in the neurosurgical literature. The exoscope consists of a high-definition or 4K video camera with

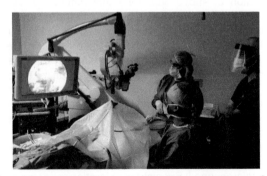

Fig. 5. Endoscopic and exoscopic-assisted retrolabyrinthine craniotomy for removal of complex skull base neoplasm. The entire procedure was performed under a barrier drape (OtoTent) to reduce particle dispersion during an AGP in April 2020.

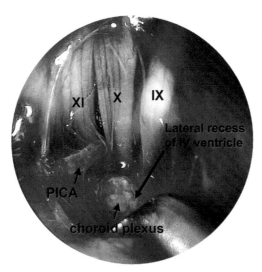

Fig. 6. Endoscopic dissection of the lateral recess of the IV ventricle following retrolabyrinthine craniotomy, left ear. A 30° endoscope was oriented posteriorly and introduced into the posterior fossa, resulting in a wide-angle view with enhanced depth of field. In contrast, the foramen of Luschka and root entry zones of cranial nerves IX, X, and XI cannot be visualized microscopically using this same approach without sacrificing the posterior canal. Endoscopes enable less-invasive auditory brainstem implant surgery for deaf patients with cochlear nerve aplasia and other cochlear anomalies. PICA, posterior inferior cerebellar artery.

optical and/or digital zoom and a fiberoptically delivered or LED light source. This system is suspended above the surgical field with a manually actuated articulating holder or robotic arm, which transmits a 2-dimensional (2-D) or 3-D image to a high-resolution monitor placed at eye level directly across from the surgeon (**see Fig. 2**B).

The exoscope has distinct advantages over the traditional binocular microscope. These include a large field of view, a longer focal length creating ample working space, and the ability to easily adjust the surgical view without anatomic constraints.[28] The microscope and the exoscope are external to the body cavity and can provide 3-D visualization of the surgical field (**see Fig. 1**). The exoscope utilizes an external video monitor, which allows the surgeon to assume a heads-up posture and allows others to share the surgeon's view.[29] A 2019 systematic review found that the exoscope was equivalent or superior to the microscope in terms of image quality, magnification, lighting, focal length, and depth of field. When a 3-D exoscope was used, stereopsis also was found to be equivalent or superior. The exoscope also was reported to be less expensive, more comfortable to use, more manageable and maneuverable, less obstructive of the surgical field, and better for teaching.[30]

Following the initial studies that demonstrated its efficacy and safety in microneurosurgery, the exoscope has been adopted by various otolaryngologic subspecialties.[28,31,32] Reports have demonstrated successful use of the exoscope in cochlear implantation, mastoidectomies, vestibular schwannoma resections, temporal lobe encephaloceles, and cholesteatomas.[27,33–35]

A disadvantage with exoscopes is lack of training opportunities. With experience, however, there does not appear to be significant differences in operating time or complication rates when comparing the exoscope to the microscope.[31,35] Other disadvantages include reduced image resolution at higher magnifications and decreased illumination in narrow surgical corridors,[27] supporting the idea that the exoscope is best suited for large surgical corridors.

In conclusion, exoscopes offer superior depth of field and ergonomics compared with microscopes at a competitive cost. Finally, a heads-up approach is compatible with full PPE (see **Fig. 5**). Future developments will include (1) a more compact working head, (2) greater optical zoom capability, and (3) improved focused illumination.

Ergonomics

Ergonomics is the study of work-related efficiency and safety. Surgical ergonomics include optimization of OR layout and body mechanics to decrease musculoskeletal pain and disability. Poor ergonomics can affect cost, efficiency, performance, and patient safety.[36] Survey studies show that 47% to 74% of otolaryngologists report work-related musculoskeletal pain attributable to poor ergonomics.[37] Among the otolaryngology subspecialties, neck and back pain commonly have been associated with otologists or those performing otologic surgery.[38,39] This phenomenon likely is due to frequent use of the operating microscope, which requires the surgeon to maintain a static *heads-down* position with the neck flexed and arms stretched forward in order to maintain a proper view through the rigid binocular eyepiece (**see Fig. 2**A). Cervical and thoracic pain have been associated with 3 or more hours of microscope usage per week.[40]

In contrast to the heads-down posture assumed during microscope use, the endoscope and exoscope utilize a video monitor placed at eye level, directly across from the user. Such eye-level displays are inspired by the heads-up display system developed for military aviation, which present data on transparent displays directly in front of the pilot.[41] Heads-up technology and eye-level displays have been adapted for the OR, allowing the surgeon to view the surgical field while maintaining proper natural neck joint alignment (see **Fig. 2**B). This posture avoids stress on the cervical and thoracic spine.[40]

The 3-D heads-up systems have been associated with a significant increase in surgeons' rating of ergonomic comfort[42] and decrease in back and eye strain[43] and may reduce asthenopia and subsequent difficulties in concentration that can accompany prolonged microscopic ocular use.

Heads-up Surgery in the Era of the Coronavirus Disease Pandemic

The COVID-19 pandemic has had an impact on PPE requirements and safety recommendations for medical providers globally. Enhanced protection is of particular importance for otolaryngologists, who are at increased risk of nosocomial spread when performing AGPs on the upper aerodigestive tract, which has a high severe acute respiratory syndrome (SARS)–coronavirus 2 (CoV-2) viral load in infected individuals.[44,45] It is not yet known if the respiratory mucosa that lines the middle ear and mastoid cells also demonstrates high viral loads, but this likely seems due to its continuity with the nasopharynx and previous reports of unspecified coronavirus present in cases of otitis media.[46] SARS–CoV-2 has been isolated from the middle ear and mastoid in a cadaveric specimens from individuals with COVID-19[47] and other respiratory viruses, including previous strains of coronavirus, have been previously identified in middle ear fluid samples.[48,49] Suctioning, cautery, and drilling on these areas with the potential for high viral loads, therefore, are considered high-risk AGPs, including mastoidectomies.[9,10,44]

Although personal respirator masks can prevent inhalation of aerosol particles, a face shield should be used to prevent ocular exposure to viral particles when performing an AGP. Otolaryngologists, therefore, are recommended to wear an N95 or FFP2/3 mask in combination with a face shield, goggles, or powered air–purifying respirator hood when operating on high-risk or COVID-19–positive patients. Eye or face PPE, however, often interferes with a surgeon's ability to use binocular eyepieces.[50,51] Endoscopes and exoscopes are ideal alternatives to the microscope due to (1) full compatibility with eye covering PPE and (2) the decreased need for mastoidectomies when performing EES.[45]

A barrier drape, or Ototent, has been shown to reduce both large and small particle dispersion during bony dissection with powered instrumentation (see **Fig. 5**).[9] A recent report described the use of a draping method with a 3-D exoscope during mastoidectomy. They found that the 3-D image was obscured when looking through 3-D glasses under a face shield but that the image was restored when the glasses placed on the outside.[52] They reported a minimal learning curve, improved ergonomics, and similar surgical time and recommend the use of transmastoid exoscopic and transcanal endoscopic approaches to perform surgery safely while wearing the necessary PPE.

SUMMARY

The binocular microscope revolutionized modern surgery, transformed the field of otology and neurotology. Despite its historical importance, the traditional operating microscope has several significant drawbacks compared with the modern endoscope and exoscope. Microscopic surgery is performed using a heads-down posture that has been associated with musculoskeletal pain and disability, and the microscopic view is limited by the size and shape of small surgical corridors.

The endoscope and exoscope are ergonomically superior to the operating microscope, overcoming many of its limitations and yielding comparable or improved outcomes. The endoscope improves access through small surgical corridors, whereas the exoscope is best suited for large surgical corridors, making them complementary modalities. In the midst of the current COVID-19 pandemic, heads-up surgery is favorable due to compatibility with face covering PPE. The endoscope provides additional protection by reestablishing the external auditory canal as a minimal access surgical corridor, thereby avoiding aerosol-generating mastoidectomies. These advantages make the endoscope and exoscope valuable tools for the modern era of otology and neurotology.

CLINICS CARE POINTS

- Endoscopes can enhance visual access through small surgical corridors such as the external auditory canal, thereby decreasing the need for extensive soft tissue dissection and aerosol generating mastoidectomies.
- Exoscopes are a viable alternative to binocular microscopy and are best suited for access through large surgical corridors.
- Endoscopes and exoscopes rely on eye-level monitors and enable surgeons to operate using a heads-up approach, with a relaxed and ergonomically superior posture compared with the binocular microscope.

DISCLOSURE

The senior author has financial relationships with 3NT Medical, Akouos, Frequency Therapeutics, Boston Pharmaceuticals, and Agilis.

REFERENCES

1. Mudry A. The history of the microscope for use in ear surgery. Am J Otol 2000; 21(6):877–86.
2. Eivazi S, Afkari H, Bednarik R, et al. Analysis of disruptive events and precarious situations caused by interaction with neurosurgical microscope. Acta Neurochir (Wien) 2015. https://doi.org/10.1007/s00701-015-2433-5.
3. Kapadiya M, Tarabichi M. An overview of endoscopic ear surgery in 2018. Laryngoscope Investig Otolaryngol 2019. https://doi.org/10.1002/lio2.276.
4. Kennedy DW. Serious misconceptions regarding functional endoscopic sinus surgery. Laryngoscope 1986;96:1170–1.
5. Kennedy DW. Functional endoscopic sinus surgery: technique. Arch Otolaryngol 1985. https://doi.org/10.1001/archotol.1985.00800120037003.
6. Kennedy DW, Zinreich SJ, Rosenbaum AE, et al. Functional endoscopic sinus surgery: theory and diagnostic evaluation. Arch Otolaryngol 1985. https://doi.org/10.1001/archotol.1985.00800110054002.
7. Ryan P, Wuesthoff C, Patel N. Getting started in endoscopic ear surgery. J Otol 2018. https://doi.org/10.1016/j.joto.2018.10.002.
8. Kozin ED, Lee DJ. Basic principles of endoscopic ear surgery. Oper Tech Otolaryngol - Head Neck Surg 2017. https://doi.org/10.1016/j.otot.2017.01.001.
9. Chen JX, Workman AD, Chari DA, et al. Demonstration and mitigation of aerosol and particle dispersion during mastoidectomy relevant to the COVID-19 era. Otol Neurotol 2020. https://doi.org/10.1097/MAO.0000000000002765.
10. Chari DA, Workman AD, Chen JX, et al. Aerosol dispersion during mastoidectomy and custom mitigation strategies for otologic surgery in the COVID-19 era. Otolaryngol Head Neck Surg 2020. https://doi.org/10.1177/0194599820941835.
11. Alp E, Bijl D, Bleichrodt RP, et al. Surgical smoke and infection control. J Hosp Infect 2006. https://doi.org/10.1016/j.jhin.2005.01.014.
12. Miller KA, Fina M, Lee DJ. Principles of pediatric endoscopic ear surgery. Otolaryngol Clin North Am 2019. https://doi.org/10.1016/j.otc.2019.06.001.
13. Marchioni D, Soloperto D, Rubini A, et al. Endoscopic exclusive transcanal approach to the tympanic cavity cholesteatoma in pediatric patients: our experience. Int J Pediatr Otorhinolaryngol 2015. https://doi.org/10.1016/j.ijporl.2014.12.008.
14. Han SY, Lee DY, Chung J, et al. Comparison of endoscopic and microscopic ear surgery in pediatric patients: a meta-analysis. Laryngoscope 2019. https://doi.org/10.1002/lary.27556.
15. Kiringoda R, Kozin ED, Lee DJ. Outcomes in endoscopic ear surgery. Otolaryngol Clin North Am 2016. https://doi.org/10.1016/j.otc.2016.05.008.
16. Hu Y, Teh BM, Hurtado G, et al. Can endoscopic ear surgery replace microscopic surgery in the treatment of acquired cholesteatoma? A contemporary review. Int J Pediatr Otorhinolaryngol 2020. https://doi.org/10.1016/j.ijporl.2020.109872.
17. Manna S, Kaul VF, Gray ML, et al. Endoscopic versus microscopic middle ear surgery: a meta-analysis of outcomes following tympanoplasty and stapes surgery. Otol Neurotol 2019. https://doi.org/10.1097/MAO.0000000000002353.
18. Tseng CC, Lai MT, Wu CC, et al. Comparison of the efficacy of endoscopic tympanoplasty and microscopic tympanoplasty: a systematic review and meta-analysis. Laryngoscope 2017. https://doi.org/10.1002/lary.26379.
19. Creighton F, Barber SR, Ward BK, et al. Underwater endoscopic repair of superior canal dehiscence. Otol Neurotol 2020. https://doi.org/10.1097/MAO.0000000000002277.

20. Carter MS, Lookabaugh S, Lee DJ. Endoscopic-assisted repair of superior canal dehiscence syndrome. Laryngoscope 2014. https://doi.org/10.1002/lary.24523.
21. Setty P, D'Andrea KP, Stucken EZ, et al. Endoscopic resection of vestibular schwannomas. J Neurol Surg Skull Base 2015. https://doi.org/10.1055/s-0034-1543974.
22. Kozin ED, Lee DJ. Staying safe during endoscopic ear surgery. Entandaudiology-newsCom 2016;25(2):3–6. Available at: https://www.entandaudiologynews.com/media/5028/ent-leekozin-2.pdf.
23. Kozin ED, Lehmann A, Carter M, et al. Thermal effects of endoscopy in a human temporal bone model: Implications for endoscopic ear surgery. Laryngoscope 2014. https://doi.org/10.1002/lary.24666.
24. Mitchell S, Coulson C. Endoscopic ear surgery: a hot topic? J Laryngol Otol 2017. https://doi.org/10.1017/S0022215116009828.
25. Aksoy F, Dogan R, Ozturan O, et al. Thermal effects of cold light sources used in otologic surgery. Eur Arch Otorhinolaryngol 2015. https://doi.org/10.1007/s00405-014-3202-4.
26. McCallum R, McColl J, Iyer A. The effect of light intensity on image quality in endoscopic ear surgery. Clin Otolaryngol 2018. https://doi.org/10.1111/coa.13139.
27. Smith S, Kozin ED, Kanumuri VV, et al. Initial experience with 3-dimensional exoscope-assisted transmastoid and lateral skull base surgery. Otolaryngol Head Neck Surg 2019. https://doi.org/10.1177/0194599818816965.
28. Mamelak AN, Danielpour M, Black KL, et al. A high-definition exoscope system for neurosurgery and other microsurgical disciplines: preliminary report. Surg Innov 2008. https://doi.org/10.1177/1553350608315954.
29. Uluç K, Kujoth GC, Başkaya MK. Operating microscopes: past, present, and future. Neurosurg Focus 2009. https://doi.org/10.3171/2009.6.FOCUS09120.
30. Ricciardi L, Chaichana KL, Cardia A, et al. The exoscope in neurosurgery: an innovative "Point of View". A systematic review of the technical, surgical, and educational aspects. World Neurosurg 2019. https://doi.org/10.1016/j.wneu.2018.12.202.
31. Mamelak AN, Nobuto T, Berci G. Initial clinical experience with a high-definition exoscope system for microneurosurgery. Neurosurgery 2010. https://doi.org/10.1227/01.NEU.0000372204.85227.BF.
32. Patel VA, Goyal N. Using a 4K-3D exoscope for upper airway stimulation surgery: proof-of-concept. Ann Otol Rhinol Laryngol 2020. https://doi.org/10.1177/0003489420905873.
33. Garneau JC, Laitman BM, Cosetti MK, et al. Repair of a temporal bone encephalocele with the surgical exoscope. Otol Neurotol 2020. https://doi.org/10.1097/MAO.0000000000002433.
34. Rubini A, Di Gioia S, Marchioni D. 3D exoscopic surgery of lateral skull base. Eur Arch Otorhinolaryngol 2020. https://doi.org/10.1007/s00405-019-05736-7.
35. Garneau JC, Laitman BM, Cosetti MK, et al. The use of the exoscope in lateral skull base surgery: advantages and limitations. Otol Neurotol 2019. https://doi.org/10.1097/MAO.0000000000002095.
36. Ramakrishnan VR, Montero PN. Ergonomic considerations in endoscopic sinus surgery: lessons learned from laparoscopic surgeons. Am J Rhinol Allergy 2013. https://doi.org/10.2500/ajra.2013.27.3872.
37. Vaisbuch Y, Aaron KA, Moore JM, et al. Ergonomic hazards in otolaryngology. Laryngoscope 2019. https://doi.org/10.1002/lary.27496.

38. Ho TVT, Hamill CS, Sykes KJ, et al. Work-related musculoskeletal symptoms among otolaryngologists by subspecialty: a national survey. Laryngoscope 2018. https://doi.org/10.1002/lary.26859.

39. Babar-Craig H, Banfield G, Knight J. Prevalence of back and neck pain amongst ENT consultants: national survey. J Laryngol Otol 2003. https://doi.org/10.1258/002221503322683885.

40. Capone AC, Parikh PM, Gatti ME, et al. Occupational injury in plastic surgeons. Plast Reconstr Surg 2010. https://doi.org/10.1097/PRS.0b013e3181d62a94.

41. MODI YS, EHLERS JP. Heads-up vitreoretinal surgery: emerging technology in surgical visualization. Retin Physician 2016;13(Jan/Feb):26–9.

42. Zhang Z, Wang L, Wei Y, et al. The preliminary experiences with three-dimensional heads-up display viewing system for vitreoretinal surgery under various status. Curr Eye Res 2019. https://doi.org/10.1080/02713683.2018.1526305.

43. Wong AK, Davis GB, Joanna Nguyen T, et al. Assessment of three-dimensional high-definition visualization technology to perform microvascular anastomosis. J Plast Reconstr Aesthet Surg 2014. https://doi.org/10.1016/j.bjps.2014.04.001.

44. Mick P, Murphy R. Aerosol-generating otolaryngology procedures and the need for enhanced PPE during the COVID-19 pandemic: a literature review. J Otolaryngol Head Neck Surg 2020;49(1):29.

45. Topsakal V, Rompaey V Van, Kuhweide R, et al. Prioritizing otological surgery during the COVID-19 Pandemic. B-ENT 2020. https://doi.org/10.5152/b-ent.2020.20126.

46. Wiertsema SP, Chidlow GR, Kirkham LAS, et al. High detection rates of nucleic acids of a wide range of respiratory viruses in the nasopharynx and the middle ear of children with a history of recurrent acute otitis media. J Med Virol 2011. https://doi.org/10.1002/jmv.22221.

47. Frazier KM, Hooper JE, Mostafa HH, et al. SARS-CoV-2 virus isolated from the mastoid and middle ear. JAMA Otolaryngol Head Neck Surg 2020. https://doi.org/10.1001/jamaoto.2020.1922.

48. Pitkaranta A, Virolainen A, Jero J, et al. Detection of rhinovirus, respiratory syncytial virus, and coronavirus infections in acute otitis media by reverse transcriptase polymerase chain reaction. Pediatrics 1998. https://doi.org/10.1542/peds.102.2.291.

49. Heikkinen T, Thint M, Chonmaitree T. Prevalence of various respiratory viruses in the middle ear during acute otitis media. N Engl J Med 1999. https://doi.org/10.1056/NEJM199901283400402.

50. Kozin AED, Remenschneider AK, Blevins NH, et al. American neurotology society, american otological society, and american academy of otolaryngology - head and neck foundation guide to enhance otologic and neurotologic care during the COVID-19 pandemic. Otol Neurotol 2020;41(9):1163–74.

51. Clamp PJ, Broomfield SJ. The challenge of performing mastoidectomy using the operating microscope with Covid-19 personal protective equipment (PPE). J Laryngol Otol 2020. https://doi.org/10.1017/s0022215120001607.

52. Gordon SA, Deep NL, Jethanamest D. Exoscope and personal protective equipment use for otologic surgery in the era of COVID-19. Otolaryngol Head Neck Surg 2020. https://doi.org/10.1177/0194599820928975. 194599820928975.

53. Mer SB, Derbyshire AJ, Brushenko A, et al. Fiberoptic endotoscopes for examining the middle ear. Arch Otolaryngol 1967. https://doi.org/10.1001/archotol.1967.00760040389009.

54. Nomura Y. Effective photography in otolaryngology-head and neck surgery: endoscopic photography of the middle ear. Otolaryngol Head Neck Surg 1982. https://doi.org/10.1177/019459988209000406.

55. Tajudeen BA, Kennedy DW. Thirty years of endoscopic sinus surgery: what have we learned? World J Otorhinolaryngol Head Neck Surg 2017. https://doi.org/10.1016/j.wjorl.2016.12.001.

56. Zinreich SJ, Kennedy DW, Rosenbaum AE, et al. Paranasal sinuses: CT imaging requirements for endoscopic surgery. Radiology 1987. https://doi.org/10.1148/radiology.163.3.3575731.

57. Kenned DW, Zinreich SJ, Kuhn F, et al. Endoscopic middle meatal antrostomy: theory, technique, and patency. Laryngoscope 1987. https://doi.org/10.1288/00005537-198708002-00001.

58. Thomassin JM, Duchon-Doris JM, Emram B, et al. Endoscopic ear surgery. Initial evaluation. Ann Otolaryngol Chir Cervicofac 1990;107(8):564–70.

59. Thomassin JM, Inedjian JM, Rud C, et al. Otoendoscopy: application in the middle ear surgery. Rev Laryngol Otol Rhinol (Bord) 1990;111(5):475–7.

60. Thomassin JM, Korchia D, Duchon-Doris JM. Cholesteatome Residuel: Sa Prevention Par La Chirurgie Sous Guidage Endoscopique. Rev Laryngol Otol Rhinol (Bord) 1991;112(5):405–8.

61. Thomassin JM, Korchia D, Doris JMD. Endoscopic-guided otosurgery in the prevention of residual cholesteatomas. Laryngoscope 1993. https://doi.org/10.1288/00005537-199308000-00021.

62. Poe DS. Transtympanic endoscopy of the middle ear. Oper Tech Otolaryngol - Head Neck Surg 1992. https://doi.org/10.1016/S1043-1810(10)80121-6.

63. Poe DS, Bottrill ID. Comparison of endoscopic and surgical explorations for perilymphatic fistulas. Am J Otol 1994;15(6):735–8.

64. Bottrill ID, Poe DS. Endoscope-assisted ear surgery. Am J Otol 1995;16(2):158–63.

65. Tarabichi M. Endoscopic management of acquired cholesteatoma. Am J Otol 1997. https://doi.org/10.1016/j.otohns.2008.05.179.

66. Tarabichi M. Endoscopic middle ear surgery. Ann Otol Rhinol Laryngol 1999. https://doi.org/10.1177/000348949910800106.

67. Tarabichi M. Endoscopic management of cholesteatoma: Long-term results. Otolaryngol Head Neck Surg 2000. https://doi.org/10.1016/S0194-5998(00)70017-9.

68. News and Announcements. Otolaryngol Neck Surg 1995. https://doi.org/10.1016/S0194-59989570264-4.

Endoscopic Ear Surgery

Redefining Middle Ear Anatomy and Physiology

Daniele Marchioni, MD, Alessia Rubini, MD,
Davide Soloperto, MD, PhD*

KEYWORDS

- Anatomy • Middle ear • Ventilation pathway • Retrotympanum • Epitympanum
- Epitympanic diaphragm

KEY POINTS

- The epitympanum is separated from the mesotympanic space by the epitympanic diaphragm. The main ventilation route of the epitympanic-mastoid compartments is through the anterior and posterior isthmus.
- The selective epitympanic dysventilation syndrome can occur with the presence of four conditions: an attic retraction pocket or attic cholesteatoma, a type A tympanogram or a normal tubal function test, complete epitympanic diaphragm, and isthmus blockage.
- The middle ear is divided into five subspaces: the mesotympanum, the retrotympanum posteriorly, the epitympanum superiorly, the protympanum anteriorly, and the hypotympanum inferiorly.

INTRODUCTION

In recent years, the use of endoscope with varied angulations has become crucial to explore all of the hidden areas that are often not visualized using a microscope, with a better comprehension of the anatomy and the pathophysiologic aspects of middle ear ventilation pathways.[1,2]

Aeration of the tympanic cavity, mastoid cells, and anatomic pathways for middle ear ventilation have been studied since the end of the nineteenth century, starting with the work of Prussak[3] in 1867. More recently, Palva and Johnsson[4,5] were the first to describe middle ear anatomy focusing on ventilation patterns and their implications for middle ear disease. The Eustachian tube (ET) plays a crucial role in maintaining middle ear aeration and atmospheric pressure. Inflammatory middle ear chronic disease is usually related to ET dysfunction caused by poor tympanic ventilation, but other anatomic factors may play important roles in ventilation of these spaces, especially for epitympanic retraction pockets.

Department of Otolaryngology-Head and Neck Surgery, Azienda Ospedaliera Universitaria Integrata Verona, Piazzale Aristide Stefani, 1, Verona 37126, Italy
* Corresponding author.
E-mail address: davidesolop@gmail.com

Otolaryngol Clin N Am 54 (2021) 25–43
https://doi.org/10.1016/j.otc.2020.09.003
0030-6665/21/© 2020 Elsevier Inc. All rights reserved.

The endoscope plays an important role in better studying the anatomy of the middle ear, especially the hidden recess. The middle ear is divided into five subspaces. The mesotympanum is the space that is possible to visualize through the external auditory canal by the use of otoscope or microscope. Posteriorly to it lies the retrotympanum, superiorly the epitympanum, anteriorly the protympanum, and inferiorly the hypotympanum (**Fig. 1**).

EPITYMPANUM

The knowledge of endoscopic anatomy of the epitympanum and the study of the principal ventilation pathway routes are mandatory for the comprehension of middle ear diseases, such as cholesteatoma or chronic otitis media.

Boundaries

- Superior: tegmen tympani
- Inferior: epitympanic diaphragm (**Fig. 2**)
- Anterior: anterior root of the zygomatic arch or tensor fold in case of a vertical tensor fold
- Posterior: confluent with the mastoid antrum
- Medial: suprageniculate fossa
- Lateral: scutum and pars flaccida of the tympanic membrane

The epitympanum represents the cranial portion of the middle ear and it is connected to the mastoid and antrum. From an anatomic point of view, this space is

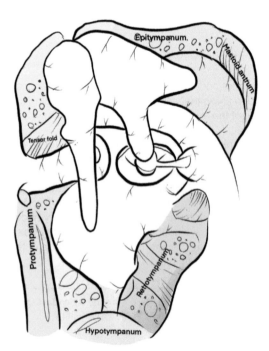

Fig. 1. Left ear. The subspaces of the middle ear: posteriorly the retrotympanum, superiorly the epitympanum, anteriorly the protympanum, inferiorly the hypotympanum, and in a central location the mesotympanum.

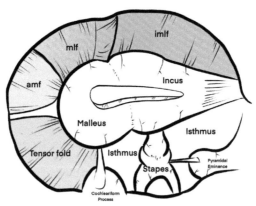

Fig. 2. Left ear. Schematic drawing that shows the epitympanic diaphragm. It is composed of three malleal ligamental folds (anterior, lateral, and posterior), the lateral and medial posterior incudal ligaments, the tensor fold, the lateral incudomalleal fold, together with the malleus and incus. The tympanic anterior isthmus is the area in between incudostapedial joint and cochleariform process, whereas the space between the pyramidal process and the short process of the incus is the tympanic posterior isthmus. Amf, anterior malleal ligamental fold; imlf, incudomalleal fold; mlf, lateral malleal ligamental fold.

mostly occupied by the ossicular chain and in particular by the incudomalleolar joint and by its ligaments and physiologic mucosal folds. In 1946 Chatellier and Lemoine[6] studied frontal histologic sections of newborn's temporal bone and described an "attico tympanic diaphragm" that results in a clear separation of the attic from the mesotympanum.

Palva and Johnsson,[4] through meticulous observations of healthy and diseased specimens, defined this further anatomically and used the term "epitympanic diaphragm" and emphasized the role of the "tympanic isthmus" in the ventilation of the attic.[4] They also described several diseased specimens in children and demonstrated pathology involving the isthmus.[5]

The epitympanum is divided into two compartments: a large posterior compartment and a smaller anterior compartment. The demarcation between the anterior and posterior epitympanum depends on the anatomic variations of important structures, such as the cog and the tensor fold. In most people, the demarcation is represented by the transverse ridge or cog. The cog is a bony septum that detaches from the tegmen tympani cranially, leading vertically toward the cochleariform process in front of the malleus head. Much of the posterior epitympanic volume is occupied by the body and short process of the incus together with the head of the malleus. The lateral portion of the posterior epitympanum is narrow and is divided by the lateral incudo-malleal fold in two further portions, the superior and inferior lateral attic, positioned separately one above the other.

The incudomalleal fold originates at the posterior extremity of the short process of incus and the lateral portion of the posterior incudal fold, continuing anteriorly between the body of the incus, the head of the malleus. and the lateral aspect of the attic. At this level, the fold bends inferiorly, joining the lateral malleal fold. The medial and inferior aspects of the Prussak space are formed, respectively, by the neck and the short process of the malleus. The superior limit is the lateral malleal fold, which also represents the floor of the superior lateral attic; this ligament inserts laterally on the medial wall of the scutum. The anterior aspect of the Prussak area is bounded by a thin, membranous fold among the tympanic membrane and the anterior ligament of the malleus, which inserts laterally on the tympanic membrane and medially on the neck and long process of the malleus. In some cases, this fold is absent, causing a further anterior ventilation trajectory to the Prussak space. The lateral aspect is represented by the Shrapnell membrane. The posterior wall is represented by a large posterior pouch (the posterior pouch of von Tröltsch), which is the ventilation rout of the Prussak space (**Fig. 3**).

The epitympanum is separated from the mesotympanic space from the epitympanic diaphragm, which consists of three malleal ligamental folds (anterior, lateral, and posterior), the lateral and medial posterior incudal ligaments, the tensor fold, the lateral incudomalleal fold together with the malleus and incus.

The tensor fold is the anatomic boundary between the protympanum and epitympanum, but in case of incomplete tensor fold, a direct communication through the membranous defect is present, so it does not functionally separate the two compartments.

The tensor fold can be complete with an intact membrane or incomplete with a membranous defect. Three different orientations of the tensor fold were observed similarly in the literature: vertical, oblique, and horizontal (**Fig. 4**).[7]

A tensor fold with vertical orientation is inserted to the cog. In case of this tensor fold morphology, the supratubal recess is large.

In most cases, the tensor fold has an oblique orientation and attached to the anterior tegmen tympani. The transverse crest served as the division plane between the anterior and the posterior epitympanic space.

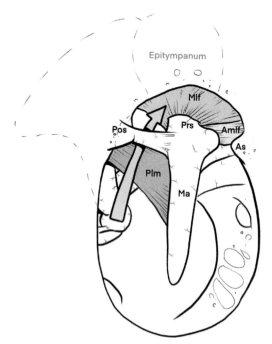

Fig. 3. Right ear. Prussak space: lateral aspect is represented by the Sharpnell membrane; the posterior wall is represented by the posterior pouch of von Tröltsch; medial and inferior aspects are formed, respectively, by the neck and the short process of the malleus; and the superior limit is the lateral malleal fold. Amlf, anterior malleal ligament fold; As, anterior tympanic spine; Ma, malleus; Mlf, lateral malleal ligament fold; Plm, posterior malleal ligament fold; Pos, posterior tympanic spine; Prs, Prussak space.

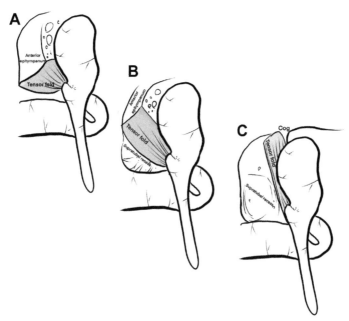

Fig. 4. Left ear. Relationship between supratubal recess and anterior epitympanic space. The drawing shows three different orientations of the tensor fold: horizontal (*A*), oblique (*B*), and vertical (*C*).

When the tensor fold has a horizontal orientation, attaching to the tensor tympani canal, the supratubal recess is small or nonexistent. In a horizontal type of tensor fold, the epitympanum is characterized by a wide space with a large anterior portion ventilated by the anterior isthmus, and it is excluded from direct ventilation from the ET when the tensor fold is complete. When the tensor fold is an incomplete membrane, the anterior epitympanic space receives additional ventilation through the ET. The case of complete tensor fold membrane and inflammatory tissue blocking the tympanic isthmus could be predisposed to more likely anterior epitympanic dysventilation with a subsequent development of anterior attic retraction (anterior epitympanic cholesteatoma).[7]

In any case, in the presence of an intact tensor fold, there is a fully formed diaphragm that separates the attic from the mesotympanum. The main ventilation route of the epitympanic-mastoid compartments (called upper unit) is through the anterior and posterior isthmus. The tympanic anterior isthmus is the area in between the incudostapedial joint and cochleariform process with the tensor tendon (Proctor anterior isthmus), whereas the space between the incudostapedial joint and the short process of the incus is the tympanic posterior isthmus (Proctor posterior isthmus).[1]

The Prussak space (lower unit) is important because it represents an independent unit. This ventilation route of the inferior epitympanic compartment through the posterior pouch of von Tröltsch is rough and narrow, especially if compared with the ventilation route through tympanic isthmus, which aerates the upper epitympanic compartment. For these reasons, the possibility of anatomic reduction of the air passage until the closing of the posterior pouch of von Tröltsch is possible, especially in case of the presence of viscous secretions within the Prussak space, which could cause a chronic sectorial dysventilation associated with a retraction of the Sharpnell membrane and its adhesion to the malleus neck, without any involvement of the compartments above the epitympanic diaphragm, as the anterior and posterior epitympanum, the aditus, and mastoid cells.

This pathophysiologic concept is important in transcanal endoscopic ear surgery, because surgical treatment is based on the restoration of ventilation of the upper unit and the lower unit, through the creation of a large tympanic isthmus and an accessory route through the tensor fold and the Prussak space (**Fig. 5**).

Based on these concepts, endoscopic ear surgery reveals that some patients affected by an epitympanic cholesteatoma often have a total isthmus blockage that completely excludes the entire epitympanum and mastoid compartments from the mesotympanum, causing a lack of ventilation that induces a progressive air resorption by the middle ear mucosa and creates a negative epitympanic pressure. In patients with this anatomic condition, it is common to observe a complete retraction of the pars flaccida with a normal conformation of the pars tensa, without pathologic signs in the mesotympanum. In addition, the function of the ET is physiologically normal in these patients. This situation is defined as "selective epitympanic dysventilation syndrome"[8] and consists of the concomitant presence of a series of complete or incomplete epitympanic diaphragms and tympanic isthmus blockage causing a negative pressure, leading to formation of a retraction pocket or cholesteatoma, with a normal ET function (**Fig. 6**). The syndrome can therefore occur with the contemporaneous presence of four conditions: (1) an attic retraction pocket or attic

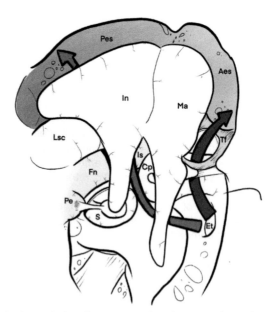

Fig. 5. Right ear. A schematic drawing representing the two independent aeration routes of the epitympanum. The major aeration route (*orange arrow*) passing through the isthmus for the large upper unit (epitympanic compartments, antrum, and mastoid cells); and the second independent aeration route (*red arrow*) for the smaller lower unit (Prussak space) passing through the posterior pouch of von Tröltsch. Aes, anterior epitympanic space; Cp, cochleariform process; Et, Eustachian tube; Fn, facial nerve; In, incus; Is, isthmus; Lsc, lateral semicircular canal; Ma, malleus; Pe, pyramidal eminence; Pes, posterior epitympanic space; S, stapes; Tf, tensor fold.

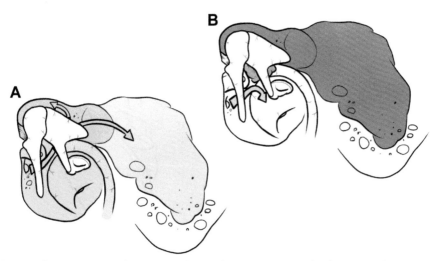

Fig. 6. Left ear. *A)* Normal anatomy. *B)* Complete epitympanic diaphragms and tympanic isthmus blockage causing a negative pressure in the upper unit (epitympanum and mastoid compartments), leading to formation of a retraction pocket or cholesteatoma, with a normal Eustachian tube function.

cholesteatoma, (2) a type A tympanogram or a normal tubal function test, (3) complete epitympanic diaphragm, and (4) isthmus blockage. As confirmed during surgery, an open ET and a good protympanic and mesotympanic mucosa appearance were found in cases of selective dysventilation. To treat this condition, and perhaps to prevent cholesteatoma formation, a surgery of the isthmus should be done restoring the ventilation pathway through this anatomic structure and a new ventilation route should be created during surgery, and this is performed by endoscopic middle ear surgery in a preserving way.

Considering that middle ear pressure seems related not only to a functioning ET, but also to transmucosal gas exchange through the mastoid mucosa, and the mucosal gas exchange is related to the degree of mastoid pneumatization,[9] even if the ET is functioning, an isthmus blockage could impair ventilation of the mastoid cells, leading to a sclerotic mastoid. The surgical solution must ensure the ventilation of all parts of the epitympanum. Three types (A, B, and C) of anatomic ventilation blockage patterns of middle ear are identified during endoscopic ear surgery.

In type A blockage of the isthmus is associated with a complete tensor fold (most of these patients presented with a selective attic retraction pocket or attic cholesteatoma without pathologic tissue in the mesotympanic spaces). In type B blockage of the isthmus is associated with an attical vertical blockage (consisting of a fold or granulation tissue involving the incudomalleal fold) separating the anterior epitympanic space from the posterior epitympanic space with or without a complete tensor fold. In these subjects a selective retraction pocket into the posterior attic was found. Type C is a complete epidermization of the attic space causing a blockage of the isthmus and a complete antral blockage excluding the mesotympanic space from the epitympanic and mastoid spaces (**Fig. 7**).

Special attention should be paid to restoring an isthmus ventilation pathway, removing inflammatory tissue, or creating a new isthmus with an ossiculoplasty; the tensor fold usually should be removed to create an accessory ventilation route to

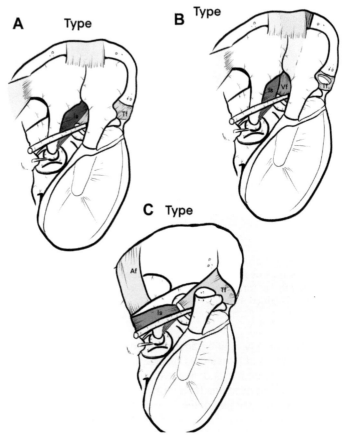

Fig. 7. Right ear. Three types of anatomic ventilation blockage patterns of the middle ear identified during endoscopic ear surgery: type A, type B, type C. Af, antral blockage; Is, isthmus; Tf, tensor fold; Vf, attical vertical blockage.

the epitympanum. These procedures are necessary for good epitympanic ventilation.[10] The use of the endoscope during surgery permits a good view of the tensor fold area and the isthmus tympani and, consequently, is really important to understand the type of dysventilation pattern.

Regarding the anatomy, to show better the other anatomic structures of the epitympanum, in particular the tympanic portion of the facial nerve, the geniculate ganglion, and the cochleariform process, it is necessary to perform an atticotomy with removal of the incus and head of the malleus. The tympanic segment of the facial nerve runs through the medial wall of the tympanic cavity and it is divided into two portions relative to the cochleariform process: precochleariform and postcochleariform segments (**Fig. 8**). The precochleariform segment is the portion of the tympanic facial nerve lying superiorly and anteriorly to the cochleariform process. It is composed of the geniculate ganglion and the greater superficial petrosal nerve. The precochleariform segment has a parallel orientation with respect to the hemicanal of the tensor tympani muscle, lying superiorly to this hemicanal. The cochleariform process represents an excellent landmark to identify the geniculate ganglion, which is located just medially and superiorly to the cochleariform process. Another

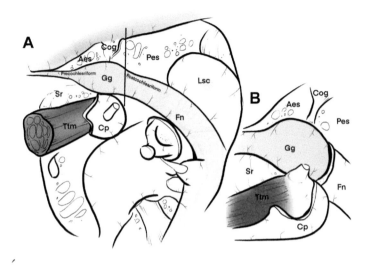

Fig. 8. Left ear. (*A*) Endoscopic anatomy of the tympanic portion of the facial nerve: precochleariform and postcochleariform segments. (*B*) Precochleariform segment of the tympanic portion of the facial nerve and the relationship between the geniculate ganglion and the tensor tympani muscle. Aes, anterior epitympanic space; Cp, cochleariform process; Fn, facial nerve; Gg, geniculate ganglion; Lsc, lateral semicircular canal; Pes, posterior epitympanic space; Sr, supratubal recess; Ttm, tensor tympani muscle.

anatomic landmark for the geniculate ganglion is the transverse crest, or "cog," which descends from the tegmen like a finger indicating the location of the geniculate ganglion, and is complete or rudimentary.[7,11]

The postcochleariform segment is parallel with respect to the lateral semicircular canal and lies posteriorly to the posterior bony limit of the cochleariform process. That is an important landmark to reach the aditus ad antrum endoscopically.

Over the tympanic portion of the facial nerve and geniculate ganglion is located the suprageniculate fossa. This fossa is a pyramidal-shaped space delimited inferiorly by the geniculate ganglion, superiorly by the middle cranial fossa dura, and posteriorly by the lateral semicircular canal. This area is considered a corridor from laterally to medially, from the geniculate fossa to the petrous apex by removing the bone along the medial aspect of the suprageniculate fossa.[12] The knowledge of this anatomy is also important to perform a total endoscopic decompression of the facial nerve, especially in the tympanic portion of the facial nerve, the geniculate ganglion, and the suprageniculate fossa (**Fig. 9**).[13]

PROTYMPANUM

The protympanic space lies anteriorly to the mesotympanum and inferiorly to the anterior epitympanic space (**Fig. 10**).

Boundaries

- Superior: tensor fold and tegmen tympani in case of a vertical tensor fold
- Inferior: the protiniculum
- Anterior: confluent with the junctional and then cartilaginous portion of the ET

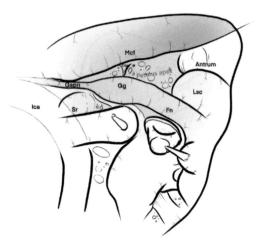

Fig. 9. Left ear. Anatomy of the suprageniculate fossa, which is delimited inferiorly by geniculate ganglion, superiorly by the middle cranial fossa dura, and posteriorly by the lateral semicircular canal. Fn, facial nerve; Gg, geniculate ganglion; Gspn, greater superficial petrosal nerve; Ica, internal carotid artery; Lsc, lateral semicircular canal; Mcf, dura mater of middle cranial fossa; Sr, supratubal recess.

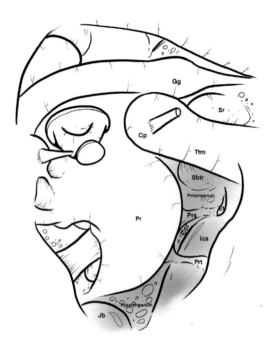

Fig. 10. Right ear. Anatomy of the protympanum. Ccr, caroticocochlear recess; Cp, cochleariform process; Et, Eustachian tube; Gg, geniculate ganglion; Ica, internal carotid artery; Jb, Jacobson nerve; Pr, promontory; Prs, protympanic spine; Prt, protiniculum; Sbtr, subtensor recess; Sr, supratubal recess; Ttm, tensor tympani muscle.

- Posterior: confluent with the mesotympanum
- Medial: lateral wall of the carotid canal, extending from the caroticocochlear recess anteriorly, with caroticotympanic vessels and nerves including anterior branches from Jacobson nerve
- Lateral: bony wall separating the space from the mandibular fossa and extending to the anterior annulus

The inferior border of the protympanum is the protiniculum, an oblique bony ridge that divides the protympanum superiorly from the hypotympanum inferiorly (**Fig. 11**).[14]

This bony ridge has three conformations: bony ridge, with no air cells passing medially (type A); bony bridge, with hypotympanic air cells extending inferiorly into the protympanum (type B); absent, no discernible protiniculum, the hypotympanum fusing with the protympanum (type C).

The protympanum is divided into two spaces: the supratubal recess superiorly, and the ET orifice inferiorly. The supratubal recess has variable size, which is related to the inclination of the tensor fold: the more vertical is the tensor fold, the wider is the supratubal recess.

When an area of pneumatization is inferomedial to the tensor tympani canal, it is called the subtensor recess. Based on the depth of the subtensor recess one can distinguish three different morphologies: flat tensor canal, absent subtensor recess (type A); raised tensor canal, shallow subtensor recess, easily visible fundus (type B); and raised tensor canal, deep subtensor recess, difficult to see limits of fundus (type C).[15]

RETROTYMPANUM
Boundaries

- Superior: superior limit of the posterior sinus

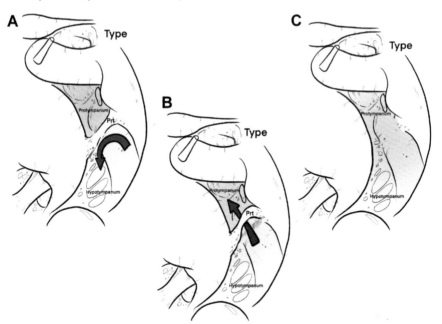

Fig. 11. Right ear. Different morphology of protiniculum: bony ridge (type A), bony bridge (type B), and absent (type C). Prt, protiniculum.

- Inferior: funiculus (a bony landmark that extends from the anterior pillar of the round window toward the jugular dome)
- Anterior: confluent with the mesotympanum
- Posterior: posterior bony wall of the posterior sinus, sinus tympani, sinus subtympanicus, facial recess, and lateral tympanic sinus
- Medial: medial bony wall of tympanic cavity
- Lateral: styloid eminence, medial aspect of the bony canal of the mastoid portion of the facial nerve and stapedius muscle

The funiculus (from Latin, "borderline") separates the retrotympanum from the hypotympanum, inferiorly. Some variations in morphology of the funiculus are noticed: it is a ridge of bone, a bridge of bone, absent, or incomplete. The inferior tympanic artery lies in this structure.

The retrotympanum lies in the posterior aspect of the tympanic cavity and it is divided into the superior and inferior retrotympanum by a small bony structure called the subiculum, a bony ridge extending from the posterior pillar of the round window niche outward to the styloid eminence (**Fig. 12**).[16]

Four spaces are identified in the superior retrotympanum: two spaces lying medially with respect to the third portion of the facial nerve and two spaces lying laterally. The pyramidal eminence is the fulcrum of the superior retrotympanum. From this structure, two bony structures arise: the chordal ridge extending outward and toward the chordal eminence, and separating the facial recess superior and laterally and the lateral tympanic sinus inferiorly; and the ponticulus, a bony structure extending inward and medially from the pyramidal eminence to the promontory, dividing the sinus tympani inferiorly and the posterior sinus superiorly (**Fig. 13**).

In most cases, a space is present under the pyramidal eminence with variable shape and depth: the subpyramidal space (**Fig. 14**). This anatomic entity is delimited laterally

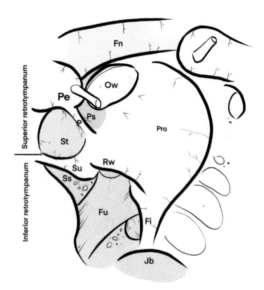

Fig. 12. Right ear. Anatomy of the retrotympanum that is divided into superior and inferior retrotympanum by the subiculum. Fi, funiculus; Fn, facial nerve; Fu, fustis; Jb, jugular bulb; Ow, oval window; P, ponticulus; Pe, pyramidal eminence; Pro, promontory; Ps, posterior sinus; Rw, round window; Ss, sinus subtympanic; St, sinus tympani; Su, subiculum.

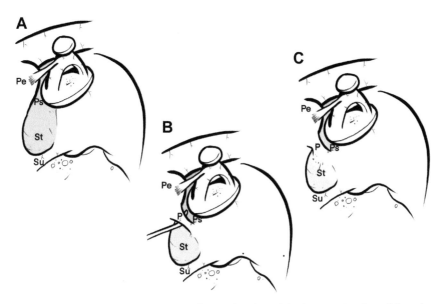

Fig. 13. Right ear. Anatomic variations of the subiculum. (*A*) Absent subiculum. (*B*) Bridge subiculum. (*C*) Ridge subiculum. P, ponticulus; Pe, pyramidal eminence; Ps, posterior sinus; St, sinus tympani; Su, subiculum.

by the medial aspect of the pyramidal eminence, and medially by the medial side of the bony wall of the retrotympanum. Posteriorly, this space is separated from the vertical tract of the bony canal of the facial nerve by a thin bony layer.

The pyramidal eminence has an independent morphology (the medial surface was completely formed and recognizable), with communicating sinus tympani and posterior sinus through a subpyramidal space. The pyramidal eminence can also show a partial morphology or a merged morphology. In this last case the medial surface was completely merged with the medial bony boundary of the retrotympanum, and no space was present under the pyramidal eminence. The subpyramidal space could potentially be a further place where the cholesteatoma could remain hidden during middle ear surgery, especially if this space is deep.[17]

In this area, it is important to understand the relationship of the pyramidal eminence and stapedius muscle to the facial nerve. The muscle runs medial to the facial nerve, contained within a bony grove in the fallopian canal. Following its course from posterior to anterior, the muscle separates itself from the facial nerve becoming anterior to it, contained in its own bony canal. From inferior to superior the stapedius muscle was medial then anterior to the facial nerve to its tendon attached to the stapes.[18]

Medially to the fallopian canal, in the superior retrotympanum there is the sinus tympani, which is the anatomic space between the subiculum and the ponticulus and it is subject to great variability in size and shape. A radiologic classification of the sinus tympani shows three different sinus tympani (**Figs. 15 and 16**). Type A presents a limited sinus tympani (the medial limit of the third portion of the facial nerve corresponded to the depth of the sinus). Type B presents a deep sinus tympani (the medial boundary of the sinus lies medially with respect to the third portion of the facial nerve and did not present a posterior extension with respect to the facial nerve). Type C is rare and presents a deep sinus tympani with a posterior extension (the medial

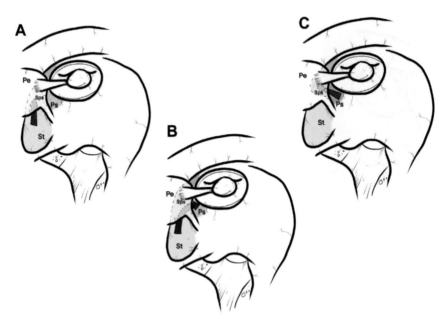

Fig. 14. Right ear. Morphology of the pyramidal eminence and subpyramidal space. (*A*) Partial morphology of the pyramidal eminence, subpyramidal space communicating with sinus tympani. (*B*) Complete morphology of the pyramidal eminence and communicating sinus tympani and posterior sinus through a subpyramidal space. (*C*) Partial morphology of the pyramidal eminence, subpyramidal space communicating with posterior sinus. Pe, pyramidal eminence; Ps, posterior sinus; Sps, subpyramidal space; St, sinus tympani.

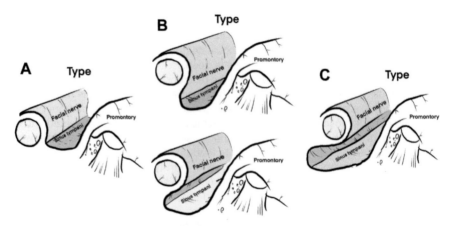

Fig. 15. Right ear. Radiologic classification of the sinus tympani. Type A: limited sinus tympani without medial and posterior extension with respect to the third portion of facial nerve. Type B: sinus tympani with medial extension without posterior extension with respect to the third portion of facial nerve. Type C: sinus tympani with posterior extension with respect to the third portion of the facial nerve.

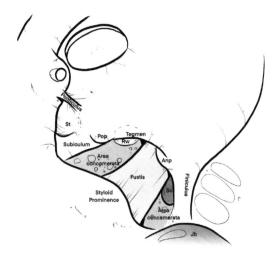

Fig. 16. Right ear. Anatomy of the round window niche. Anp, anterior pillar; Jb, jugular bulb; Pop, posterior pillar; Rw, round window; Sc, subcochlear canaliculus; St, sinus tympani.

boundary of the sinus lies medially and posteriorly with respect to the third portion of the facial nerve). In these cases, the sinus tympani is large and deep and it is not always possible to have good control of the sinus tympani; in these cases, a posterior retrofacial approach is suggested.[19]

The inferior retrotympanum is formed by the sinus subtympanicus (medial to the third portion of the facial nerve) and the round window region.

The sinus subtympanicus was defined as an anatomic space between the subiculum superiorly and the funiculus inferiorly, developing medially with respect to the styloid prominence, forming a deep space into the retrotympanum below the sinus tympani.

Anterior to the sinus subtympanicus there is the round window chamber, which is a three-dimensional space lying between the round window niche and round window membrane and confluent posteriorly and laterally to the inferior retrotympanum.

The round window niche was formed in a triangular shape by the posterior pillar, the tegmen, and the anterior pillar at the apex of this triangular shape was the round window membrane whose internal aspect opened into the tympanic scala of the basal turn of the cochlea.

The floor of the round window chamber is represented by the fustis, a smooth bony structure that seems to indicate the round window membrane. This structure links the styloid prominence with the basal turn of the cochlea. The Proctor area concamerata was defined as an anatomic area composed by bony cells developed around the fustis bone.

Two unique anatomic conformations of the fustis were identified (**Fig. 17**). In type A the fustis coursed in an oblique direction from the styloid prominence posteriorly and inferiorly to the round window niche anteriorly and superiorly, pointing like a finger to the round window membrane. In Type B the fustis was arising from the styloid prominence posteriorly and passes under the round window membrane anteriorly, in particular the anterosuperior limit of the fustis seemed to delimit the anterior edge of the round window membrane. The fustis is an important landmark for the surgeon to

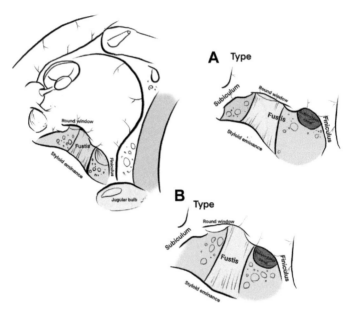

Fig. 17. Right ear. Anatomic variations of the fustis. Type A: the fustis courses in an oblique direction from the styloid prominence posteriorly and inferiorly to the round window niche anteriorly and superiorly, pointing like a finger to the round window membrane. Type B: the fustis arising from the styloid prominence posteriorly and passes under the round window membrane anteriorly, the anterosuperior limit of the fustis seemed to delimit the anterior edge of the round window membrane.

find the correct site for the insertion of a cochlear implant electrode array when it is difficult to correctly identify the round window niche and the scala tympani, such as in case of malformed ears or when cochlear ossification is found.[20]

Between the fustis and the funiculus, a subcochlear canaliculus is often seen, which is a tunnel/pneumatization that connects the round window chamber to the petrous apex (**Fig. 18**).

There are three types of conformations of the round window chamber related to the relationship between the fustis, area concamerata, and the funiculus bone. In type A between the fustis and the funiculus, a deep subcochlear canaliculus is present with extension to the petrous apex cells lying below the cochlea. In type B is when between the fustis and the funiculus a small hole is present, the connection between this hole and the apex. Type C is when the fustis and the area concamerata are fused with the funiculus and anterior pillar without any connection between the round window chamber and the petrous apex.

It is important to keep in mind, especially in children, that a wide subcochlear canaliculus (type A) extending to the petrous apex lying below the promontory is expected in most cases, and this anatomic area could be infiltrated by cholesteatoma.[21]

HYPOTYMPANUM
Boundaries

- Superior: confluent to the mesotympanum
- Inferior: bony wall, which separates the tympanic cavity from the jugular bulb

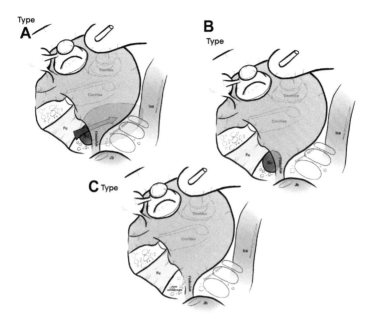

Fig. 18. Right ear. Anatomic variations of the subcochlear canaliculus. Type A: the subcochlear canaliculus is a deep extension to the petrous apex cells lying below the cochlea. Type B; the subcochlear canaliculus is a small hole, the connection between this hole and the apex is not recognizable endoscopically because of the dimensions of this area. Type C: the subcochlear canaliculus is absent. The fustis and the area concamerata are fused with the funiculus and anterior pillar, without any connection between the round window chamber and the petrous apex. Fu, fustis; Ica, internal carotid artery; Jb, Jacobson nerve; Sc, subcochlear canaliculus.

- Anterior: petrous bone that extends from its floor to the protiniculus; sometimes is compact, usually is pneumatized (infratubal pneumatic cells), and in some cases the front wall is formed by the bony canal of the horizontal petrous internal carotid artery
- Posterior: funiculus
- Medial: medial bony wall of the tympanic cavity
- Lateral: lateral bony wall of the tympanic cavity

The hypotympanum is the inferior area of the tympanic cavity from the funiculus to the protiniculus anteriorly. The inferior bony aspect of the hypotympanum separates the tympanic cavity from the jugular bulb, but in 25% of cases the jugular bulb protrudes into the tympanic cavity.[22]

SUMMARY

Endoscopic ear surgery is an innovative surgical technique. It offers a direct visualization of the retrotympanum and surrounding structures, such as the ossicular chain, chorda tympani, facial nerve, round and oval window niches, improving the anatomic and physiologic knowledge of the middle ear. It is also a "mastoid sparing" surgery, avoiding unnecessary mastoid bone and functional healthy mucosa removal. Thanks to the endoscope, new concepts were developed in the surgical treatment of middle ear pathologies, especially cholesteatoma.

CLINICS CARE POINTS

- Endoscopic ear surgery is an innovative surgical technique.
- Direct visualization of hidden areas, such as retrotympanum and surrounding structures, epitympanum and protympanum.
- It improvs the anatomic and physiologic knowledge of the middle ear.
- Functional surgery, preserving healthy mucosa of the middle ear and mastoid.

DISCLOSURE

The authors have nothing to disclose.

REFERENCES

1. Marchioni D, Mattioli F, Alicandri-Ciufelli M, et al. Endoscopic evaluation of middle ear ventilation route blockage. Am J Otolaryngol 2010;31(6):453–66.
2. Marchioni D, Alicandri-Ciufelli M, Grammatica A, et al. Lateral endoscopic approach to epitympanic diaphragm and Prussak's space: a dissection study. Surg Radiol Anat 2010;32(9):843–52.
3. Prussak A. Zur Anatomie des menschlichen Trommelfells. Arch Augenheilkd 1867;3:255–78.
4. Palva T, Johnsson LG. Epitympanic compartment surgical considerations: reevaluation. Am J Otol 1995;16(4):505–13.
5. Palva T, Johnsson LG, Ramsay H. Attic aeration in temporal bones from children with recurring otitis media: tympanostomy tubes did not cure disease in Prussak's space. Am J Otol 2000;21(4):485–93.
6. Chatellier HP, Lemoine J. Le diaphragme interatticotympanique du nouveau-ne. Ann Otolaryngol Chir Cervicofac 1946;13:534–66.
7. Li B, Doan P, Gruhl RR, et al. Endoscopic anatomy of the tensor fold and anterior attic. Otolaryngol Head Neck Surg 2018;158(2):358–63.
8. Marchioni D, Alicandri-Ciufelli M, Molteni G, et al. Selective epitympanic dysventilation syndrome. Laryngoscope 2010;120(5):1028–33.
9. Tanabe M, Takahashi H, Honjo I, et al. Gas exchange function of the middle ear in patients with otitis media with effusion. Eur Arch Otorhinolaryngol 1997; 254(9–10):453–5.
10. Marchioni D, Piccinini A, Alicandri-Ciufelli M, et al. Endoscopic anatomy and ventilation of the epitympanum. Otolaryngol Clin North Am 2013;46(2):165–78.
11. Marchioni D, Soloperto D, Rubini A, et al. Endoscopic facial nerve surgery. Otolaryngol Clin North Am 2016;49(5):1173–87.
12. Marchioni D, Rubini A, Nogueira JF, et al. Transcanal endoscopic approach to lesions of the suprageniculate ganglion fossa. Auris Nasus Larynx 2018;45(1): 57–65.
13. Soloperto D, Di Maro F, Le Pera B, et al. Surgical anatomy of the facial nerve: from middle cranial fossa approach to endoscopic approach. A pictorial review. Eur Arch Otorhinolaryngol 2020;277(5):1315–26.
14. Jufas N, Rubini A, Soloperto D, et al. The protympanum, protiniculum and subtensor recess: an endoscopic morphological anatomy study. J Laryngol Otol 2018; 132(6):489–92.
15. Jufas N, Marchioni D, Tarabichi M, et al. Endoscopic anatomy of the protympanum. Otolaryngol Clin North Am 2016;49(5):1107–19.
16. Marchioni D, Alicandri-Ciufelli M, Piccinini A, et al. Inferior retrotympanum revisited: an endoscopic anatomic study. Laryngoscope 2010;120(9):1880–6.

17. Marchioni D, Alicandri-Ciufelli M, Grammatica A, et al. Pyramidal eminence and subpyramidal space: an endoscopic anatomical study. Laryngoscope 2010; 120(3):557–64.
18. Rubini A, Jufas N, Marchioni D, et al. The endoscopic relationship of the stapedius muscle to the facial nerve: implications for retrotympanic surgery. Otol Neurotol 2019;41(1):e64–9.
19. Marchioni D, Mattioli F, Alicandri-Ciufelli M, et al. Transcanal endoscopic approach to the sinus tympani: a clinical report. Otol Neurotol 2009;30(6):758–65.
20. Marchioni D, Soloperto D, Colleselli E, et al. Round window chamber and fustis: endoscopic anatomy and surgical implications. Surg Radiol Anat 2016;38(9): 1013–9.
21. Marchioni D, Alicandri-Ciufelli M, Pothier DD, et al. The round window region and contiguous areas: endoscopic anatomy and surgical implications. Eur Arch Otorhinolaryngol 2015;272(5):1103–12.
22. Presutti L, Marchioni D. Endoscopic ear surgery. Principles, indications, and techniques, vol. 4. Thieme. Thieme Publishers Stuttgard; 2015. p. 7.

Getting Started with Endoscopic Ear Surgery

Elliott D. Kozin, MD[a],*, Daniel J. Lee, MD[a], Natasha Pollak, MD[b]

KEYWORDS

- Endoscopic ear surgery • Neurotology • Cholesteatoma • Endoscope • EES
- Otology • Transcanal surgery

KEY POINTS

- Endoscopes allow for improved visualization of the operative field, as the light emanates from the distal tip of the instrument, with specialized optics designed to offer a wide perspective.
- Essential equipment for endoscopic ear surgery includes a (1) light source, for example, xenon, halogen, or light-emitting diode; (2) selection of rigid endoscopes, for example, 14 cm in length and 3 mm in diameter; (3) high-definition (HD) 3-chip camera; and (4) HD video monitor.
- A 0° endoscope should be used initially, as it provides a safe view of the surgical field without "blind spots" of angled endoscopes.
- Because of the potential for tissue desiccation and thermal injury, light source intensity should be no greater than 50%.
- Nearly all standard otologic instruments can be used with EES.
- Once proficiency is gained in EES, additional curved instruments may be incorporated.
- Meticulous vasoconstriction is essential in EES cases given the need for one-handed dissection.

INTRODUCTION

Otologic surgery has progressed rapidly over the past century. In the first half of the twentieth century, ear surgery was generally completed with loupes or without magnification. With the introduction of the binocular operating microscope by Karl Zeiss and Hans Littmann in 1953, otologic surgery entered its modern era.[1–3] The operative microscope has been essential for otologic surgery, as it provides excellent illumination, depth perception, adjustable magnification, and ability to work with 2 hands. The

[a] Department of Otolaryngology, Massachusetts Eye and Ear Infirmary, Harvard Medical School, 243 Charles Street, Boston, MA 02114, USA; [b] Department of Otolaryngology–Head and Neck Surgery, Lewis Katz School of Medicine, 7604 Central Avenue, Friends Hall, Suite 100, Philadelphia, PA 19111, USA
* Corresponding author.
E-mail address: Elliott_Kozin@meei.harvard.edu

Otolaryngol Clin N Am 54 (2021) 45–57
https://doi.org/10.1016/j.otc.2020.09.009
0030-6665/21/© 2020 Elsevier Inc. All rights reserved.

microscope, however, is limited when constrained by small surgical corridors, such as the external auditory canal. In these cases, soft tissue dissection (eg, endaural or post-auricular approaches) or bone removal (eg, canalplasty, atticotomy, removal of ossicles, and canal up or down mastoidectomy) are often needed in order to visualize and access middle ear disease.

Paralleling the introduction of endoscopes for sinus surgery by David Kennedy in 1985, otology is undergoing a similar paradigm shift. The use of endoscopy to visualize the middle ear was discussed as early as the 1940s and more practically trialed in the late 1960s.[4,5] (**Fig. 1**) Unfortunately, poor image resolution limited its widespread application.[3,4] With the introduction of the Hopkins rod endoscope, cold light sources, 3-phase charge-coupled device (3-CCD) cameras, and h-gh definition video monitors, contemporary surgical endoscopy systems can provide brilliant high-resolution images of the ear that rival or surpass those of operative microscopes.

Advocates of endoscopic ear surgery (EES) appreciate the wide field of view, magnification, and the ability to "look around corners" (**Fig. 2**). Transcanal endoscopic ear surgery (TEES) approaches transform the external auditory canal into a minimally invasive surgical portal to access middle ear (and inner ear) disease. It is important to emphasize that the endoscope is not a "microscope replacement" but may serve a specialized purpose in select cases (**Table 1**). In this article the authors discuss (1) rationale for EES, (2) terminology and classification, (3) surgical indications, (4) essential equipment, (5) surgical ergonomics, and (6) practical steps to safely incorporate EES into practice.

RATIONALE FOR ENDOSCOPIC EAR SURGERY

Rigid endoscopes were initially used in the ear as an adjunct to hand-held otoscopes and microscopes for diagnostic purposes.[6,7] Early adopters quickly realized that the wide-angle view of endoscopes can reveal recesses of the tympanic cavity not

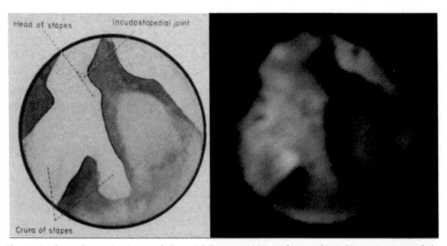

Fig. 1. Early endoscopic views of the middle ear, 1967. Left panel: endoscopic view of the stapes and incudostapedial joint. Right panel: cadaveric view of stapes and incudostapedial joint using a custom built rigid endoscope with roughly 2.5 mm diameter. (*Reproduced with permission from* Mer SB, Derbyshire AJ, Brushenko A, Pontarelli DA. Fiberoptic endotoscopes for examining the middle ear. Arch Otolaryngol. 1967 Apr;85(4):387-93. Copyright © 1967 American Medical Association. All rights reserved.)

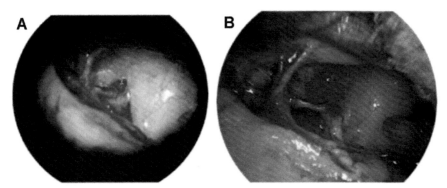

Fig. 2. Microscopic and endoscopic views of the right middle ear. This patient presented with right-sided conductive hearing loss and normal otoscopy. Intraoperative findings were consistent with spontaneous erosion of the incus. (*A*): Microscopic view of the right middle ear (patient is in supine position), taken at highest magnification with an HD 3 CCD video camera. (*B*): Endoscopic view of the same ear, demonstrating a wide field view that has greater detail, depth, and clarity (0° endoscope, held in the RIGHT hand). (*Adapted from* Kozin ED, Kiringoda R, Lee DJ. Incorporating Endoscopic Ear Surgery into Your Clinical Practice. Otolaryngol Clin North Am. 2016 Oct;49(5):1237-51 https://doi.org/10.1016/j.otc.2016.05.005.)

generally visible with the microscope. Early studies focused on descriptions of middle ear anatomy more easily seen with endoscopes. In the 1990s, investigators extended these studies to middle ear pathology, and applied endoscopes as observational tools and operative tools in cholesteatoma cases to detect "hidden" disease that would have been missed by a microscope.[8–13] Studies over the past 15 to 20 years have demonstrated that the endoscope may be a reasonable alternative and/or adjunct

Table 1
Basic differences between endoscopic and microscopic ear surgery

	Endoscope	Microscope
Number of Hands Available for Dissection	One-handed	Two-handed
Typical Surgical Approach	Transcanal (can be postauricular for combined cases as well as via the antrum following canal up mastoidectomy)	Transcanal with speculum ± endaural incision or postauricular
Resolution	High	High
Binocular Vision	No	Yes
Field of View	Wide	Narrow
Ability to Look Around Corners	Yes (0°–70°)	No
Portal needed for visualization	Narrow	Wide

to the microscope to perform a wide range of otologic procedures. Benefits of endoscopes in otologic surgery include the following[14]:

1. *Endoscopes let the surgeon see better*—the wide field of view provided by endoscopes allows for improved visualization of the tympanic cavity and its recesses. This enhanced surgical view enables more robust understanding of middle ear structures and their spatial relationships.
2. *Endoscopes allow the surgeon to complete more work transcanal*—EES transforms the external auditory canal into a minimally invasive portal for middle ear surgery (and inner ear surgery in selected cases). This reduces the need to dissect bone and soft tissue solely for exposure. Often, postauricular incisions and canalplasties can be avoided. This may reduce associated morbidity and improve wound healing.
3. *Endoscopes may reduce cholesteatoma recidivism rates and other ear surgery complications*—studies over the past 15 years have shown either equivalent outcomes or decreased residual disease using an endoscope, also minimal complications when using the microscope.[15–17]

It is also necessary to point out some potential drawbacks of EES:

1. Significant time and practice are needed to gain proficiency with EES
2. Challenges with one-handed dissection
3. Reliance on motion parallax to assess depth perception. Slight movement of the endoscope tip improves depth perception.

Although some investment of time and effort is needed to gain a level of proficiency, the endoscope is emerging as a valuable adjunct to the binocular microscope, and in some cases, the sole means for visualization for many routine and complex otologic and skull base procedures for experienced surgeons (**Fig. 3**). Although challenges exist in the adoption and development of EES, the benefits of a minimally invasive approach with improved visualization are convincingly pushing ear surgeons toward adopting this technique.

Endoscopic Ear Surgery Terminology and Classification Systems

Over the past half-century, various terminologies have been applied to describe the use of the endoscopes to visualize ear anatomy. Standardized terminology is necessary to communicate with colleagues and patients.

- *Otoendoscopy:* use of the endoscope for inspection of the outer ear, middle ear, mastoid, or lateral skull base. Otoendoscopy may be used in the clinical setting to inspect the tympanic membrane or middle ear through a perforation and can be used in the operating room setting to look around corners and assess for residual disease.
- *EES:* use of the endoscope for simultaneous visualization and dissection of the outer ear, middle ear, and/or mastoid. Typically, the endoscope is held in the nondominant hand, whereas the dissecting instrument is applied with the dominant hand.
- *TEES:* refers to EES techniques in which the external auditory canal is used as the primary surgical portal to access the tympanic membrane, middle ear, and in very specialized cases, the inner ear and lateral aspect (fundus) of the internal auditory canal.

A classification system by Cohen and colleagues[18] for EES has been developed to facilitate communication among physicians, patients, and researchers (**Table 2**).

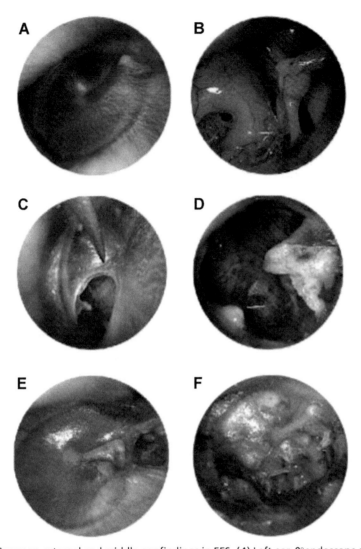

Fig. 3. Common external and middle ear findings in EES. (*A*) Left ear, 0°endoscope showing a normal tympanic membrane in a patient with conductive hearing loss. (*B*) Left ear, 0° endoscope showing the ossicular chain, facial nerve, and cochlea following elevation of tympanomeatal flap from Panel A. This patient was found to have stapes fixation from otosclerosis (subtle white plaque seen anterior to stapes, in fissula ante fenestrum). (*C*) Left ear, 0° endoscope showing an inferior central perforation of the tympanic membrane, an ideal pediatric case for the beginning endoscopic ear surgeon (courtesy of Michael Cohen, MD). (*D*) Left ear, 0° endoscope showing a child with a subtotal tympanic membrane perforation with cholesteatoma—this patient underwent a transcanal endoscopic lateral graft tympanoplasty with resection of disease. (*E*) Left ear, 0° endoscope showing attic cholesteatoma, an ideal indication for EES. (*F*) Left ear, 0° endoscope showing a thin dimeric tympanic membrane with complex retraction and perforation, incus erosion, and myringostapediopexy. This case is better suited for an experienced endoscopic ear surgeon or open approach. (*Adapted from* Kozin ED and Lee DJ. Basic Principles of Endoscopic Ear Surgery. Operative Techniques in Otolaryngology. – Head and Neck Surgery. 28(1): 2-10 2017; needs permission.)

Table 2		
Transcanal endoscopic ear surgery classification system		
Class	**Description**	**TEES vs Non-TEES**
0	Operative microscope alone	Non-TEES
1	Endoscope used for inspection/observation-only; no dissection	
2A	Mixed microscopic/endoscopic dissection; minority (<50%) of dissection with endoscope	
2B	Mixed microscopic/endoscopic dissection; majority (>50%) of dissection with endoscope	
3	Endoscope-only	TEES

Adapted from Cohen MS, Basonbul RA, Barber SR, Kozin ED, Rivas AC, Lee DJ. Development and validation of an endoscopic ear surgery classification system. Laryngoscope 2018; 128:967-970.

Class 0 cases only use a microscope and may be considered as use of "traditional" approaches. Class 1 cases use the endoscope for visualization but not dissection. Class 2 cases are a "mixed cases" with use of both the endoscope and microscope for dissection. Finally, class 3 refers to cases in which the endoscope is used from start to finish. Class 3 cases are synonymous with TEES.

INDICATIONS AND CONTRAINDICATIONS FOR ENDOSCOPIC EAR SURGERY

Otologic cases performed via microscopic techniques may generally be assisted by use of an endoscope. The endoscope may be used to replace the microscope for purposes of dissection or used to augment microscopic visualization given wide field of view and ability to look around corners. The application of the endoscope to perform otologic surgery is growing, and new surgical approaches are being refined (**Table 3**). There are no known absolute contraindications to EES. Potential complications of EES are identical to that of traditional microscopic ear surgery, including damage to surrounding structures, such as ossicular chain, bony labyrinth and, facial nerve. There are no studies that directly compare immediate surgical complications from microscope-based approaches with endoscope-based approaches.

Table 3	
Basic indications for endoscopic ear surgery	
External Ear	• Cholesteatoma • Exostosis repair • Canalplasty • Debridement and biopsy
Middle Ear	• Myringotomy • Myringoplasty • Medial graft tympanoplasty • Lateral graft tympanoplasty • Tympanic membrane retraction • Acquired cholesteatoma • Congenital cholesteatoma • Neoplasms of middle ear (eg, glomus tympanicum) • Ossiculoplasty

Still, there is no reason to believe that complications for EES are higher than for microscope-based approaches. The authors recommend that adopters of EES attend a dedicated course to practice techniques before incorporating them into practice. The surgical views vary dramatically from microscope-based otologic cases, and transcanal techniques take practice to learn. Practice with one-handed dissection in the controlled environment of a temporal bone laboratory is important. If unable to attend a course, the authors encourage use of fresh cadaveric tissue, rather than fixed tissue, which better replicates the pliable feel of the external auditory canal.

ESSENTIAL INSTRUMENTATION FOR ENDOSCOPIC EAR SURGERY

Essential equipment for endoscopic middle ear surgery includes (1) a light source, (2) rigid endoscopes (0° and 30°), (3) a high-definition (HD) 3-phase charge-coupled device (3-CCD) camera, and (4) HD video monitor.

Light Sources and Camera Systems

Light sources of varying brightness and temperature are readily available, including xenon, light-emitting diode, and halogen. Endoscope camera systems are available from a variety of vendors. The main requirement for camera systems is a 3-CCD camera. Single-chip cameras tend to become saturated and "red out" when used in a small area that contains bleeding and are therefore unacceptable. Light source and camera systems are identical to that of endoscopic sinus surgery.

Endoscopes

The Hopkins rod is a popular choice among otolaryngologists for endoscopic surgery. Endoscopes of varying diameters, lengths, and angles are available. As the diameter expands, the image quality generally improves as more light is transmitted to the operative field and back. Wider diameter endoscopes, however, decrease the working space available for additional instruments. The rigid endoscope diameters commonly used for ear surgery are 2.7 mm, 3 mm, and 4 mm (**Fig. 4**). EES can be performed with 4 mm diameter scopes if the external canal is large enough; however, it may be difficult to place an instrument alongside the scope. Typical endoscope shaft lengths in EES are 11 cm, 14 cm, and 18 cm. The authors generally recommend endoscopes that are approximately 3 mm in diameter and ~14 cm in length. Both 0° and 30° endoscopes are routinely used for most of the EES cases.[14,16,19]

Additional Instruments

Most of the standard otologic instruments may be used for EES (**Table 4**). Several manufacturers offer EES-specific instruments. These are not necessary to begin EES but are useful, as surgeons gains greater proficiency with this new technique. As surgeons become more experienced, additional curved instruments may be used, including curved suctions and dissectors, that take advantage of the endoscope's wide field of view.

ERGONOMICS FOR ENDOSCOPIC EAR SURGERY

Proper surgical ergonomics are crucial to reduce the frustration and added operative time needed to develop proficiency with endoscopic cases. Proper body mechanics for EES is different from microscopic cases, as surgeons perform "heads up surgery" and watch a monitor instead of using the binocular eyepieces of the microscope. Before the patient is brought into the room, surgeon, anesthesia, and ancillary

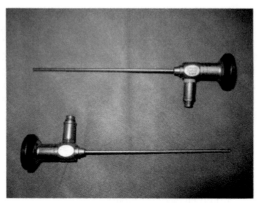

Fig. 4. Endoscopes designed for EES. 0° (*top*) and 30° (*bottom*), 3-mm diameter, 14-cm length rigid endoscopes. (*Adapted from* Kozin ED, Kiringoda R, Lee DJ. Incorporating Endoscopic Ear Surgery into Your Clinical Practice. Otolaryngol Clin North Am. 2016 Oct;49(5):1237-51 https://doi.org/10.1016/j.otc.2016.05.005.)

operating staff must discuss the optimized room layout. In case the microscope is needed, it should be readily accessible (**Figs. 5** and **6**).

Operating Room Setup

The patient's head should be placed directly on the pad of the operating room table. One should avoid placing the head on a dedicated elevated headrest, such as a surgical donut, unless there is limited neck extension, as this will limit the ability to turn the head and rapidly use the microscope, if needed. To ensure minimal neck strain of the surgeon, the video tower (or boom-mounted video screen) should be directly across from the surgeon and placed as close to eye level as possible (see **Fig. 6**). The microscope should be placed in the corner of the room that allows for easy access.[16,19]

Hand Positioning and Placement of the Endoscope

An otologic chair with armrests may be helpful for additional support while holding an endoscope, decreasing fatigue, and reducing physiologic tremor. Both forearms/elbows should rest either on the table, patient shoulder, or armrest to maintain stability and minimize fatigue. The endoscope may be held in a similar fashion as endoscopic sinus surgery, which is partly along the shaft and camera head. The endoscope is

Table 4		
Differences between endoscopic and microscopic ear surgery equipment		
	Endoscope	**Microscope**
Source of visualization	Endoscope, 3 CCD camera, HD monitor	Microscope
Basic instrumentation	Standard otologic instrument set	Standard otologic instrument set
Additional instruments	Suction dissector, curved suction tips	None

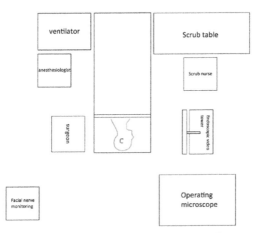

Fig. 5. EES room setup. The surgeon should be directly across from the endoscopic video tower (or ceiling-mounted video screen), which should be placed close to eye level to avoid neck strain. The scrub table can be placed at the foot of the bed to accommodate the video system. Layout may vary based on the constraints of a particular operating room; however, certain principles are always maintained, such as keeping the video tower opposite the surgeon, near eye level. (*Adapted from* Kozin ED, Kiringoda R, Lee DJ. Incorporating Endoscopic Ear Surgery into Your Clinical Practice. Otolaryngol Clin North Am. 2016 Oct;49(5):1237-51 https://doi.org/10.1016/j.otc.2016.05.005.)

proximally stabilized gently along the cartilaginous meatus. Note that any significant torque on the endoscope will bend the fiberoptic cable and reduce image quality.

Left Versus Right Ears

Although EES reduces the visual limitations imposed by the anterior overhang of the external auditory canal, it does make it more difficult to instrument the middle ear.

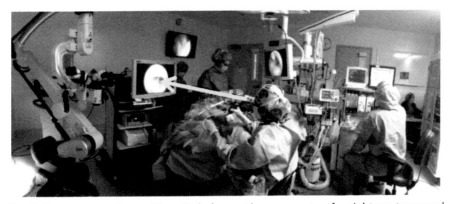

Fig. 6. Surgeon—monitor position. Typical operating room setup for right ear transcanal EES. Note the operating microscope positioned near the head of the patient, in case needed. The monitor is placed directly across from the surgeon at eye level. The surgical assistant (scrub) is also across from the patient to facilitate instrument transfer. (*Adapted from* Kozin ED and Lee DJ. Basic Principles of Endoscopic Ear Surgery. Operative Techniques in Otolaryngology. – Head and Neck Surgery. 28(1): 2-10 2017; needs permission.)

The right-handed surgeons are recommended to start with left ear cases because dissection of routine and complex middle ear disease is easier in the left than the right ear. The 2 reasons for this are that the anterior canal overhang does not limit access with dissection instruments and that the trajectory of the endoscope is biased toward the superior portion of the tympanic cavity to allow for visualization of the ossicles and facial nerve as well as access to most of the middle ear diseases. The authors recommend using the dominant hand for dissection in both left and right ear cases.

INTRODUCING ENDOSCOPIC EAR SURGERY INTO PRACTICE

After taking an EES course, the authors recommend a *3-step process* to introduce EES into your operative routine:

1. Use the endoscope during chronic ear surgery *after* the microscope-based dissection to
   - Look for hidden disease
   - Perform a complete 360° endoscopic survey of the middle ear cleft with a 30° endoscope
   - Assess the ossicular chain and round window
2. Perform a "basic" transcanal procedure, including
   - Endoscopic examination under anesthesia of the external canal and tympanic membrane before your microscopic dissection to document pathology
   - Cerumen removal
   - Tympanostomy tube placement
   - Myringoplasty (without drum elevation)
3. Use the microscope to begin raising the tympanomeatal flap, then complete elevation with EES techniques
   - Switch to a 0° endoscope before dissection of the annulus and then complete your tympanotomy endoscopically

At the onset, do not expect to be able to perform a case from beginning to end using an endoscope. Use the endoscope for limited aspects of cases. As you gain proficiency, do less with the microscope and more with the endoscope. Indeed, do not be concerned if you need to transition to a microscopic case, which is very common when starting EES and is encouraged. After fluency in basic EES techniques is achieved, you may begin to consider more advanced instrumentation, such as curved suctions (**Fig. 7**).

Pearls and Pitfalls

The following are some pearls and pitfalls for new endoscopic ear surgeons:

- *Proper trimming of ear hair is critical before the start of EES.* The endoscope will likely be placed into the ear canal many times during a routine case. Hair will smudge the lens, and the endoscope will require constant wiping. The authors use curved iris scissors under endoscopic guidance to ensure atraumatic hair removal.
- *A microwipe saturated with saline and defog pad may be placed near the head of the patient for easy access.* Animal studies have indicated potential ototoxicity of defog solution, a combination of ethyl alcohol and surfactant.[20] The authors advise wiping the endoscope after application of defog with a saline-saturated microwipe or sponge to avoid introducing excessive defog solution into the middle ear. Avoid placing the defog pad near the patient's eye.

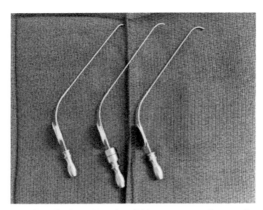

Fig. 7. Curved suctions. The ideal suction should have a manufactured curved tip and swivel connector for tubing to reduce twisting during delicate maneuvers. Traditional otologic suctions can also be bent by the surgeon to achieve similar results; however, bending often crimps the lumen of the suction, reducing suctioning power and causing premature blockage. A wire stylet can be placed before bending but this only minimally reduces crimping. For most applications, only a minimally curved or bent suction tip is needed. A more exaggerated curved suction is difficult to manipulate and can increase the risk of injuring ossicles, facial nerve, or tympanic tegmen. (*Adapted from* Kozin ED, Kiringoda R, Lee DJ. Incorporating Endoscopic Ear Surgery into Your Clinical Practice. Otolaryngol Clin North Am. 2016 Oct;49(5):1237-51 https://doi.org/10.1016/j.otc.2016.05.005.)

- *Avoid endoscope holders.* We generally do not recommend the use of an endoscope holder.[21] If the patient moves during surgery, a fixed endoscope in the external or middle ear could irreversibly damage critical structures. In addition, most ear canals are unable to easily accommodate 3 simultaneous instruments.
- *Hemostasis is critical.* Injection of a mixture of lidocaine and dilute epinephrine with a 27-gauge bent needle may assist in hemostasis when raising a tympanomeatal flap. A small cotton ball soaked in epinephrine may also be helpful to place in the ear canal near the edge of the flap. Continuous surgical count of cotton balls during surgery is crucial to avoid leaving these items in the middle ear. Also, gently elevating the upper body may result in decreased bleeding. It is also important to communicate with the anesthesiologist regarding blood pressure maintenance. Safely avoiding high blood pressure will help reduce bleeding.
- *Keep the light source at less than 50% power.* Several studies have demonstrated the potential for high temperatures in the middle ear associated with radiant energy from the endoscope.[22–25] For this reason, the authors recommend keeping the power of the light source no greater than 50% and a safe distance (>5 mm) away inner ear structures. Frequently taking the endoscope out of the middle ear, along with occasional suction and saline irrigation, is important for cooling the middle ear space.

SUMMARY

The experienced ear surgeon who wishes to include the intraoperative use of rigid endoscopes into his or her surgical practice may readily do so with only minimal additional equipment and setup. Essential equipment for EES includes a light source, rigid endoscopes, HD camera, and an HD video monitor, equipment already available in operating rooms where endoscopic sinus surgery is done. In order to successfully use endoscopic ear techniques, it is important to have good optics. Endoscopes gradually and insidiously degrade in optical quality and have to be replaced. Mishandling endoscopes during sterile processing may degrade the optics rapidly. High-quality camera systems and HD monitors are needed to proceed with EES in a stress-free manner. Several good ear surgeons have grown frustrated and abandoned EES solely due to limitations in optical quality of their equipment.

One should not expect to be able to perform surgery from beginning to end using an endoscope while learning EES. Initially, use the endoscope for limited aspects of cases. There is no need to be concerned if one needs to transition back to a microscopic case, which is very common when starting EES. As the surgeon gains experience with EES, he or she may do less with the microscope and more with the endoscope, while gradually incorporating the use of angled instruments.

CLINICS CARE POINTS

- Studies have demonstrated equivlanet and/or improved outcomes of endoscopic ear surgery compared to standard operative microscopy.
- Endoscopes allow improved visualization of the middle ear.
- Endoscopes are increasingly part of routine otologic procedures.

DISCLOSURES

None.

CONFLICT OF INTEREST

None.

REFERENCES

1. Uluc K, Kujoth GC, Baskaya MK. Operating microscopes: past, present, and future. Neurosurg focus 2009;27:E4.
2. Mudry A. The history of the microscope for use in ear surgery. Am J Otol 2000;21: 877–86.
3. N. P.. Introduction to endoscopic ear surgery. In: Pollak N, editor. Endoscopic ear surgery. San Diego (CA): Plural Publishing; 2013.
4. Mer S, Derbyshire J, Brushenko A, et al. Fiberoptic endotoscope for examing the middle ear. Arch Otolaryngol 1967;85:61–7.
5. Bekesy G. Suggestions for determining the mobility of the stapes by means of an endotoscope for the middle ear. Laryngoscope 1950;60:97–100, illust.
6. Nomura Y. Effective photography in otolaryngology-head and neck surgery: endoscopic photography of the middle ear. Otolaryngol Head Neck Surg 1982; 90:395–8.
7. Takahashi H, Honjo I, Fujita A, et al. Transtympanic endoscopic findings in patients with otitis media with effusion. Arch Otolaryngol Head Neck Surg 1990; 116:1186–9.
8. Yung M. The use of rigid endoscopes in cholesteatoma surgery. J Laryngol Otol 1994;108:307–9.
9. Thomassin J, Korchia D, Doris J. Endoscope-guided otosurgery in the prevention of residual cholesteatomas. Laryngoscope 1993;103:939–43.

10. Rosenberg S, Silverstein H, Hoffer M, et al. Use of endoscopes for chronic ear surgery in children. Arch Otolaryngol Head Neck Surg 1995;121:870–2.
11. Good G, Isaacson G. Otoendoscopy for improved pediatric cholesteatoma removal. Ann Otol Rhinol Laryngol 1999;108:893–6.
12. Haberkamp T, Tanyeri H. Surgical techniques to facilitate endoscopic second-look mastoidectomy. Laryngoscope 1999;109:1023–7.
13. Kozin ED, Gulati S, Kaplan AB, et al. Systematic review of outcomes following observational and operative endoscopic middle ear surgery. Laryngoscope 2015;125:1205–14.
14. Pollak N. Endoscopic and minimally-invasive ear surgery: a path to better outcomes. World J Otorhinolaryngol Head Neck Surg 2017;3:129–35.
15. Cohen MS, Landegger LD, Kozin ED, et al. Pediatric endoscopic ear surgery in clinical practice: lessons learned and early outcomes. Laryngoscope 2016;126:732–8.
16. Kozin ED, Kiringoda R, Lee DJ. Incorporating endoscopic ear surgery into your clinical practice. Otolaryngol Clin North Am 2016;49:1237–51.
17. Cohen MS, Basonbul RA, Kozin ED, et al. Residual cholesteatoma during second-look procedures following primary pediatric endoscopic ear surgery. Otolaryngol Head Neck Surg 2017;157:1034–40.
18. Cohen MS, Basonbul RA, Barber SR, et al. Development and validation of an endoscopic ear surgery classification system. Laryngoscope 2018;128:967–70.
19. N. P. Instrumentation and operating room setup. In: Pollak N, editor. Endoscopic ear surgery. San Diego (CA): Plural Publishing; 2014.
20. Nomura K, Oshima H, Yamauchi D, et al. Ototoxic effect of Ultrastop antifog solution applied to the guinea pig middle ear. Otolaryngol Head Neck Surg 2014;151:840–4.
21. Kozin ED, Remenschneider AK, Shah P, et al. In response to: letter to the editor. Am J Otolaryngol 2015;36:844–5.
22. Aksoy F, Dogan R, Ozturan O, et al. Thermal effects of cold light sources used in otologic surgery. Eur Arch Otorhinolaryngol 2014;272(10):2679–87.
23. Kozin E, Lehmann A, Carter M, et al. Thermal effects of endoscopy in a human temporal bone model: implications for endoscopic ear surgery. Laryngoscope 2014;124:E332–9.
24. MacKeith S, Frampton S, Pothier D. Thermal properties of operative endoscopes used in otorhinolaryngology. J Laryngol Otol 2008;122:711–4.
25. Tomazic P, Hammer G, Gerstenberger C, et al. Heat development at nasal endoscopes' tips: danger of tissue damage? A laboratory study. Laryngoscope 2012;122:1670–3.

Otoendoscopy in the Office and Operating Room

Michal Preis, MD

KEYWORDS

- Otoendoscopy • Otology • Endoscopic ear surgery • Patient-centered care
- Pediatric otolaryngology • Transcanal

KEY POINTS

- Otoendoscopy offers superior view to anatomic structures of the middle ear.
- Using the endoscope reduces need for soft tissue and bone removal.
- Otoendoscopy improved outcomes in cholesteatoma surgery.
- Endoscopy is safe in pediatric populations.
- Otoendoscopy improves patient-centered care.
- Portable endoscopic units provide flexibility of care in remote locations.

Ear disease is one of the commonest reasons for pediatric and adult physician visits. Ear examination is a required routine in almost any sick child visit and in most adult visits. The first written descriptions of ear examinations date as early as the 1300s. Peter de la Cerlata (sixteenth century) was the first to use a speculum for widening the external auditory canal for purposes of inspection. Rivinus (Germany 1717) believed that there is a natural opening in the tympanic membrane as a constant anatomic condition. This theory ignited a heated debate among anatomists at that time, prompting close inspection of the tympanic membrane of cadavers with the use of a magnifying glass. This debate was eventually solved by Valsalva who declared that orifices only exist in diseased ears.[1]

For the purpose of detailed inspection of the external auditory canal and tympanic membrane Dr Newbourg in 1827 recommended an instrument that is the origin of the tubular ear specula now in use, later shortened by Dr Gruber of Vienna, and introduced to the profession by Sir William Wilde in 1844. Once the canal was dilated using the speculum, light was thrown into it by means of the otoscope or reflector of Von Tröltsch (1855), reflecting daylight, sunlight, lamp light, gas light, or that of a candle. Introduced into the practice of New York Eye and Ear Infirmary in 1863 the speculum

Department of Otolaryngology, Maimonides Medical Center, State University of NY Downstate, 919 49th Street, Brooklyn, NY 11219, USA
E-mail address: mpreis@maimonidesmed.org

Otolaryngol Clin N Am 54 (2021) 59–64
https://doi.org/10.1016/j.otc.2020.09.004
0030-6665/21/© 2020 Elsevier Inc. All rights reserved.

was modified by Blake of Boston in 1870 to add an attached prism giving it the advantage of an "operating head."

In the middle of the nineteenth century, in Germany, the modern otoscope began to take shape. Wilhelm Kramer, a German otologist, developed a steel ear speculum with a funnel on the end. Kramer's speculum, as it became to be known, was the primary device used by physicians until 1881, when A. Hartmann created a design that mostly resembles today's look. The otoscope has remained unchanged since its invention albeit sleeker and more lightweight.

After being introduced, the handheld otoscope became the instrument of choice for ear evaluation in the hands of otolaryngologists and primary care physicians alike. Nonetheless, otoscopes have intrinsic limits because of limited illumination, limited magnification, and lack of three-dimensional image. To this must be added difficulty with young patients who will not hold still or who have narrow or cerumen-occluded ear canals. Furthermore, most otoscopes today do not save images for record keeping. From the patient and family's perspective, otoscopy is a "black box" and they are excluded from viewing or discussing the results.

No branch of medical science has perhaps been altered more profoundly, advanced more rapidly, and benefited more completely from the use of the binocular microscope than has otologic surgery. The use of monocular ear microscopy is first described by Carl Olof Nylen in 1921.[2] One year later, the binocular microscope produced by the Zeiss factory was used for the first time by Gunnar Holmgren while performing ear surgery.[3] The binocular microscope was improved between 1922 and 1953 when the Zeiss Opmi I operating otomicroscope was introduced. Binocular otomicroscopy gained popularity among otolaryngologists and has been used in the office setting and in the operating room. The microscope enables examination and manipulation of the external auditory canal in the office and is used for performing procedures on the external auditory canal, tympanic membrane, middle ear, mastoid, and petrous bone in the operating room. The use of the binocular microscope was undoubtedly one of the most important developments in the history of otology.[4]

OTOENDOSCOPY IN THE OFFICE

In the past decade there has been an increased incorporation of using rigid endoscopes in the office setting. Otoendoscopy, defined as using endoscopes for examining the ear, offers the advantage of a wide-angle, bright, and highly magnified view. If connected to an image capture system, it allows archiving and comparing examinations through the follow-up period. In-office otoendoscopy may enable inspection of the depth of retraction pockets that are traditionally impossible to visualize using the otomicroscope, impacting the decision making for surgical intervention.[5] For example, a 30° endoscope may show that posterior epitympanic retraction does not travel into the mastoid antrum, an ability that may be impossible with the line-of-sight microscope. The otoendoscope also allows better visualization of anterior tympanic perforations because it can bypass anterior external ear canal bulges. This can enable the surgeon to offer in-office surgical treatment. In-office endoscopy of the middle ear through an existing tympanic perforation as part of the preoperative evaluation provides useful information on the continuity of the ossicular chain. Otoendoscopy of a canal wall down mastoid cavity offers an advantage in cases of anatomic barriers to the microscopic visualization, namely stenotic meatoplasty, high facial ridge, and low tegmen. Freire and colleagues[6] showed that in-office examination of postoperative open mastoid cavities using an endoscope exposed areas that were not visualized under the microscope in more than half of the cases, and in two-thirds of the cases endoscopy enabled removal of material that could not be cleared under the microscope. However, this may require specialized angled instruments. Office-based endoscopic examination of the middle ear through a myringotomy[7] was described as an alternative to exploratory tympanostomy in conductive hearing loss. Finally, otoendoscopy can be performed on hospital inpatients as demonstrated by Coticchia[8] in a study on preterm neonates where 73% were found to have otitis media.

Because most otolaryngology offices already contain equipment for sinus endoscopy, including the endoscopes (rigid, 14–18 cm length and 3–5 mm diameter, 0–30°), cameras, light sources, and high-definition monitor, the incorporation of otoendoscopy in the office setting may require no additional cost. In a pediatric office 2.7-mm diameter endoscopes might allow better examination of narrow ear canals.

OTOENDOSCOPY IN THE OPERATING ROOM

The first description of an operative middle ear examination using an endoscope was published in the English literature in 1967,[9] stating improved visualization of deeper recesses in the middle ear while avoiding the necessary soft tissue retraction or bone removal that is required for microscopic "in line" view. With the advancement of technology Poe in 1992[10] described transtympanic otoendoscopy of the middle ear. Two-millimeter diameter rigid and flexible endoscopes were introduced through a strategically placed myringotomy or an existing perforation to perform exploration of the middle ear as an in-the-office procedure. This technique was recommended as an adjunct in the diagnostic evaluation of patients with suspected middle ear conditions with the goal of avoiding middle ear exploration and to improve planning of definitive surgery based on the endoscopic findings. Tarabichi in 1997[11] described middle ear surgery performed exclusively under endoscopic guidance. Otoendoscopy was originally described in use in the operating room either as an adjunct during primary resection where 16% to 76% of residual disease was identified following microscopic resection,[12] or for second-look endoscopic explorations. Cases that used the endoscope in primary procedure had decreased cholesteatoma found during the second look. Ayache in 2008[13] determined that the contribution of otoendoscopy in the surgical management of cholesteatoma of the middle ear is in significantly reducing the frequency of open tympanoplasty, and offering a superior view of locations that require looking "around the corner" (sinus tympani, facial recess, attic, and anterior epitympanum).

Haidar[14] describes additional benefit to otoendoscopy in the operating room using a transattic endoscopic examination of the ossicular prosthesis following cholesteatoma surgery. Using this approach, they report a decreased risk of immediate ossiculoplasty failure and improvement of functional outcome of ossicular chain reconstruction in cholesteatoma surgery.

Otoendoscopy in pediatric ear surgery has been shown to be safe.[15] The detection and removal of cholesteatoma in difficult to visualize anatomic locations using the endoscope is in line with the trend toward less invasive surgery enabling preservation of the posterior ear canal and single-stage ossiculoplasty.[16] In the pediatric population, similar to adults, otoendoscopy as an adjunct to microscopic surgery was shown to detect incompletely removed cholesteatoma in 24% of the cases. Cohen[17] showed that use of the endoscope during primary cholesteatoma resection led to a lower rate of mastoidectomy for cases with similar disease extent. Rosenberg described 100% correlation between endoscopic second-look examination of the mastoid and middle ear and open mastoidectomy findings,[18,19] thus suggesting that open second-look mastoidectomy may be avoided if no recurrent cholesteatoma is found during the endoscopic exploration.

PATIENT-CENTERED CARE AND ENDOSCOPY

Medical practice is evolving from a paternalistic approach toward one characterized by shared patient/caregiver decision making. The concepts of patient-centeredness and patient empowerment offer opportunities for clinicians to allow patients to increase their autonomy and involvement in their care and treatment. This has been shown to result in better disease management, better objective medical outcomes, and reduced diagnostic test expenditure. High patient satisfaction has a positive effect on medical outcome and patient compliance.

There is a paucity of studies on the benefit of otoendoscopy for patient satisfaction and education; however, one can learn from the experience of video-otoscopy. Video-otoscopy, defined as a traditional-style otoscope that contains a camera and outputs an image to a monitor, has equal or better accuracy compared with traditional video-otoscopy with the reference being an experienced otologist's diagnosis using microscopy.[20] Children may allow examination of the ear more readily if they can see an image on a screen. video-otoscopy offers the examiner the possibility to show and explain to the patient or caregiver about the findings. video-otoscopy has been found to be suitable for educational purposes. Studies have shown higher patient centeredness and parental satisfaction with video-otoscopy than traditional video-otoscopy. These results can naturally be extrapolated to otoendoscopy, although otoendoscopy would be expected to have an even superior image.

Further study is needed to evaluate the patient satisfaction and treatment outcome when using office-based otoendoscopy compared with standard video-otoscopy or otomicroscopy without image display.

OTOENDOSCOPY AND RESIDENT EDUCATION

Since the implementation of endoscopic sinus surgery in the 1990s, otolaryngology residents have received ample training in operative endoscopy. These residents look at endoscopic ear surgery as a natural continuum of their endoscopic training and are generally not intimidated by the use of single-handed surgery. With increasing implementation of endoscopic ear surgery and otoendoscopy in academic centers around the world,[21] residency programs should offer in-residency exposure and training on ear endoscopy.[22] In cases where that is not feasible, they should encourage residents to join endoscopic ear surgery cadaver courses.

In a randomized controlled study by Anschuetz[23] comparing the acquisition of basic ear surgery skills using endoscopic and microscopic technique, the endoscopic approach provided a reduction of damage to surrounding tissues with similar operating times for both techniques. The study subjects, medical students, residents, and fellows, performed significantly faster when first taught with the endoscopic technique.

The added visibility offered by the endoscope allows for a better understanding of the middle ear anatomy by the trainee. The ease of instructing a resident while pointing at the exact location on the screen is incomparable with instruction under the microscope without the ability to accurately demonstrate the desired action. Another study by Anschuetz[24] compared microscopic and endoscopic methods for teaching middle ear anatomy. The conclusion was that the endoscopic approach to the middle ear anatomy education is associated with improved gain in knowledge when compared with the microscopic approach.

PORTABILITY OF THE OTOENDOSCOPE

Advancement in technology has allowed portable endoscopic units that contain the light source, screen, and capturing system all in a conveniently transportable box. These portable units have an obvious advantage in remote locations. One example is medical mission trips. There is great inconvenience of bringing a large, heavy, mechanically sensitive operating microscope halfway across the globe. Furthermore, there will not be any professional to service its delicate components should it require maintenance or repair. This obstacle limits the availability of otologic surgery services in remote areas. The availability of the otoendoscopic portable unit allows examination and surgical procedures to be performed in a rural setting. Another goal of medical mission trips to remote locations is educating the local staff by demonstrating the findings and procedures on the portable screen and training of the local professionals. This improves the continuity of care, self-sufficiency of the local staff, and the success of the mission. In a study by Salisu[25] before the use of an otoendoscope the patients that were suitable for ear surgery were referred to an urban-based tertiary institution but 94% failed to proceed on the referral. With the introduction of endoscopic ear surgery at the rural location[26] 78% of the surgical candidates proceeded to undergo the recommended procedure, and of those referred, 5% proceeded on the referral.

DISCLOSURE

The author has no funding, financial relationships, or conflicts of interest to disclose.

REFERENCES

1. St, John Roosa DB, editors. A practical treatise on the diseases of the ear including the anatomy of the organ. New York: William Wood & Company; 1873.
2. Nylen CO. An oto microscope. Acta Otolaryngol 1923;5:414–7.
3. Holmgren G. Operations on the temporal bone carried out with the help of the lens and the microscope. Acta Otolaryngol 1922;4:386–93.
4. Mudry A. The history of the microscope for use in ear surgery. Am J Otol 2000;21: 877–86.
5. Fina M. Office based otology procedures. Otolaryngol Clin North Am 2019;52(3): 497–507.
6. Freire GSM, Sampaio ALL, Lopes RAF, et al. Does ear endoscopy provide advantages in the outpatient management of open mastoidectomy cavities? PLoS One 2018;13(1):e0191712.
7. Kakehata S. Office-based endoscopic procedure for diagnosis in conductive hearing loss cases using OtoScan laser assisted myringotomy. Laryngoscope 2004;114(7):1285–9.
8. Coticchia J. Frequency of otitis media based on otoendoscopic evaluation in preterm infants. Otolaryngol Head Neck Surg 2014;151(4):692–9.
9. Mer S. Fiberoptic endotoscopes for examining the middle ear. Arch Otolaryngol 1967;85(4):387–93.
10. Poe DS. Transtympanic endoscopy of the middle ear. Laryngoscope 1992; 102(9):993–6.
11. Tarabichi M. Endoscopy middle ear surgery. Ann Otol Rhinol Laryngol 1999; 108(1):39–46.
12. Badr-el-Dine M. Value of ear endoscopy in cholesteatoma surgery. Otol Neurotol 2002;23(5):631–5.

13. Ayache S. Otoendoscopy in cholesteatoma surgery of the middle ear: what benefits can be expected. Otol Neurotol 2008;29(8):1085–90.
14. Haidar H. The benefit of trans-attic endoscopic control of ossicular prosthesis after cholesteatoma surgery. Laryngoscope 2019;129(12):2754–9.
15. Bottril I. In vitro and in vivo determination of the thermal effect of middle ear endoscopy. Laryngoscope 1994;106:213–6.
16. Luu K. Updates in pediatric cholesteatoma: minimizing intervention while maximizing outcomes. Otolaryngol Clin North Am 2019;52(5):813–23.
17. Cohen M. Residual cholesteatoma during second-look procedures following primary pediatric endoscopic ear surgery. Otolaryngol Head Neck Surg 2017; 157(6):1034–40.
18. Rosenberg SI. Use of endoscopes for chronic ear surgery in children. Arch Otolaryngol Head Neck Surg 1995;121(8):870–2.
19. Betnnett M. Comparison of middle ear visualization with endoscopy and microscopy. Otol Neurotol 2016;37(4):362–6.
20. Rimon O. -otoscopy in children and patient centered care: a randomized, controlled study. Int J Pediatr Otorhinolaryngol 2015;79:2286–9.
21. Tarabichi M. Principles of endoscopic ear surgery. Curr Opin Otolaryngol Head Neck Surg 2016;24(5):382–7.
22. Guy J. Comparison of microscopic and endoscopic views in cadaveric ears. Eur Arch Otorhinolaryngol 2020;277(6):1655–8.
23. Anschuetz L. Acquisition of basic ear surgery skills: a randomized comparison between endoscopic and microscopic techniques. BMC Med Educ 2019; 19(1):357.
24. Anschuetz L. Assessment of middle ear anatomy teaching methodologies using microscopy versus endoscopy: a randomized comparative study. Anat Sci Educ 2019;12(5):507–17.
25. Salisu AD. Extending otology services to rural settings: value of endoscopic ear surgery. Ann Afr Med 2016;15(3):104–8.
26. Clark MPA. Endoscopic ear surgery in the ear camp setting; forward thinking or folly? J Laryngol Otol 2018;132(1):68–70.

Teaching Endoscopic Ear Surgery

Samuel R. Barber, MD[a], Divya A. Chari, MD[b], Alicia M. Quesnel, MD[b],*

KEYWORDS

- Endoscopic ear surgery • Simulation • Education • Training

KEY POINTS

- Teaching endoscopic ear surgery presents unique challenges because of specialized skill sets with a steep learning curve.
- Endoscopic procedures are becoming more common as the endoscope garners widespread use, yet many surgical trainees and practicing otolaryngologists have limited exposure and opportunities to learn endoscopic techniques.
- Physical and virtual task trainers and simulators have been developed and may facilitate skill acquisition outside of the operating room.
- As minimally invasive, endoscopic approaches to the lateral skull base continue to develop, there is an impetus to develop additional training tools to master increasingly complex concepts.

INTRODUCTION

Endoscopic ear surgery (EES) is a rapidly evolving field. Although the basic principles and advantages of endoscopes for otologic surgery were introduced several decades ago,[1–3] more widespread use of the endoscope in place of, or in addition to, the microscope has become popularized only in recent years.[4] Advancements in endoscope image resolution, camera quality, and surgical techniques, and a growing pool of published outcome studies, have led to a steady growth in the incorporation of EES into many clinical practices. Nevertheless, exposure to EES varies widely in clinical practice and residency training. Even experienced otolaryngologists may not have used an endoscope for otologic surgery.[5] Given the relative inexperience of many practitioners and operating room staff with EES, incorporation of new devices and surgical techniques may present new challenges.

[a] Department of Otolaryngology–Head and Neck Surgery, University of Arizona College of Medicine, 1501 North Campbell Avenue, Tucson, AZ 85724, USA; [b] Department of Otolaryngology–Head and Neck Surgery, Massachusetts Eye and Ear, Harvard Medical School, 243 Charles Street, Boston, MA 02114, USA
* Corresponding author.
E-mail address: alicia_quesnel@meei.harvard.edu

Otolaryngol Clin N Am 54 (2021) 65–74
https://doi.org/10.1016/j.otc.2020.09.005
0030-6665/21/© 2020 Elsevier Inc. All rights reserved.
oto.theclinics.com

CHALLENGES IN LEARNING ENDOSCOPIC EAR SURGERY

It is not uncommon to describe the process of EES training as involving a "steep learning curve." The most fundamental hurdle to overcome is the one-handed surgical technique. As in endoscopic sinus surgery, one hand is used for all dissection (typically the dominant hand), while the other hand holds the endoscope, providing visualization. This one-handed dissection technique may be challenging initially, particularly if the surgeon only has experience with two-handed dissection methods. Compared with two-handed dissection, one of the most difficult aspects of the endoscopic approach is achieving hemostasis. Controlling bleeding without a suction in a second operative hand is a skill that can only be learned in live surgery, because bleeding is difficult to recreate accurately in cadaver courses and task trainers. Additionally, the narrow corridor of the external auditory canal creates inherent limitations for surgical access. Moreover, endoscopic dissection in the right ear tends to be more difficult than the left for right-dominant surgeons. This is caused by anatomic constraints of the anterior bony canal overhang and a less optimal view of the epitympanum.[6]

When these fundamentals are mastered, the surgeon is rewarded with unparalleled visualization of the middle ear. Compared with a microscope that collimates light at a specific focal length along a linear axis, the endoscope's fisheye-style lens captures a wide field of view in the region of interest (**Fig. 1**). The resolution of detail achieved is such that individual red blood cells may be seen traveling through middle ear vessels. Additionally, the zero-degree endoscope alone provides a superior view compared with the microscope, including visualization of the tympanic membrane in its entirety and more definitive identification of pathology within the middle ear. **Fig. 2** illustrates the comparison of detail for a congenital ossicular anomaly.

Further exploration of the tympanic cavity is made possible through the use of an angled rigid endoscope. However, this technique is more challenging for the novice operator because the orientation and projection of critical landmarks may appear

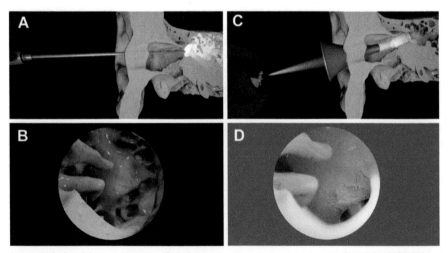

Fig. 1. Side-by-side comparison of endoscopic versus microscopic visualization. (*A*) With an endoscope, the distal nature of the lens and light source fully illuminates the middle ear. (*B*) The result is a wide field of view without obstruction of critical structures. (*C*) With a microscope, light collimates on a specific point to identify structures in one region of interest. (*D*) A narrow view with a shallow depth of field is obscured by prominent landmarks.

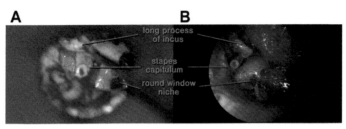

Fig. 2. Side-by-side comparison of (A) microscopic versus (B) endoscopic visualization of a congenital stapes anomaly. Labeled structures and their anatomic relationships are appreciated in higher definition and finer, intricate details with the endoscope.

distorted and unfamiliar to one accustomed to binocular microscopy. It should be noted that endoscopic dissection relies on monocular cues, and therefore lacks true depth perception. As a result, this may make surgeries that are already technically demanding, such as stapedectomy, more challenging for the novice endoscopic ear surgeon. With EES experience, however, surgeons learn to judge depth through the parallax effect with movement of the endoscope, and excellent outcomes are achieved with endoscopic stapedectomy.[7] Lastly, visualization of the middle ear is more challenging when there is a suboptimal view, such as when the rigid endoscope lens is not clear or adequate hemostasis is not achieved.[8] Any combination of the aforementioned factors has the potential to discourage a surgeon who may otherwise be skillful with traditional microscopic approaches.

Reports over the last decade demonstrate that surgical outcomes are no different between endoscopic and microscopic approaches.[5,9–12] However, the endoscope offers certain advantages over the microscope, such as the ability to access anatomic locations in a minimally invasive fashion.[2,13,14] Dissection is performed around corners and in otherwise hidden spaces with the use of angled endoscopes, often necessitating less bony dissection with a curette or otologic drill. As a result, EES has been associated with less postoperative pain and a decreased need for mastoidectomy procedures.[11,14]

The specialized skill set required to gain competency in EES has implications for surgical training. Although some microscopic surgery skills translate to EES, there are clearly approaches and techniques that are unique to EES. In this article, we discuss available resources for learning EES, physical and virtual task trainers and simulators, and novel endoscopic approaches to aid with surgical education.

ENDOSCOPIC EAR SURGERY AS A TEACHING TOOL
Endoscopic Ear Surgery and Surgical Training

EES training is becoming increasingly prevalent across otolaryngology residency programs. One study reported resident perspectives on EES in Singapore, noting overall positive reactions to EES and optimism among residents.[15] However, residents also reported that exposure to EES may have adversely affected their training, because there was a sense that this was caused by residents' operative time being lost to attending physicians tended to who performed more aspects of endoscopic procedures to gain competency themselves. In another study comparing acquisition of basic skills for endoscopic and microscopic approaches to the ear, medical students, residents, and practicing consultants were evaluated on surgical performance in a cadaver model after standardized training. Medical students were found to perform significantly better when taught first with an endoscopic technique, with a lower incidence of iatrogenic injury to the ossicular chain occurring in the endoscopic arm for all groups.[16] The time required to complete tasks differed only with level of training, not surgical approach. Of note, however, because a cadaveric temporal bone was used, this model did not factor in variables, such as hemostasis or other operative and perioperative steps of a surgery for a fully endoscopic procedure. Lastly, trainees reported subjective preference of the endoscopic technique for educational purposes. This finding highlights the benefit of emphasizing endoscopic ear anatomy during EES training.[13,17]

For experienced surgeons who were not exposed to EES during training, competency may be readily achieved after a sufficient volume of cases and operative time.[5] Even for experienced microscopic surgeons, EES training should follow a measured and graduated approach to minimize risk to patients, optimize outcomes, ensure appropriate time management in the operating room, and avoid frustration. In a single report evaluating performance on type I tympanoplasty, one surgeon with no prior EES experience ultimately demonstrated equivalent performance when using the endoscope compared with the microscope after 30 endoscopic cases, and even had a shorter operative time after 60 endoscopic cases. This study is consistent with other reports suggesting that some procedures may be faster when performed with the endoscope compared with the microscope, and may be attributed to time saved from less bony dissection required during canaloplasty.[18,19]

Endoscopic-Assisted Approaches as a Teaching Tool to Visualize Anatomic Variations

The incorporation of endoscopes for surgery of the middle ear began with endoscopic assistance, rather than a full replacement for the microscope.[20] Although exclusively endoscopic approaches may be viable alternatives to common procedures, many traditional otologic surgeries may be enriched through endoscopic assistance.[4,6] One example is via transcanal, endoscopic visualization of structures surrounding the oval window for stapes surgery. Multiple reports have demonstrated equivalent outcomes to the microscope, with more clearly defined anatomy and less posterior bony canal dissection.[7,9,11] Additionally, a transmastoid endoscopic-assisted approach to cochlear implantation has been described.[21] The nuances of round window anatomic variation and its surrounding landmarks are identified with a greater appreciation for detail. Benefits of endoscopic visualization have also been demonstrated for middle fossa approaches, such as repair of superior semicircular canal dehiscence. With the use of the endoscope, one may identify the arcuate eminence defect more easily or blue-lined canals, which is most helpful particularly when pathology is located medially along the posterior limb or abutting the superior petrosal sinus.[22] Regardless of approach, angled endoscopes may be used as a teaching tool to appreciate lateral skull base anatomy that would otherwise be challenging to visualize from traditional approaches.

TEACHING ENDOSCOPIC EAR SURGICAL SKILLS

Learning the fundamental surgical techniques of EES is critical at the onset of training. There are benefits to learning basic techniques in a controlled environment outside of the operating room. Formal endoscopic dissection courses are strongly recommended, and encompass equipment setup, endoscopic anatomy, and a stepwise approach to dissection.[6,23,24] Fresh cadavers are preferred over fixed specimens to recreate more accurate soft tissue properties for stabilizing the endoscope, and rehearsal of tasks, such as raising a tympanomeatal flap. Additionally, a recent review article by Kapadiya and Tarabichi[25] reported survey data collected from members of the American Academy of Otolaryngology-Head and Neck Surgery in 2010 and 2018. Compared with 19% of participating otologists attending any educational event on EES in 2010, 86% attended an EES lecture, cadaveric dissection course, or both, in 2018. This dramatic shift over the last decade illustrates the perceived need for training when new surgical techniques are introduced, including dissection courses and other training modalities that may improve the future of surgical education.

Skills Trainers and Surgical Simulators

Surgical simulation has a broad range of applications in surgical training for otolaryngologists.[26,27] A decrease in operative time for trainees because of institutional pressures for operative efficiency and work hour restrictions,[28] combined with a scarcity of cadaver dissection courses, make for an abrupt transition from classroom to operating room. Simultaneously, recent advances in consumer technology have enabled the recreation of high-fidelity anatomic models and procedures using three-dimensional (3D) printing and virtual reality (VR). In a review of otolaryngology simulation surgery, otology was described as the most developed out of the subspecialties.[26] Many of these studies involve surgical simulation exercises related to temporal bone drilling, but some focus on myringotomies and tube placements.[26,27,29]

EES simulators are not as widely available as those targeted at mastoidectomy or myringotomy, but a rise in interest for dedicated EES trainers over recent years is likely in response to rising popularity of EES. Simulation exercises for EES require new designs to be built from scratch. Most existing models are not repurposed easily for two main reasons: the lack of a soft tissue auricle incorporated into existing temporal bone models, and the lack of skills assessment for one-handed dissection using specialized surgical instruments. Over the last half decade, novel simulators have been designed and tested. A pilot study by Dedmon and colleagues[30] described a physical task trainer with a transcanal endoscopic approach using a cadaver model with the addition of artificial bleeding and cholesteatoma dissection. Of the participants (n = 6), median responses on a Likert scale were 4.5 out of 5 for realism, and all subjects strongly agreed that the temporal bone model would improve their surgical skills. The original model was redesigned using a 3D-printed approach by Barber and colleagues[31] to better simulate the surgical experience. The standalone task trainer did not require biologic tissue, and components were reusable. A pilot study evaluated time for task completion for moving donuts and pegs within a middle ear testing platform (**Fig. 3**). Differences were noted in completion time between the first and last trials. Evidence for construct validity was demonstrated with significant differences between level of training for junior and senior residents. Dedmon and colleagues[32] continued development toward a modular EES skills trainer that assessed part-task skills related to one-handed dissection. These findings were validated in a follow-up study with medical students (n = 5).[33] Significant decreases in time to completion were observed in tasks including placing beads on a wire, placing simulated prostheses, and navigating a pattern with a surgical tool. With repetition, subjective comfort with holding an endoscope and otologic instruments increased from 0% to 80%. In the latter study, students without any prior surgical experience showed significant improvement in EES-specific skills through repetitive practice. Skills training may have a role in surgical education through rehearsal in a safe environment.

Additionally, two other EES-specific simulators offer diverse advantages and have been reported in the literature. Anschuetz and colleagues[34] reported suitability in ex vivo ovine models for EES training. In this study, 20 ovine middle ears underwent endoscopic procedures, such as canaloplasty and ossiculoplasty. Tissue quality

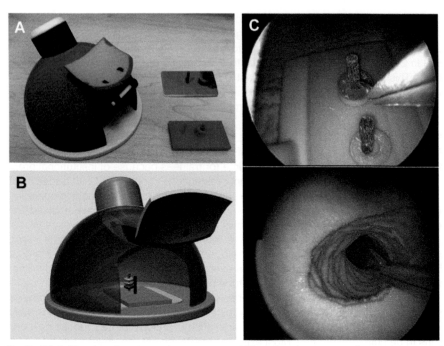

Fig. 3. (*A*) A 3D printed endoscopic ear surgery skills trainer incorporated a model external auditory canal based on anthropometric data, along with a modular middle ear testing platform. (*B*) A virtual render reveals the donut and peg task inside a dome. (*C*) Endoscopic views of the donut and peg task (*top*), along with an early iteration of the external auditory canal prototype (*bottom*). (*From* Barberab SR, Kozinab ED, Dedmonab M, et al. 3D-printed pediatric endoscopic ear surgery simulator for surgical training. International Journal of Pediatric Otorhinolaryngology 2016; 90 113-118. https://doi.org/10.1016/j.ijporl.2016.08.027; with permission.)

and learning experience, among other variables, were rated highly. An ideal simulator is one that has high fidelity but low cost. Clark and colleagues[35] described an endoscopic ear trainer for the low-resource setting that showed improvements of trainees in efficiency of instrument movement, steadiness of camera view obtained, overall global rating of task, and performance time.

Improved EES simulation models are needed. Distinct challenges unique to EES necessitates novel simulator designs based on known difficulties encountered when learning fundamental techniques. Difference in surgical technique in the right and left ears requires a more complete simulator to have the capability to recreate a test environment with either side. A validated physical simulator with realistic soft tissue properties to replicate the pinna and cartilaginous canal is also lacking. With increasing accessibility of training programs to 3D printing, future task trainers designed specifically for EES will simulate endoscopic approaches more completely.

Future Directions: Next-Generation Teaching Tools

Lateral skull base surgery requires mastery of 3D visuospatial relationships between critical anatomic landmarks. In minimally invasive endoscopic approaches to the skull base, it is necessary to know the relative location of critical structures no matter which trajectory is taken. As EES procedures for the inner ear and lateral skull base become more prevalent, the technical skill required increases.[8,36] A study by Anscheutz and colleagues[37] investigated the advantages and disadvantages of two-dimensional and 3D endoscopy in EES. Their results demonstrated a preference for the 3D technique, which was associated with a statistically shorter duration of eye fixation compared with the two-dimensional technique in the consultant group. A higher cognitive workload was reported in the resident group using both techniques.

If more complex skull base anatomy could be studied before surgery, translational skills and confidence may accelerate learning when embarking on these novel approaches. VR and augmented reality technologies have been applied to surgical training since the late 1990s.[38] However, these technologies have become accessible to a larger population of individuals in the past few years and may play a larger role in improving surgical education in the future. Through virtualization, 3D anatomy of the middle ear and skull base is projected in ways not possible in a cadaver model. A recent study by Lubner and colleagues[39] described a novel transcanal reformatted computed tomography series in the plane of the external auditory canal. Compared with preoperative planning using traditional axial and coronal views, novel radiographic landmarks are appreciated with more surgically relevant relationships (**Fig. 4**). Lastly, virtual surgical planning provides patient-specific imaging, allowing the surgeon to predict anatomic constraints and appreciate variation on an individual level. In a pilot study integrating physical and virtual modalities, augmented reality and 3D printed models of a temporal bone from a patient with a large petrous apex cyst were made before surgery.[40] These models predicted the observed relative locations of the internal carotid artery, jugular bulb, and basal turn of the cochlea through a subcochlear window in the actual surgery.

Lessons are learned from other subspecialties for educational opportunities in otology and neurotology. Within the anterior skull base, Cagiltay and colleagues[41] showed improvement of endoscopic surgical skills in a computer-based simulation environment. Dual haptic stylus controllers were combined with a display, and significant improvements in trainees were observed over repetitive trials for time to completion and

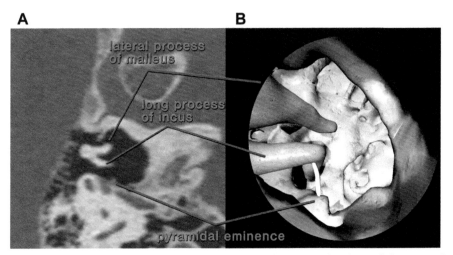

A **B**

lateral process
of malleus

long process
of incus

pyramidal eminence

Fig. 4. (*A*) Transcanal reformatted computed tomography slice in the plane of the external auditory canal. Labeled structures are projected in the same orientation is in surgery. (*B*) A virtually rendered 3D endoscopic view suggests how adjacent radiographic landmarks would represent intraoperative findings.

measures of accuracy and efficiency of coordinated hand movements. Also developed for the anterior skull base, a mixed-reality simulator was designed and validated for tracking accuracy that allows trainees to learn the fundamentals of nasal endoscopy in a fully immersive, VR environment.[42] Training modules involving virtual endonasal approaches show promise for exciting applications within the EES domain.

SUMMARY

EES requires a deep understanding of complex anatomy and incorporation of EES-specific techniques to efficiently perform one-handed dissection for otologic and neurotologic surgeries. The learning curve may be challenging because of some lack of translational skills from microscope-based otologic surgery. Although dissection courses and anatomic atlases provide a foundation for knowledge, task trainers and simulation training may serve an important role in endoscopic skill acquisition. There is a need for more accurate simulation of EES that takes into consideration soft tissue properties of the pinna and lateral external auditory canal.

With ongoing progress toward novel, minimally invasive lateral skull base endoscopic approaches that are potentially more technically challenging, preparing surgeons outside the operating room with a combination of simulations, physical task trainers, and hands-on surgical training courses becomes an even more important adjunct to operating room experience.

CLINICS CARE POINTS

- Trainees and experienced otolaryngologists alike have the capability to gain competency in EES through repetition and rehearsal of unique tasks.[5,16] Despite a steep learning curve, outcomes are the same for otologic procedures using endoscopic and microscopic approaches.[9–12,17,18]
- Endoscopic-assisted approaches provide an opportunity to increase fund of knowledge and appreciate endoscopic anatomy on a higher level of detail.[13,17] Procedures, such as cochlear implantation and repair of superior canal dehiscence, can benefit from superior visualization provided by rigid endoscopes.[21,22]
- Dissection courses on cadaver models are advised for more optimal training before live surgery.[4] Fresh specimens are preferred over fixed to retain more accurate properties of soft tissue.
- EES simulators are different from traditional temporal bone models because they require modules that facilitate skill development for one-handed dissection using specialized surgical instruments. Simulator types have a broad range from low-cost trainers to animal tissue models.[34,35]
- Physical task trainers are available to help surgeons develop endoscopic skills.[31,32] Validation studies of task trainers have demonstrated improved performance on EES skill acquisition.[33] However, to date, there is not currently a simulator that addresses all aspects of EES with high fidelity.

DISCLOSURE

The authors have nothing to disclose.

REFERENCES

1. Rosenberg SI, Silverstein H, Willcox TO, et al. Endoscopy in otology and neurotology. Am J Otol 1994;15:168–72.

2. Bowdler DA, Walsh RM. Comparison of the otoendoscopic and microscopic anatomy of the middle ear cleft in canal wall-up and canal wall-down temporal bone dissections. Clin Otolaryngol Allied Sci 1995;20:418–22.
3. Bottrill ID, Poe DS. Endoscope-assisted ear surgery. Am J otology 1995;16: 158–63.
4. Golub JS. Building an endoscopic ear surgery program. Curr Opin Otolaryngol Head Neck Surg 2016;24:395–401.
5. Dogan S, Bayraktar C. Endoscopic tympanoplasty: learning curve for a surgeon already trained in microscopic tympanoplasty. Eur Arch Otorhinolaryngol 2017; 274:1853–8.
6. Kozin ED, Kiringoda R, Lee DJ. Incorporating endoscopic ear surgery into your clinical practice. Otolaryngol Clin North Am 2016;49:1237–51.
7. Isaacson B, Hunter JB, Rivas A. Endoscopic stapes surgery. Otolaryngol Clin North Am 2018;51:415–28.
8. Alicandri-Ciufelli M, Marchioni D, Pavesi G, et al. Acquisition of surgical skills for endoscopic ear and lateral skull base surgery: a staged training programme. Acta Otorhinolaryngol Ital 2018;38:151–9.
9. Sproat R, Yiannakis C, Iyer A. Endoscopic stapes surgery: a comparison with microscopic surgery. Otol Neurotol 2017;38:662–6.
10. Tseng CC, Lai MT, Wu CC, et al. Comparison of the efficacy of endoscopic tympanoplasty and microscopic tympanoplasty: a systematic review and meta-analysis. Laryngoscope 2017;127:1890–6.
11. Manna S, Kaul VF, Gray ML, et al. Endoscopic versus microscopic middle ear surgery: a meta-analysis of outcomes following tympanoplasty and stapes surgery. Otol Neurotol 2019;40:983–93.
12. Kiringoda R, Kozin ED, Lee DJ. Outcomes in endoscopic ear surgery. Otolaryngol Clin North Am 2016;49:1271–90.
13. Tarabichi M, Marchioni D, Presutti L, et al. Endoscopic transcanal ear anatomy and dissection. Otolaryngol Clin North Am 2013;46:131–54.
14. Cohen MS, Landegger LD, Kozin ED, et al. Pediatric endoscopic ear surgery in clinical practice: lessons learned and early outcomes. Laryngoscope 2016;126: 732–8.
15. Ng CL, Ong W, Ngo RYS. Otolaryngology residents' perceptions of endoscopic ear surgery during surgical training. J Laryngol Otol 2020;134:233–40.
16. Anschuetz L, Stricker D, Yacoub A, et al. Acquisition of basic ear surgery skills: a randomized comparison between endoscopic and microscopic techniques. BMC Med Educ 2019;19:357.
17. Anschuetz L, Presutti L, Marchioni D, et al. Discovering middle ear anatomy by transcanal endoscopic ear surgery: a dissection manual. J Vis Exp 2018;(131): 56390.
18. Choi N, Noh Y, Park W, et al. Comparison of endoscopic tympanoplasty to microscopic tympanoplasty. Clin Exp Otorhinolaryngol 2017;10:44–9.
19. Emre IE, Cingi C, Bayar Muluk N, et al. Endoscopic ear surgery. J Otol 2020;15: 27–32.
20. Kozin ED, Gulati S, Kaplan AB, et al. Systematic review of outcomes following observational and operative endoscopic middle ear surgery. Laryngoscope 2015;125:1205–14.
21. Jain A, Sharma R, Passey JC, et al. Endoscopic visualisation of the round window during cochlear implantation. J Laryngol Otol 2020;134:219–21.
22. Cheng YS, Kozin ED, Lee DJ. Endoscopic-assisted repair of superior canal dehiscence. Otolaryngol Clin North Am 2016;49:1189–204.

23. Pollak N. Endoscopic and minimally-invasive ear surgery: a path to better outcomes. World J Otorhinolaryngol Head Neck Surg 2017;3:129–35.
24. Ryan P, Wuesthoff C, Patel N. Getting started in endoscopic ear surgery. J Otol 2020;15:6–16.
25. Kapadiya M, Tarabichi M. An overview of endoscopic ear surgery in 2018. Laryngoscope Investig Otolaryngol 2019;4:365–73.
26. Javia L, Sardesai MG. Physical models and virtual reality simulators in otolaryngology. Otolaryngol Clin North Am 2017;50:875–91.
27. Musbahi O, Aydin A, Al Omran Y, et al. Current status of simulation in otolaryngology: a systematic review. J Surg Educ 2017;74:203–15.
28. Reznick RK, MacRae H. Teaching surgical skills: changes in the wind. N Engl J Med 2006;355:2664–9.
29. Chen G, Jiang M, Coles-Black J, et al. Three-dimensional printing as a tool in otolaryngology training: a systematic review. J Laryngol Otol 2020;134:14–9.
30. Dedmon MM, Kozin ED, Lee DJ. Development of a temporal bone model for transcanal endoscopic ear surgery. Otolaryngol Head Neck Surg 2015;153:613–5.
31. Barber SR, Kozin ED, Dedmon M, et al. 3D-printed pediatric endoscopic ear surgery simulator for surgical training. Int J Pediatr Otorhinolaryngol 2016;90:113–8.
32. Dedmon MM, O'Connell BP, Kozin ED, et al. Development and validation of a modular endoscopic ear surgery skills trainer. Otol Neurotol 2017;38:1193–7.
33. Dedmon MM, Xie DX, O Connell BP, et al. Endoscopic ear surgery skills training improves medical student performance. J Surg Educ 2018;75:1480–5.
34. Anschuetz L, Bonali M, Ghirelli M, et al. An ovine model for exclusive endoscopic ear surgery. JAMA Otolaryngol Head Neck Surg 2017;143:247–52.
35. Clark MPA, Nakku D, Westerberg BD. An endoscopic ear trainer for the low-resource setting. J Laryngol Otol 2019;133:571–4.
36. Presutti L, Nogueira JF, Alicandri-Ciufelli M, et al. Beyond the middle ear: endoscopic surgical anatomy and approaches to inner ear and lateral skull base. Otolaryngol Clin North Am 2013;46:189–200.
37. Anschuetz L, Niederhauser L, Wimmer W, et al. Comparison of 3- vs 2-dimensional endoscopy using eye tracking and assessment of cognitive load among surgeons performing endoscopic ear surgery. JAMA Otolaryngol Head Neck Surg 2019. https://doi.org/10.1001/jamaoto.2019.1765.
38. Tang SL, Kwoh CK, Teo MY, et al. Augmented reality systems for medical applications. IEEE Eng Med Biol Mag 1998;17:49–58.
39. Lubner RJ, Barber SR, Knoll RM, et al. Transcanal computed tomography views for transcanal endoscopic lateral skull base surgery: pilot cadaveric study. J Neurol Surg B.
40. Barber SR, Wong K, Kanumuri V, et al. Augmented reality, surgical navigation, and 3D printing for transcanal endoscopic approach to the petrous apex. OTO Open 2018;2. 2473974x18804492.
41. Cagiltay NE, Ozcelik E, Isikay I, et al. The effect of training, used-hand, and experience on endoscopic surgery skills in an educational computer-based simulation environment (ECE) for endoneurosurgery training. Surg innovation 2019;26:725–37.
42. Barber SR, Jain S, Son YJ, et al. Virtual functional endoscopic sinus surgery simulation with 3d-printed models for mixed-reality nasal endoscopy. Otolaryngol Head Neck Surg 2018;159:933–7.

Endoscopic Myringoplasty and Type I Tympanoplasty

Zachary G. Schwam, MD*, Maura K. Cosetti, MD

KEYWORDS

- Myringoplasty • Tympanoplasty • Endoscopic ear surgery • TEES

KEY POINTS

- Endoscopic tympano/myringoplasty has equivalent audiometric outcomes and rates of graft success when compared with the microscopic approach.
- A variety of grafts and techniques have been used to good effect. There are no high-quality data supporting one graft or technique over others.
- Endoscopic tympano/myringoplasty is a safe procedure, with less pain and a rapid return to work expected.
- The endoscopic approach may be favored in those with particular concerns regarding cosmesis or operative times.

INTRODUCTION

Myringoplasty and tympanoplasty have a long history, with the first documented attempt to close a tympanic membrane (TM) perforation occurring in 1640, with Banzer placing a graft consisting of elkhorn wrapped in porcine bladder.[1,2] With the advent of surgical microscopes and a wide array of instrumentation, various otologic procedures were developed and refined. In the 1950s, Wullstein[3] published his tympanoplasty classification system, which categorized the reconstruction of the middle ear based on the status of the TM and ossicular chain into 5 types. Type I consisted of a simple TM perforation with normal ossicles, and type V involved stapes footplate fixation with lateral semicircular canal fenestration.[3] Although there has been some degree of variation in the literature with respect to nomenclature, many investigators refer to a type I tympanoplasty as lifting a formal tympanomeatal flap (TMF), whereas a myringoplasty does not include this step.[4] This review focuses primarily on type I tympanoplasty for dry perforations, as a detailed discussion on the management of ossicular pathology and cholesteatoma are beyond the scope of this article.

Icahn School of Medicine of Mount Sinai, Department of Otolaryngology-Head and Neck Surgery, 1 Gustave L. Levy Place, Box 1189, New York, NY 10029, USA
* Corresponding author.
E-mail address: zachary.schwam@mountsinai.org

Otolaryngol Clin N Am 54 (2021) 75–88
https://doi.org/10.1016/j.otc.2020.09.010
0030-6665/21/© 2020 Elsevier Inc. All rights reserved.

Although otoendoscopy has become increasingly popular since the 1990s, it was first reported in 1967 and later in 1982, when Mer and colleagues[5,6] and Nomura[7] used endoscopes through TM perforations to evaluate the middle ear and ossicular chain. At the time of this writing, transcanal endoscopic ear surgery (TEES) has been used for a variety of procedures, including myringoplasty, tympano-ossiculoplasty, tympanomastoidectomy, stapedotomy/stapedectomy, and lateral skullbase surgery. In this review, we seek to inform the reader, whether an otolaryngology resident or practicing otologist, of the current landscape with respect to endoscopic myringoplasty and type I tympanoplasty. Although the literature is rather extensive on this topic, there is a dearth of randomized, prospective data regarding techniques, nuances, patient criteria, and graft materials.[8]

DISCUSSION
Goals and Steps of Myringoplasty and Tympanoplasty

Regardless of approach, tympano/myringoplasty seeks to create an intact TM with aerated middle ear, ensure continuity of the air-conduction mechanism from TM to inner ear, preserve hearing with minimal air-bone gap (ABG), and to eliminate pathology.[8–10] In placing a graft to act as a scaffold for epithelial migration, steps include optimizing hemostasis, harvesting an autologous graft (or in some cases using a xenograft), preparing the TM and middle ear, eradicating pertinent pathology, reconstructing the ossicular chain, and opening ventilation routes as necessary, and placing the graft.[9] We have outlined the pertinent steps for performing type I tympanoplasty with a chondroperichondrial underlay graft accompanied by operative images from one of our own patients (**Figs. 1–5**).

Improved Visualization With Endoscopy and Its Downstream Effects

Using computed tomography (CT)-based models of temporal bones, Bennett and colleagues[11] demonstrated that a 0° endoscope had superior visualization as compared with a microscope for every subsite examined, and that the visual field was augmented with higher degrees of angulation. Only the mesotympanum could be adequately seen with a straight-line microscopic view, and bony overhangs or tortuous canals may preclude visualizing the entire TM, particularly the anterior aspect.[12–16] With an endoscope, one can inspect the TM for epithelial ingrowth,[13]

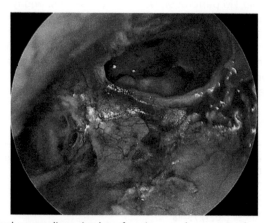

Fig. 1. Preoperatively, a medium-sized perforation can be seen in the anterosuperior and posterosuperior quadrants of the patient's left ear.

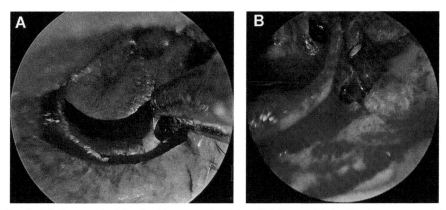

Fig. 2. (A) Once an incision had been made with a #72 Beaver blade, the tympanomeatal flap was raised with a suction-round knife. (B) Once the flap had been raised to the interface of the bony and fibrous annulus, a suction-Rosen was used to enter the middle ear space.

detect stapedial and light reflexes through a perforation,[17] and evaluate various crevices in the retro-, epi-, pro-, and hypotympanum for cholesteatoma.[18,19] It is also more difficult to tear the TMF endoscopically as the surgeon may see both surfaces thereof while dissecting.[17]

Due to superior circumferential visualization with an endoscopic approach, rates of canalplasty are exceedingly low and frequently nil,[12–14,20–26] as compared with the microscopic approach, which ranges from 4.0% to 33.3%.[12,23–27] In a meta-analysis by Manna and colleagues[27] examining 21 studies encompassing 1323 ears undergoing tympanoplasty, canalplasty rates were significantly lower in endoscopic cases (0% vs 18%, $P < .0001$).

As the visual field is significantly wider when using endoscopes, not only is the rate of canalplasty minimized, but so is that of a postauricular approach.[20,21] In using the

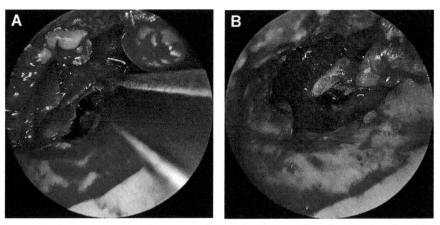

Fig. 3. (A) The tympanic membrane was dissected off the malleus handle sharply with a endoscopic microscissor. (B) Once the malleus was skeletonized, the middle ear was packed with Gelfoam.

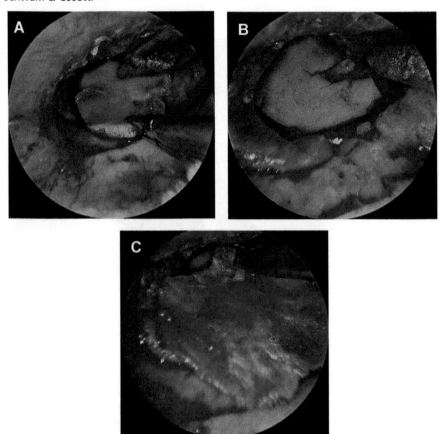

Fig. 4. (*A*) A cartilagenous shield graft with cutout for the malleus handle was introduced and (*B*) put in position. (*C*) A tragal perichondrial graft was placed lateral to it.

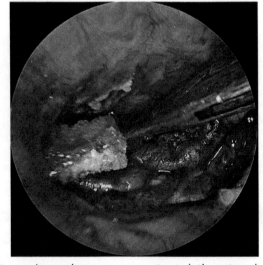

Fig. 5. Once the tympanic membrane was reconstructed, the external canal was carefully packed with Gelfoam to stabilize the graft.

endoscope, Tarabichi and colleagues[17,28] were able to decrease their rate of postauricular incisions for middle ear procedures from 42% to 0%. With a more minimally invasive approach, there were expected improvements in cosmesis, pain, and time to return to work. With a postauricular incision, not only is there a scar, hypoesthesia, and palpable depression, but also changes to the auriculomastoid angle, which may result in a protruding pinna. In several series, an endoscopic approach was found to have a superior cosmetic profile to a postauricular incision.[9,12,13,24,27,29] In the report of Harugop and colleagues[24] of 50 endoscopic and 50 microscopic myringoplasties, 100% of endoscopic patients were found to have an "excellent" cosmetic result, whereas 20% and 50% of the microscopic group were found to have a poor or satisfactory cosmetic outcome, respectively. Similarly, endoscopic patients were found to have significantly less pain and have a shorter admission or time period to return to work as compared with their counterparts undergoing microscopic approaches.[13,21,23–26,30–32] In the series of Tseng and colleagues,[21] endoscopic patients took pain medications for a mean of 2.0 days, and resumed normal activity within 1.0 day. In the report of Harugop and colleagues,[24] the endoscopic and microscopic groups returned to normal activity in 2.4 and 5.4 days, respectively. The rigorous pain study of Kakehata and colleagues[32] involved keeping all patients undergoing middle ear surgery as inpatients for a period of 1 week to eliminate recall bias and enhance data collection. They found that mean pain scores were significantly lower in the endoscopic group at every time point, and that significantly less pain medication was consumed as compared with the patients undergoing postauricular approaches.[32]

Shorter Operative Times With an Endoscopic Approach

As a consequence of better visualization, saving time in not making or closing a postauricular incision, and largely avoiding a canalplasty, most reports document shorter operative times for equivalent procedures when using the endoscope.[21,25,27,30,31,33–35] Some series did not compare their times to that of a conventional postauricular approach but did document times of approximately an hour or less for a variety of techniques.[14,20,21,36,37] Although this was most reports, it was not uniform; both Gaur and colleagues[29] and Harugop and colleagues[24] documented longer operative times with the endoscopic approach while performing myringoplasties.

Endoscopic Learning Curve

Although rigid endoscopy has been a mainstay of rhinologic procedures, it has only recently come into favor in the otologic community. As one might expect with any newer procedure, there is an associated learning curve. Dogan and Bayraktar[38] estimated that the learning curve for an experienced tympanoplasty surgeon would be 60 procedures to achieve the same outcomes and operative times. Tseng and colleagues[4] demonstrated a shortening operative time between their 10th (75 minutes) and 150th patients (55 minutes) and an accompanying increase in graft success rate from 75% to 95%. The graft success rate plateaued at patient number 50 and fluctuated between 85% to 100%. There was a positive correlation between perforation size and the time required to repair it as well as an inverse correlation between perforation size and closure of the postoperative ABG.[4] In the report of Zhu and colleagues[39] of endoscopic ossiculoplasty for pediatric congenital stapes malformations, operative times decreased from 110.4 minutes for their first 5 cases to 70.67 minutes for their last 3. In their examination of the learning curve for endoscopic stapes surgery, Iannella and Magliulo[40] showed a similar improvement in operative times, with the last 10 endoscopic and microscopic cases in his series having similar operative times. In looking at microscopic approaches, Liu and colleagues[41] tracked residents longitudinally as they became attendings, and found that it took 5 years to reach a plateau in speed, with no differences in surgical success and complication rates between years 3 and 7.

Tips for making the learning curve less steep include incremental addition of techniques, trimming ear hair, starting on left ears if the surgeon is right-handed (with the opposite being the case if the pathology is inferior), using flexible suction tubing, adept hemostasis, and having a variety of suction instruments available.[42,43] In addition, starting with easier cases or smaller perforations and attending a training course may be useful.[4]

Cost

The literature with respect to cost of endoscopic versus microscopic tympanoplasty is scant. In Kuo and Wu's[30] comparison of endoscopic and microscopic tympanoplasty, they found that the average cost of an endoscopic case was 645 euros as compared with 1170 euros for the microscopic approach. Patel and colleagues[44] examined totally endoscopic versus canal-wall-up tympanomastoidectomies and found an overall savings of 2978.89AUD when taking into account operative time, anesthesia setup, and other resources used. Both Migirov and colleagues[18] and Harugop and colleagues[24] maintain that the cost of their 2 approaches was comparable, but did not provide concrete figures. Any facility in which endoscopic sinus surgery is performed is expected to have a high-definition multichip camera and endoscopic tower; startup costs may include 3 mm endoscopes 14 to 18 cm in length and specialty endoscopic instruments. Although most of the cases can be completed using standard otologic instruments, certain specialty instruments such as a suction-enabled round knife or Rosen pick are very helpful.

Education

Although there are no formal data in the literature, anecdotally endoscopic ear surgery is appreciated by trainees for its common field of view and demonstration of anatomic relationships.[12,13] For an attentive assistant, anticipation of next steps and observing how instruments are used and in what order may provide invaluable training.

Disadvantages of Endoscopic Ear Surgery

The disadvantages of endoscopic ear surgery include 1-handed surgery, frequent lens fogging, difficulty with hemostasis, loss of binocular vision, and the potential for unintentional heat injury.

Although otologists may initially decry the loss of one hand to holding the endoscope, some investigators believe that tympano/myringoplasty is simple enough that it should not be a large impediment.[13] Use of a suction-round-knife or suction-Rosen may also obviate the need for a second hand while raising the TMF or entering the middle ear space. Most published articles report not having to convert to a microscopic approach, but it is occasionally done when removing sclerotic plaques or releasing adhesions.[16,18] Although we do not recommend use of an endoscope holder due to the possibility of patient movement causing unintentional damage,[43] there are reports of its successful use during myringoplasty; it may be more amenable to this procedure as opposed to cholesteatoma surgery as there is less of a need for a dynamic field of view.[45]

Maintaining visualization with frequent fogging and controlling bleeding may be difficult for the beginner otoendoscopist. Frequently wiping the scope on defogging solution (and thereafter warm saline as the defogging solution may be ototoxic) may ensure image clarity but also control heat emission from the tip of the scope. To maintain hemostasis, tips include reverse Trendelenburg of approximately 15°, using suction dissectors, avoiding hypertension (and even maintaining slight hypotension), using total intravenous anesthesia, and frequent use of topical epinephrine.[9,12,15,19,43]

The potential for heat injury and desiccation of the chorda tympani and middle ear structures has always been a concern, as maximum temperatures can quickly reach 44.1° to 46.0°C using a 4 mm endoscope and a xenon light source at maximum intensity.[46] By using a smaller diameter scope with light intensity of less than 40%, frequent repositioning and irrigation, and keeping the tip of the endoscope as lateral as is feasible, unintentional damage can be avoided without compromising visualization or outcomes.[9,39,43,46]

Although the loss of binocular vision may be initially disorienting, many investigators find that the loss of depth perception is compensated for by experience and a higher fidelity view.[16–18,28] Due to the fish-eye design of all endoscopes, the center of the field is slightly less magnified than the periphery; therefore, to make a TMF of adequate length, the lateral cut should be made a bit further out than anticipated.[47]

Equivalent Audiometric Outcomes and Tympanic Membrane Closure Rates

In the literature reviewed, audiometric outcomes were equivalent or in some cases superior with an endoscopic approach. Other articles reported high success rates in their endoscopic-only series.[4,12,14,20,25,27,30,34,35,48,49] When analyzed in aggregate by Manna and colleagues[27] in their meta-analysis, the audiometric outcomes were also comparable between the 2 techniques. As with the microscopic approach, results will depend on primary versus revision surgery, concomitant pathology, reconstructive technique, and status of the middle ear.

In the large microscopic series of Nardone and colleagues[50] of 1040 myringoplasty patients, his overall 10-year graft success rate was 78% with a significant recurrence rate for chronic otitis media. In the Common Otology Database of the United Kingdom, myringoplasty data are collected for 33 otolaryngologists, and their overall primary microscopic closure rate was 90.6%, compared with 84.2% for revisions.[51] Many of the endoscopic series document shorter-term graft success rates greater than 80%, typically in the mid-80s to low-90s, which compare favorably to their respective microscopic numbers.[4,10,12,13,15,20,21,23–27,29,31,49,51] Select series show superior rates for their microscopic myringoplasties; Dundar and colleagues[33] had a 1-year failure rate of 12.5% for endoscopic type I tympanoplasty as compared with 5.71% for identical microscopic procedures with the caveat that the endoscopic group had on average larger perforations. In their report of 60 myringoplasties, Maran and colleagues[35] noted higher success rates for microscopic approaches for larger central perforations and a negligibly higher rate for medium-sized perforations. This is in contrast to the article of Tseng and colleagues,[20] which noted no difference in larger or even marginal perforations.

The Pediatric Population

Pediatric tympano/myringoplasty has classically been thought of as less successful than adult surgery due to more middle ear infections, prominent adenoid tissue, and eustachian tube dysfunction.[9] However, the endoscopic literature has shown excellent results in this group. Although the bony ear canal is narrower in young children and grows with time,[19] the shorter, straighter conformation of the canal is considered advantageous in an endoscopic approach, allowing increased angulation and range.[14] Various investigators suggest a canal size of at least 4.5 mm to make an endoscopic approach feasible.[19,52] Typically, a 3-mm endoscope should provide adequate visualization and working room for other instruments. A protected drill shaft and curved burr allow for nontraumatic canalplasty should the need arise.[26] Awad and Hamid[37] stratified his pediatric cohort into those older and younger than 10 years and noted similarly high rates of graft uptake between the groups. Although some groups note successful use of a tragal chondroperichondrial underlay graft,[33] James[26] found less success with a tragal perichondrial underlay or push-through graft than in using a lateral graft with either autologous tissue or a xenograft. In addition, it is important to note that in small children, the tragus may be of insufficient size to harvest an adequate graft.[26]

Graft Materials

The full gamut of grafting material, from autologous to xenograft, has been reported in the endoscopic literature. Due to the various approaches and pathology across reports, recommendations cannot be made with respect to the most effective grafting material for a given location or perforation type. Although temporalis fascia is often the graft material of choice in a postauricular approach, many endoscopic investigators tend to harvest tragal chondroperichondrial grafts, as the cartilage provides rigid support against negative middle ear pressures, its location within the surgical field, the expediency with which it can be harvested, and minimal effect on cosmesis as long as the lateral cap is left intact.[9,21,31,50] Tragal cartilage also has acceptable acoustic transfer, does not stimulate an inflammatory response, and has prolonged viability should wound healing prove slow. The tragus has 2 layers of perichondrium, with the undersurface being thinner and perhaps more suited to primary TM reconstruction, with the anterior layer preferred for composite grafting in scutum reconstruction.[9] In addition, if one is planning concurrent ossiculoplasty, the graft can be placed on top of a titanium prosthesis to prevent extrusion and improve the frequency response of the TM.[53,54]

Fat, which is typically taken from the lobule of the pinna, may be used as an inlay graft for smaller perforations, and may be done in the office or in the operating room. Adipose tissue promotes neovascularization and tissue repair via the secretion of angiogenic growth factors.[9,55] Its use was first reported by Ringenberg in 1962,[56] with recent reports documenting success rates between 76% and 92%.[1,9]

In recent years, xenografts, particularly Biodesign® (Cook Group, Bloomington, IN), a multilayered product derived from porcine intestinal submucosa, has been used to good effect in the tympano/myringoplasty literature. De Zinis and colleagues[45] used it with a 100% success rate in 10 children, noting savings in operative time and surgical morbidity. Similarly, James[26] used it in his endoscopic cases when there was insufficient autologous tissue, allowing him to repair larger perforations. Yawn and colleagues[57] evaluated its utility in 37 adults and children with a mix of endoscopic and microscopic approaches, harvesting a concomitant cartilage graft in most cases. The overall success rate of the graft material was 86.5%, with a significant improvement noted in those undergoing concurrent cartilage graft.[57]

Specific Techniques

A range of grafting techniques have been used successfully in the endoscopic literature, with the selected technique at the discretion of the surgeon; there is a paucity of data with respect to randomized trials comparing techniques or approaches. The following seeks to highlight some of the possibilities in one's armamentarium.

The butterfly chondroperichondrial inlay graft has been used extensively by various investigators with very high success rates and fast operative times.[9,20,36,58] It can be used to reconstruct a wide variety of perforations, with particular utility in anterior perforations.[17,58] Because of the reduced vascular supply, relatively poor visualization (particularly when using the microscope), and lack of support, anterior perforations are characteristically more difficult to repair.[9,20] Butterfly grafts are best for small to medium-sized perforations and rely on the strength of the surrounding remnant TM; subtotal or marginal perforations, or cases in which a remnant has significant tympanosclerosis, are not ideal situations in which to use this technique.[36,59] Eren and colleagues[58] reported using an otologic compass to measure the size of the tympanic membrane perforation (TMP) and to size their graft accordingly. In Gülşen and Erden's[59] randomized control trial of small and medium anterior TMPs, they compared an endoscopic butterfly inlay graft to an endoscopic push-through graft and noted comparable success rates greater than 90%. However, the butterfly graft took approximately 10 minutes less and required no middle ear packing.[59]

The push-through method has also been used successfully in other series, and avoids raising a TMF.[9,20] Although raising the TMF allows one to fully explore the middle ear and remove disease, it may not be necessary in simple perforations with low likelihood of concurrent pathology as determined by physical examination, audiometry, and preoperative imaging.[4,9,20] In his series of 91 endoscopic myringoplasties, Tseng and colleagues[21] raised a TMF only when the perforation was greater than 50% and noted no difference in audiometric or graft-take outcomes. However, in James'[26] pediatric series, he found push-through myringoplasty the least successful of his techniques, with a success rate of only 68%. In not raising a TMF, the vascular strip is untouched; preserving the malleolar and radial arterial blood supply may theoretically contribute to faster wound healing.[14]

Whether to choose an underlay or lateral graft largely depends on surgeon and regional preferences; both are effective and have similar outcomes when used properly.[50] Lateral grafts may be favored particularly in the case of a subtotal or anterior perforation. Although lateral grafts have been placed successfully in several endoscopic series,[17,22,23,26] the endoscopic view may lead one to underestimate the depth of the anterior sulcus and subsequently lead to blunting.[17] It is also considerably more tedious and may take significantly longer. Some investigators make use of an interlay technique, in which the graft is placed between the squamous and fibrous layers of the TM and the fibrous annulus is not raised.[9,26] In the exclusively microscopic series of 1040 tympanoplasties by Nardone and colleagues,[50] lateral grafts were more successful in revision surgery, and were typically used in anterior or subtotal perforations. Wick and colleagues[60] performed 34 lateral endoscopic chondroperichondrial grafts in both children and adults with total or near-total perforations or myringitis; their initial success rate was 88.2% and 79% achieved a postoperative ABG less than 20 dB.[50]

Poor Prognostic Factors

Poor predictors of success include otorrhea,[20,50] large or subtotal perforations,[13,14,50,61] significant myringosclerosis,[13] marginal or anterior perforations,[14,37,48,50,58] and concurrent ossicular pathology.[61] In Awad and Hamid's[37] pediatric series, patient age, eustachian tube dysfunction, and previous adenotonsillectomy were interestingly not found to be predictive of success rates.

However, attention should be paid to the status of the contralateral ear when risk-stratifying patients for risk of recurrence.[50]

Complications

The most common complication of tympanoplasty is residual perforation or graft failure, the rates of which vary with operative technique as well as the size and location of the perforation. To prevent iatrogenic cholesteatoma, it is necessary to evaluate the medial side of the TM for inappropriate epithelial migration.[62] Even in taking the proper precautions, superficial cholesteatomas or epithelial pearls in the TM are possible.[1,15,23] Although this is theoretically lower in endoscopic cases due to enhanced visualization, James[26] had similar rates between the 2 approaches. Overall, the complication rate in an endoscopic approach is low and comparable to the microscopic approach, without the risk of soft tissue complications from a postauricular approach. External canal stenosis is, however, possible and documented in one report. For a tympano/myringoplasty, rates of hearing deterioration or facial nerve injury were found to be rare or did not occur.[10,46] If there is graft take and an intact ossicular chain, lack of improvement in hearing may be from the altered structure of the neotympanic membrane.[50] Both Marchioni and colleagues[46] and Glikson and colleagues[63] documented their complication rates in resecting middle ear cholesteatomas and in endoscopic ear surgery, respectively. Glikson and colleagues[63] had minor and major complication rates of 16.6% and 6.0%, respectively, with a 3.3% rate of stapes footplate fracture, 5.0% sensorineural hearing loss (SNHL), 3.3% labyrinthitis, and 3.3% superficial surgical site infection of the tragal graft site. Marchioni and colleagues[46] had the following complications: 1.9% chorda tympani injury, 0.2% transient facial palsy, 1.2% SNHL, 0.1% ossicular disruption, and one footplate fracture. Caution must be used when evaluating the middle ear and retrotympanum with an angled scope for potential cholesteatoma; ossicular subluxation may occur and requires immediate repair.[15] A myringoplasty/type I tympanoplasty is expected to have a lower complication profile than more complex procedures.

SUMMARY

Endoscopic tympano/myringoplasty is both feasible and safe, with comparable success rates to a microscopic approach. In many cases using an endoscopic approach may obviate the need for a postauricular incision and its attendant morbidity, even in the case of an anterior perforation or a stenotic/tortuous canal. A variety of grafts and techniques have been used successfully, with the decision of which to use based on surgeon preference and specific pathology.

CLINICS CARE POINTS

- Endoscopic tympano/myringoplasty has equivalent audiometric outcomes and rates of graft success when compared with the microscopic approach in both adults and children.
- A variety of grafts and techniques have been used to good effect. There are no high-quality data supporting one graft or technique over others.
- Endoscopic tympano/myringoplasty is a safe procedure, with less pain and a rapid return to normal activity expected.
- The endoscopic approach may be favored in those with particular concerns regarding cosmesis or operative times.

DISCLOSURE

Z.G. Schwam: none. M.K. Cosetti has received travel grants from Med-El, Cochlear, Stryker, educational research grants from Advanced Bionics, and has done clinical research with Advanced Bionics, Cochlear, and Otonomy.

REFERENCES

1. Ayache S, Braccini F, Facon F, et al. Adipose graft: an original option in myringoplasty. Otol Neurotol 2003;24:158–64.
2. Banzer M. Disputatio de auditione laesa. Trans Am Acad Ophthalmol Otolaryngol 1963;67:233–59.
3. Wullstein H. Theory and practice of tympanoplasty. Laryngoscope 1956;66: 1076–93.
4. Tseng CC, Lai MT, Wu CC, et al. Comparison of endoscopic transcanal myringoplasty and endoscopic type I tympanoplasty in repairing medium-sized tympanic perforations. Auris Nasus Larynx 2017;44:672–7.
5. Mer SB, Derbyshire AJ, Brushenko A, et al. Fiberoptic endoscopes for examining the middle ear. Arch Otolaryngol 1967;85:387–93.
6. Kakehata S, Futai K, Sasaki A, et al. Endoscopic transtympanic tympanoplasty in the treatment of conductive hearing loss: early results. Otol Neurotol 2006; 27:14–9.
7. Nomura Y. Effective photography in otolaryngology-head and neck surgery: endoscopic photography of the middle ear. Otolaryngol Head Neck Surg 1982; 90:395–8.
8. De Vos C, Gersdorff M, Gerard JM. Prognostic factors in ossiculoplasty. Otol Neurotol 2007;28:61–7.
9. Anzola JF, Nogueira JF. Endoscopic techniques in tympanoplasty. Otolaryngol Clin North Am 2016;49:1253–64.
10. Hunter JB, O'Connell BP, Rivas A. Endoscopic techniques in tympanoplasty and stapes surgery. Curr Opin Otolaryngol Head Neck Surg 2016;24:388–94.
11. Bennett ML, Zhang D, Labadie RF, et al. Comparison of middle ear visualization with endoscopy and microscopy. Otol Neurotol 2016;37:362–6.
12. Lade H, Choudhary SR, Vashishth A. Endoscopic vs microscopic myringoplasty: a different perspective. Eur Arch Otorhinolaryngol 2014;271:1897–902.
13. Furukawa T, Watanabe T, Ito T, et al. Feasibility and advantages of transcanal endoscopic myringoplasty. Otol Neurotol 2014;35:140–5.
14. Marchioni D, Gazzini L, De Rossi S, et al. The management of tympanic membrane perforation with endoscopic type i tympanoplasty. Otol Neurotol 2020;41: 214–21.
15. Ayache S. Cartilaginous myringoplasty: the endoscopic transcanal procedure. Eur Arch Otorhinolaryngol 2013;270:853–60.
16. Migirov L, Wolf M. Transcanal microscope-assisted endoscopic myringoplasty in children. BMC Pediatr 2015;15:32.
17. Tarabichi M, Ayache S, Nogueira JF, et al. Endoscopic management of chronic otitis media and tympanoplasty. Otolaryngol Clin North Am 2013;46:155–63.
18. Migirov L, Shapira Y, Horowitz Z, et al. Exclusive endoscopic ear surgery for acquired cholesetatoma. Otol Neurotol 2011;32:433–6.
19. James AL. Endoscopic middle ear surgery in children. Otolaryngol Clin North Am 2013;46:233–44.

20. Tseng CC, Lai MT, Wu CC, et al. Endoscopic transcanal myringoplasty for anterior perforations of the tympanic membrane. JAMA Otolaryngol Head Neck Surg 2016;142:1088–93.

21. Tseng CC, Lai MT, Wu CC, et al. Short-term subjective and objective outcomes of patients receiving endoscopic transcanal myringoplasty for repairing tympanic perforations. Otolaryngol Head Neck Surg 2018;158:337–42.

22. Creighton FX Jr, Kozin E, Rong A, et al. Outcomes following transcanal endoscopic lateral graft tympanoplasty. Otol Neurotol 2019;40:989–92.

23. Plodpai Y, Paje N. The outcomes of overlay myringoplasty: endoscopic versus microscopic approach. Am J Otolaryngol 2017;38:542–6.

24. Harugop AS, Mudhol RS, Godhi RA. A comparative study of endoscope assisted myringoplasty and micrsoscope assisted myringoplasty. Indian J Otolaryngol-head Neck Surg 2008;60:298–302.

25. Choi N, Noh Y, Park W. Comparison of endoscopic tympanoplasty to microscopic tympanoplasty. Clin Exp Otorhinolaryngol 2017;10:44–9.

26. James AL. Endoscope or microscope-guided pediatric tympanoplasty? Comparison of grafting technique and outcome. Laryngoscope 2017;127:2659–64.

27. Manna S, Kaul VF, Gray ML, et al. Endoscopic versus microscopic middle ear surgery: a meta-analysis of outcomes following tympanoplasty and stapes surgery. Otol Neurotol 2019;40:983–93.

28. Tarabichi M. Endoscopic middle ear surgery. Ann Otol Rhinol Laryngol 1999;108:39–46.

29. Gaur RS, Tejavath P, Chandel S. Comparative study of microscopic-assisted and endoscopic-assisted myringoplasty. Indian J Otol 2016;22:177.

30. Kuo CH, Wu HM. Comparison of endoscopic and microscopic tympanoplasty. Eur Arch Otorhinolaryngol 2017;274:2727–32.

31. Kaya I, Sezgin B, Sergin D, et al. Endoscopic versus microscopic type 1 tympanoplasty in the same patients: a prospective randomized controlled trial. Eur Arch Otorhinolaryngol 2017;274:3343–9.

32. Kakehata S, Furukawa T, Ito T, et al. Comparison of postoperative pain in patients following transcanal endoscopic versus microscopic ear surgery. Otol Neurotol 2018;39:847–53.

33. Dundar R, Kulduk E, Soy FK, et al. Endoscopic versus microscopic approach to type I myringoplasty in children. Int J Pediatr Otoloaryngol 2014;78:1084–9.

34. Huang TY, Ho KY, Wang LF, et al. A comparative study of endoscopic and microscopic approach Type 1 tympanoplasty for simple chronic otitis media. J Int Adv Otol 2016;12:28–31.

35. Maran RK, Jain AK, Haripriya GR, et al. Microscopic versus endoscopic myringoplasty: A comparative study. Indian J Otolaryngol Head Neck Surg 2018. https://doi.org/10.1007/s12070-018-1341-4.

36. Özgür A, Dursun E, Terzi S, et al. Endoscopic butterfly cartilage myringoplasty. Acta Otolaryngol 2016;136:144–8.

37. Awad OG, Hamid KA. Endoscopic type 1 tympanoplasty in pediatric patients using tragal cartilage. JAMA Otolaryngol Head Neck Surg 2015;141:532–8.

38. Dogan S, Bayraktar C. Endoscopic tympanoplasty: Learning curve for a surgeon already trained in microscopic tympanoplasty. Eur Arch Otorhinolaryngol 2017;274:1853–8.

39. Zhu VF, Kou YF, Lee KH, et al. Transcanal endoscopic ear surgery for the management of congenital ossicular fixation. Otol Neurotol 2016;37:1071–6.

40. Iannella G, Magliulo G. Endoscopic versus microscopic approach in stapes surgery: are operative times and learning curve important for making the choice? Otol Neurotol 2016;37:1350–7.

41. Liu CY, Yu EC, Shiao AS, et al. Learning curve of tympanoplasty type I. Auris Nasus Larynx 2009;36:26–9.

42. Cohen MS, Landegger LD, Kozin ED, et al. Pediatric endoscopic ear surgery in clinical practice: lessons learned and early outcomes. Laryngoscope 2016;126: 732–8.

43. Kozin ED, Kiringoda R, Lee DJ. Incorporating endoscopic ear surgery into your clinical practice. Otolaryngol Clin North Am 2016;49:1237–51.

44. Patel N, Mohammadi A, Jufas N. Direct cost comparison of totally endoscopic versus open ear surgery. J Laryngol Otol 2018;132:122–8.

45. De Zinis LR, Berlucchi M, Nassif N. Double-handed endoscopic myringoplasty with a holding system in children: preliminary observations. Int J Pediatr Otorhinolaryngol 2017;96:127–30.

46. Marchioni D, Rubini A, Gazzini L, et al. Complications in endoscopic ear surgery. Otol Neurotol 2018;39:1012–7.

47. Pothier DD. Introducing endoscopic ear surgery into practice. Otolaryngol Clin North Am 2013;46:245–55.

48. Nassif N, Berlucchi M, de Zinis LO. Tympanic membrane perforation in children: endoscopic type I tympanoplasty, a newly technique, is it worthwhile? Int J Pediatr Otorhinolaryngol 2015;79:1860–4.

49. Jyothi AC, Shrikrishna BH, Kulkarni NH, et al. Endoscopic myringoplasty versus microscopic myringoplasty in tubotympanic CSOM: a comparative study of 120 cases. Indian J Otolaryngol Head Neck Surg 2017;69:357–62.

50. Nardone M, Sommerville R, Bowman J, et al. Myringoplasty in a simple chronic otitis media: critical analysis of long-term results in a 1,000-adult patient series. Otol Neurotol 2012;33:48–53.

51. Phillips JS, Yung MW, Nunney I. Myringoplasty outcomes in the UK. J Laryngol Otol 2015;129:860–4.

52. Kobayashi T, Gyo K, Komori M, et al. Efficacy and safety of transcanal endoscopic ear surgery for congenital cholesteatomas: a preliminary report. Otol Neurotol 2015;36:1644–50.

53. Gardner EK, Jackson CG, Kaylie DM. Results with titanium ossicular reconstruction prostheses. Laryngoscope 2004;114:65–70.

54. Murbe D, Zahnert T, Matthias B, et al. Acoustic properties of different cartilage reconstruction techniques of the tympanic membrane. Laryngoscope 2002; 112:1769–76.

55. Teh BM, Marano RJ, Shen Y, et al. Tissue engineering of the tympanic membrane. Tissue Eng B Rev 2013;19:116–32.

56. Ringenberg JC. Fat graft tympanoplasty. Laryngoscope 1962;72:188–92.

57. Yawn RJ, Dedmon MM, O'Connell BP, et al. Tympanic membrane perforation repair using porcine small intestinal submucosal grafting. Otol Neurotol 2018; 39:332–5.

58. Eren SB, Tugrul S, Ozucer B, et al. Endoscopic transcanal inlay myringoplasty: alternative approach for anterior perforations. Otolaryngol Head Neck Surg 2015;153:891–3.

59. Gülşen S, Erden B. Comparison of endoscopic butterfly-inlay versus endoscopic push-through myringoplasty in repairing anterior perforations of the tympanic membrane. J Laryngol Otol 2020;22:1–7.

60. Wick CC, Arnaoutakis D, Kaul VF, et al. Endoscopic lateral cartilage graft tympanoplasty. Otolaryngol Head Neck Surg 2017;157:683–9.
61. Albu S, Babighian G, Trabalzini F. Prognostic factors in tympanoplasty. Am J Otol 1998;19:136–40.
62. Karhuketo TS, Puhakka HJ. Technique of endoscope-aided myringoplasty. Otol Neurotol 2002;23:129–31.
63. Glikson E, Yousovich R, Mansour J, et al. Transcanal endoscopic ear surgery for middle ear cholesteatoma. Otol Neurotol 2017;38:41–5.

Novel Radiologic Approaches for Cholesteatoma Detection

Implications for Endoscopic Ear Surgery

Alexander J. Saxby, MB BChir, MA (Cantab), FRACS[a],*,
Nicholas Jufas, MBBS, BSc (Med), FRACS, MS[b],
Jonathan H.K. Kong, MBBS, FRACS, FRCS, MS[a],
Allison Newey, MBBS, FRANZCR[c],
Alexander G. Pitman, MBBS, BMedSc, MMed, FRACR[d],
Nirmal P. Patel, MBBS, FRACS, MS[b]

KEYWORDS

- Endoscopic ear surgery • Otoendoscopy • Cholesteatoma • Computed tomography
- Magnetic resonance imaging • Diffusion-weighted imaging • Cone beam CT
- Fusion imaging

KEY POINTS

- Imaging plays a vital role in cholesteatoma management offering benefits for diagnosis, planning, patient counseling, and recidivism surveillance. Furthermore, radiology provides a teaching aid and research tool to better understand the disease.
- Computed tomography (CT) imaging remains the gold standard for preoperative imaging but can be augmented by fusion with non–echo-planar (EPI) diffusion-weighted (DWI) imaging, especially to avoid overestimation of mastoid involvement.
- Non-EPI DWI remains the gold standard for postoperative surveillance imaging. When used as an alternative to second-look surgery, surgeons should consider fusion imaging with CT, which improves the specificity.

Continued

[a] Department of Otolaryngology-Head and Neck Surgery, Royal Prince Alfred Hospital, Camperdown, NSW 2050, Sydney, Australia; [b] Department of Otolaryngology-Head and Neck Surgery, Royal North Shore Hospital, 1 Reserve Road, St. Leonards, NSW 2065, Sydney, Australia; [c] Department of Radiology, Royal North Shore Hospital, 1 Reserve Road, St. Leonards, NSW 2065, Sydney, Australia; [d] Department of Radiology, Northern Beaches Hospital, 105 Frenchs Forest Road W, Frenchs Forest, NSW 2086, Sydney, Australia
* Corresponding author.
E-mail address: saxbyaj@gmail.com

Otolaryngol Clin N Am 54 (2021) 89–109
https://doi.org/10.1016/j.otc.2020.09.011
0030-6665/21/© 2020 Elsevier Inc. All rights reserved.

Continued

- Fusion CT/MRI may increase sensitivity and specificity close to 100% for disease spread at the antrum. Fusion images hold promise in identifying disease medial to the ossicles, which may help the endoscopic ear surgeon in planning ossicle-preserving surgery.
- Further development and research are required to know the clinical potential of new technologies such as dual-energy CT (DECT), optical coherence tomography (OCT), and augmented reality (AR) in cholesteatoma surgery.
- Low-dose CT protocols are important to minimize radiation exposure in children. Parental counseling can focus on comparison with normal daily life radiation exposure when discussing risk and benefit.
- Successful imaging in cholesteatoma relies on a close collaboration between surgeon and radiologist. A feedback loop and common language between the 2 parties will improve the sensitivity and specificity of all imaging modalities.

ESTABLISHED PROTOCOLS
Computed Tomography

Modern computed tomography (CT) scanners are capable of very high-resolution imaging of the temporal bone and middle ear structures. In addition to clinical examination of cholesteatoma, CT scanning helps delineate potential extent of disease, erosion of bony structures, precise anatomic location, and potential complications of cholesteatoma.

CT produces a radiographic tissue density map of the volume of tissue imaged. In all modern scanners, native slice thickness (1 mm or less) is ample for clinical needs of cholesteatoma detection and monitoring. CT is the only modality (compared with MRI-based methods) to demonstrate bone directly: bony structures have a distinctly higher radiographic density than all other tissues. CT accurately differentiates bone from air and soft tissue on this basis. It is consequently the reference standard modality for detection and characterization of bony erosion by cholesteatoma.

Radiographic density (also called CT density or Hounsfield density) represents the underlying physical property of X-ray absorption by tissue, which is in turn determined by atomic number of the elements in the path of the X-ray beam and the spatial density of the atoms. It varies for X-ray beams of different energy (the more energetic the beam, the less absorption). This property is exploited by current efforts in dual-energy CT. Tissue density in CT is expressed in terms of Hounsfield units (HU). HU is a relative scale, calibrated for each scanner model so that water density is 0 and room air density is −1000. Very dense cortical bone has HU of 1500 to 2000. All native human tissues fall somewhere in this scale.

Human fat has CT density distinctly below that of water, and is characterizable in its own right (HU density of −10 or lower). All other soft tissue types cluster between HU of approximately 0 and approximately 100, so that complex effusions, exudates, scar, and proteinaceous debris all have overlapping CT densities. The cost of accurate characterization of tissue density ("contrast resolution") is higher radiation dose (undesirable), and the 2 competing needs result in a daily clinical trade-off. CT is therefore unable to easily differentiate cholesteatoma from other soft tissue (such as granulation or fibrosis) or fluid.[1,2] Small-volume disease is also subject to statistical noise of tissue density measurement which obscures the underlying average tissue density so that, at clinical radiation doses, tissue characterization through its CT density becomes more problematic for small soft tissue clumps, such as cholesteatoma.

MRI

MRI produces a density map of hydrogen atoms (protons) in the volume of tissue imaged. Since its inception, MRI has also been able to produce volumetric maps of 2 other fundamental physical magnetic properties of tissue, called "T1 relaxivity" and "T2 relaxivity"; however, discussion of the nature of these properties is beyond the scope of this article. Clinical MRI does not produce pure T1 or T2 maps; rather, it produces predominantly T1 or predominantly T2 maps, correspondingly titled "T1 weighted" (T1W) and "T2 weighted" (T2W).

Air (with its minimal density of hydrogen atoms compared with solids) produces no MRI signal. The hydrogen atoms in cortical bone are tightly chemically bound and so also do not generate an MRI signal. As a result, the dense cortical bone of the otic capsule and temporal bone does not produce any clinically detectable MRI signal and is not distinguishable from air. Consequently, MRI is fundamentally unable to detect boundaries of the mesotympanum when aerated. Effusions, cholesterol granulomas, scar tissue and cholesteatoma all produce detectable signal. Spatial resolution of MRI at its best approaches CT (1 mm or less) and MRI is subject to similar difficulties to CT in tissue characterization with smaller target sizes.

MRI (but not CT) has the contrast resolution capabilities to detect contrast enhancement within small soft tissue masses. This has led to attempts to differentiate vascularized scar from all other soft tissue in the middle ear. However, contrast enhancement does not assist in differentiating non-vascularized soft tissue including cholesteatoma and complex effusions.[3] Speed of MRI acquisition is considerably slower than speed of CT (except for echo-planar techniques) creating vulnerability to motion artifact.

Diffusion-Weighted Imaging

Diffusion-weighted imaging (DWI) uses detection of water molecule Brownian motion to differentiate more freely diffusible water molecules (in this setting, effusions) from "bound water" (in this setting, cholesteatoma). Discussion of the physics is again beyond the scope of this article. Clinical sequences generate an isotropic volumetric diffusion sequence (DWI map) and a derived parametric map of apparent diffusion coefficient (ADC map). Tissues with abnormally restricted diffusion have higher DWI signal and a reduced ADC. DWI maps are contaminated by high T2W signal (T2 shine-through), such that high DWI signal must always be validated by comparison to the ADC map and T2W image in the same position.

Conventionally, cholesteatoma will display high restriction of diffusion (hyperintensity) measured by b-factors of 800 to 1000 s/mm^2.[4,5] ADC maps are less essential if this b factor threshold is used in DWI map interpretation.[6] Hyperintensity of cholesteatoma is thought to be due to restricted molecular diffusion but may also reflect a T2 "shine-through" effect.[7] The true mechanism remains debated. DWI can be either echo-planar (EPI DWI), or non–echo-planar (non-EPI DWI).

Echo-Planar Diffusion-weighted Imaging

This rapid acquisition "single-shot" technique, regularly used for cerebral infarct detection, is unfortunately prone to interface edge artifacts and anatomic distortion, limiting its usefulness in cholesteatoma detection, with poor resolution of disease <5 mm.[5,8] Newer EPI protocols such as REadout Segmentation of Long Variable Echo trains (RESOLVE)-DWI may improve spatial resolution and reduced slice thickness (2–3 mm) with the added possibility of coronal DWI images. Sensitivity and specificity for cholesteatoma detection (88% and 96% respectively)[9] approaches that of non-EPI techniques.

Non–Echo-planar Diffusion-weighted Imaging

This technique uses multiple excitation pulses with a longer echo time to provide a higher signal-to-noise ratio, producing fewer distortions or artifacts, better spatial resolution, and thinner slices.[6] Superiority of non-EPI DWI was demonstrated in a recent metanalysis of 575 studies (727 patient episodes) showing a significant difference in pooled sensitivity for EPI and non-EPI (71.8% ± SD 24.5% and 89.8% ± SD12.1, respectively [P = .02]).[10] Pooled data for specificity, positive predictive value (PPV) and negative predictive value (NPV) was 94.57, 96.50, and 80.46, respectively. Increased magnetic field strength (3T vs 1.5T) has not been shown to improve detection of cholesteatoma.[11,12]

NOVEL IMAGING TECHNIQUES
Multimodality Fusion Imaging

Multimodality fusion imaging is not a new form of image acquisition, but rather uses established modalities and overlays one over the other to gain additional benefit. Its application for cholesteatoma was first published in 2010 in a pediatric study using non-EPI DWI fused to CT imaging which described excellent correlation between preoperative localization and intraoperative findings.[13] Five years later the first study using non-EPI DWI images fused to heavily T2-weighted datasets (MR Cisternography) and to T1-weighted MRI images[14] was published. This reported accurate detection of cholesteatoma more than 3 mm and found the additional T1 dataset overlay reduced false positives due to cholesterol granuloma. Subsequent cholesteatoma fusion studies have all reverted back to using CT to provide the anatomic detail, most using the technique in postoperative surveillance for residual disease.[15–19]

Fusion of the non-EPI DWI dataset to either CT or MRI datasets, attempts to capitalize on the high specificity (and high PPV) of the DWI sequence combined with accurate visibility of anatomic landmarks to guide surgery (**Fig. 1**). MRI-DWI fusion avoids the disadvantage of patients needing to be scanned twice in 2 machines. If both MRI and DWI sequences are acquired without patient movement and with the same spatial reference points, fusion of the 2 datasets can be achieved with the basic inherent fusion software of most MR scanners. It still requires manual operator actions, yet has low chance of mis-registration error with correctly set protocols. Limitations are the absence of bony anatomic landmarks or knowledge of aeration, particularly relevant in the postoperative ear. Other standard limitations of MRI (implantables, edge susceptibility, metal and movement artifact) apply.

The more common use of CT as the anatomic base on which to fuse the DWI dataset, overcomes these limitations and provides optimal information for surgical planning as the isocenter and margins of the cholesteatoma can be related accurately to bony landmarks. However, the technique faces the challenge of combining 2 datasets acquired on 2 different gantries, requiring active and complex operator intervention to produce meaningful results. The 2 datasets need to share sufficient unequivocal anatomic fiducial points to enable optimal manual fusion. There is no single best choice; the authors use the endosteal calvarial table (CT) and surface of the cerebral and cerebellar cortices (MRI). The manual fusion is undertaken by best-fit in 6° of freedom. Once fused, level and window must be manually set to make the cholesteatoma margins visible, using a color scale for the DWI dataset. A limitation of CT-DWI Fusion is the learning curve required and the time-consuming nature of its

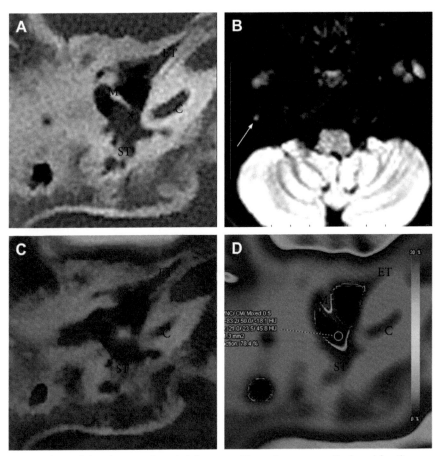

Fig. 1. Multimodal Fusion Imaging. Axial temporal bone images are displayed for the same patient showing images acquired using (A) CT, (B) non-EPI DWI, (C) CT-DWI Fusion, and (D) DECT. This 9-year-old patient had totally endoscopic resection of the cholesteatoma which was filling the retrotympanum and eroding the ossicular chain. (A, C, D) CT, CT-DWI Fusion, and DECT all demonstrate a zoomed image of the right temporal bone centered on the mesotympanum, whereas (B) the DWI image shows the whole brain. White arrow in (B) and asterisk in (A) indicate position of cholesteatoma. ET, Eustachian Tube; C, Basal turn of cochlear; M, Malleus handle; ST, Sinus Tympani.

creation. Institutions well accustomed to the technique require at least 20 minutes of extra time to produce the fused map.

Summating the strengths of 2 modalities has been shown to improve overall specificity. In a recent pediatric study, sensitivity was minimally affected by fusion (CT alone 87%; DWI 84%; CT-DWI Fusion 85%) whereas specificity was significantly improved after fusion (CT alone 46%; DWI 76%; CT-DWI Fusion 97%).[19] The confidence of diagnosis also appears improved by fusion, illustrated in a separate study by increased reliability scores in blinded radiologist assessment of preoperative CT and CT-DWI Fusion images (60% intraclass correlation in fusion dataset vs 52% with CT alone).[20]

Cone-Beam Computed Tomography

Cone-beam CT (CBCT) uses a solid-state plate detector instead of the ring of individual detectors of a traditional CT gantry. The machines have evolved from orthopantomogram (OPG) dental scanners, usually with an upright rotating gantry. CBCT proposed advantage is a reduced radiation dose, better spatial resolution of 75 to 150 μm (compared with 300–600 μm for multidetector CT [MDCT]), and less distortion from metal artifact (**Fig. 2**). Its other main differentiator is substantially lower cost and the ability to be installed in a surgeon's office.

Disadvantage is the long acquisition time (up to 40 seconds), which can lead to movement artifact resulting in the need to repeat the study.[21] The patient needs to be extremely well immobilized which is more difficult with the patient sitting or standing. Newer machines are beginning to offer supine imaging.

A number of papers have used CBCT to characterize anatomic features within the middle ear,[22–28] some specific to cholesteatoma describing how the size and shape of the Eustachian tube[29] or the characterization of Prussak's space[30] differed between cholesteatoma and non-cholesteatoma CBCT scans. No statistical differences were found in either study, but this highlights how imaging is beginning to play an increasing role in our investigation of disease pathophysiology as opposed to solely diagnosis. A retrospective study of 554 children[31] emphasized the main advantages being lower radiation and very fast acquisition times, both particularly relevant to the pediatric cohort. This study was not exclusively for cholesteatoma (20% of the cohort) but within the images acquired of the lateral skull base, the limitations of CBCT were listed as motion artifact and blurred image requiring repetition of the scan in 5.5% and alternative imaging in 3.8%[31]

Dual-Energy Computed Tomography

Dual-energy CT (DECT) offers the possibility of CT-only improved soft tissue differentiation. It uses 2 spectrally different polychromatic X-ray beams (typically a high kVp heavily low-end filtered beam and a low kVp conventionally low-end filtered beam) either from dual CT tubes at right angles or by rapid focal point switching. This produces 2 spatially concordant volumetric maps of X-ray beam attenuation for the 2 different beams, translated to 2 "apparent CT density values," one for each beam, for each voxel in the dataset (see **Fig. 1**).

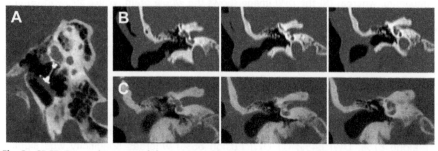

Fig. 2. CBCT. Coronal images of the temporal bone are presented. (*A*) CBCT image showing a titanium total ossicular reconstruction prosthesis (TORP) positioned between cartilage tympanoplasty and footplate, illustrating the resolution achievable at low radiation dose and the lack of artifact from metallic components. (*B,C*) Data from a second patient showing in upper row (*B*) images acquired using a conventional high-resolution CT and for comparison in the lower row (*C*) the same patient scanned using CBCT.

Tissue characterization is typically derived from preexisting knowledge of "apparent CT density" values for different tissue types. The technique is manufacturer dependent, limited to narrow clinical applications based on proprietary in vitro and in vivo databases for that tissue type. Current clinical applications include diagnosis of gouty tophi, renal stones and masses, pulmonary embolism, liver disease and malignancy.[32]

Clinical use in cholesteatoma diagnosis will depend on development of a robust algorithm to delineate keratin rich pathology from adjacent effusion or granulation tissue. The use of DECT in liver imaging is perhaps the most analogous and promising on the basis that cholesterol granuloma has a similar fat density to fatty liver and cholesteatoma (keratin debris) is comparable in DECT appearance to nonfatty liver soft tissue while effusions although variable in density remain closest to water. Although still in a developmental stage, it requires significant operator processing and interpretation to make clinical sense of the acquired CT density values. DECT protocols can be set up to deliver equivocal or lower patient radiation dose than equivalent conventional structural CT, while providing no loss of anatomic detail in the final (2 beam fused) structural CT dataset.

To date, only 1 study has published on DECT use in cholesteatoma, comparing postoperative recidivism using DECT versus non-EPI DWI in 19 patients. The investigators reported similar sensitivity and specificity, PPV, and NPV for each modality (DECT: 87.5, 87.5, 93.3, 87.5; DWI: 93.7, 87.5, 93.7, 87.5) with good intraobserver and interobserver agreement.[33]

Optical Coherence Tomography

Initially commercialized for application in ophthalmology, this probe-based imaging modality has application for middle ear diagnosis.[34,35] Analogous to ultrasound imaging, but not requiring a transduction medium, it works by using the time-of-flight information of light waves to visualize tissue microstructure at high resolution. It can achieve very high resolution (5–15 μm), compared with CT, MRI, and ultrasound (400 μm, 300 μm, and 150 μm, respectively). Depth of penetration is only up to 3 mm with a field of view of up to 15 mm.[35] Recent clinical studies have concentrated on otitis media,[36,37] and none have specifically addressed use in cholesteatoma. Although still at a research stage, it holds promise for transcanal real-time imaging of the mesotympanum (**Fig. 3**), potentially offering intraoperative information to the surgeon. This could be particularly useful with the endoscopic approach.

Augmented Reality

AR combines computer-generated images to enhance real-world visualization. It is a rapidly developing technology with increasing application to otolaryngology.[38] Various platforms have been developed and the technology lends itself well to the endoscope using CT or MRI data for the virtual input. Ex vivo prototypes have promise for future clinical intraoperative application.[39] It also offers potential preoperative benefits to the surgeon allowing practice run-throughs in preparation for complex approaches.[40]

Preoperative Implications

The main reasons for imaging in the preoperative setting are for diagnosis, strategic operative planning and informed patient counseling. As a diagnostic tool in a de novo case, imaging will generally only be useful in combination with the clinical findings. CT imaging is more useful in aiding diagnosis when there are erosive changes, such as blunting of the scutum, or ossicular erosion. Non-EPI DWI in the preoperative setting has a diagnostic role when the tympanic membrane is intact, either due to

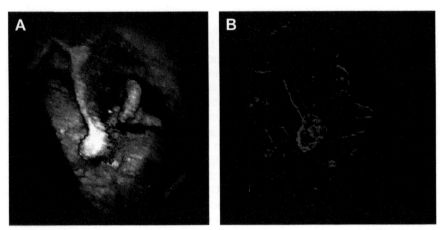

Fig. 3. OCT. OCT view of tympanic membrane rendered from 2D to 3D with software and layers stripped back (*A*) and then converted to mesh overlay to better define middle ear structures (*B*).

congenital cholesteatoma or in acquired cases where the opening of the retraction pocket has sealed over, entrapping a covert cholesteatoma.[41]

Once the diagnosis is made, preoperative imaging plays a key role in planning the surgical resection with CT imaging currently the gold standard modality, given its superior ability to delineate bony structures. Diagnosing erosion of the ossicular chain, otic capsule, fallopian canal or tegmen can help the surgeon predict potential complications and give more accurate and realistic patient counseling.[42] With respect to endoscopic access, CT can give valuable information about the size limitations of the canal, particularly pertinent to the pediatric population (see section entitled "Pediatric Considerations" below). Three dimensional (3D) reconstruction of preoperative CT images enables an enhanced visualization of the anatomic structures, termed "virtual endoscopy." Several studies have reported enhancement in the visualization of complex anatomic regions such as the sinus tympani,[43] ossicular chain,[44] and epitympanum[45] and described advantages as a teaching tool.[46] With the emergence of the endoscopic technique, 3D reconstruction (virtual endoscopy) may prove a valuable addition in predicting limitations of access and the need for canal-widening procedures.

Determining the boundaries of cholesteatoma extent is another major benefit of preoperative imaging. CT imaging used alone, suffers from the inability to distinguish extensive mastoid involvement from sequestered mastoid fluid or granulation tissue. With the increasing use of transcanal endoscopic approaches, it is helpful for surgeons to know the likelihood of cases requiring mastoidectomy. The ability of non-EPI DWI and multimodality fusion imaging to more accurately predict cholesteatoma extent has relevance for preoperative counseling of patients and time management of the operating room.

CT alone will overestimate the degree of mastoid involvement. Blinded preoperative assessment of CT versus CT-DWI Fusion has shown, when CT demonstrates opacification into the mastoid, almost half (45%) will have cholesteatoma that does not extend beyond the posterior border of the lateral semicircular canal[47] (**Fig. 4**). This study suggested limited disease, amenable to total transcanal endoscopic removal, was possible in 60% (35 of 58 cases), when predicted by CT-DWI Fusion, as opposed to 28% when assessed using CT alone.[47] From this the investigators proposed that

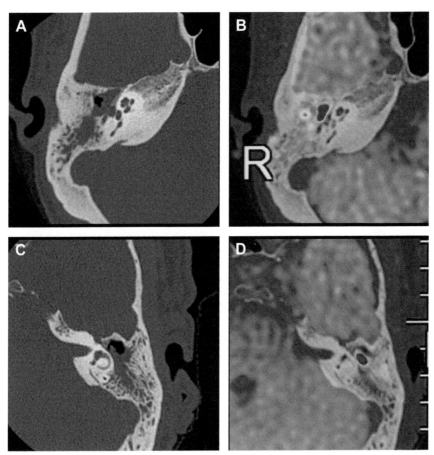

Fig. 4. Mastoid interpretation with fusion imaging. (*A,C*) Axial CT images of the temporal bones of 2 different patients demonstrating opacification extending throughout the mastoid. (*B,D*) Corresponding CT-DWI Fusion maps illustrating cholesteatoma occupying only the middle ear with the remainder of the mastoid filled with fluid or granulation tissue.

when a CT-MRI Fusion scan is not available, the case should still be commenced via an endoscopic transcanal approach in the first instance, only converting to mastoidectomy if necessary. This notion has been supported by others reporting a mastoid conversion rate of 36% (19 cases of 52) when commencing all cases endoscopically.[48] Features on the preoperative CT scan that predicted conversion were tegmen erosion, malleus or incus erosion and opacification of the aditus ad antrum, antrum, or mastoid cavity (*P*<.05).[48]

In clinical practice, patients may present with a CT already performed and so the benefits of re-imaging a patient for fusion purposes is harder to justify. Access to a radiology department with fusion capabilities, radiologists skilled in the technique and available time resources also present real-world limitations on what is available.

Postoperative Implications

Utilization of imaging for postoperative surveillance of cholesteatoma recidivism as an alternative to second-look surgery is becoming more popular. Indications where imaging may be preferable to surgery include patient preference, young children, elderly patients, or those with significant comorbidities. Findings at the first operation, confidence of disease removal and necessity for staged ossicular chain reconstruction will also dictate a surgeon's preference.

A recent cost-saving analysis showed a benefit for non-EPI DWI MRI over traditional surgical approaches. This may apply to the universal healthcare model available for the country it was analyzed in, but remains a consideration within the context of local facilities and resources.[49]

Increased utilization of endoscopic ear surgery to manage cholesteatoma has resulted in a substantial paradigm shift in recent years. Minimally invasive surgery at the initial operation behoves avoidance of further invasiveness where possible. Imaging can provide this option, offering an alternative to further surgery, particularly given the low rate of residual and recurrent cholesteatoma found at second look.[50]

The risk of relying on imaging to diagnose recidivism is defined by the false negative and false positives rate (**Fig. 5**). Given that the alternative to imaging is an operation, the false positive rate, although undesirable, results in the default option of having to re-open the ear, but the false negative rate is potentially much more serious. With an NPV of 80.46,[10] use of non-EPI DWI will result in missing residual disease in as many as 1 in 5 patients. Some may argue that serial imaging would detect growth in subsequent imaging, but loss to follow-up remains a problem. A demonstrated increase in specificity from 76% to 97% when fusing the surveillance imaging, at least in a pediatric dataset is therefore relevant.[19]

In cases in which false positives occur, reported findings at surgery include cholesterol granuloma, abscess, bone pate, wax, cartilage graft, encephalocele, squamous cell carcinoma and no obvious cause.[6,15,51–55] Inflamed mucosa or granulation at the

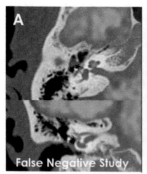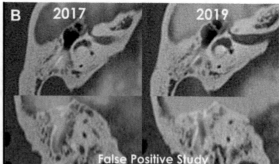

Fig. 5. False positive and negative results with fusion imaging. CT-DWI Fusion images in an axial plane (*top row*) and coronal plane (*bottom row*) of the temporal bones of 2 separate patients. (*A*) False negative case: This patient underwent a second-look procedure to perform an ossicular chain reconstruction revision. The cartilage tympanoplasty and tip of the previous partial ossicular reconstruction prosthesis can be seen in the coronal view. The asterisk marks the discovered cholesteatoma at surgery, wrapped around the stapes superstructure and footplate. Failure of the CT-MRI was presumed due to the small size of this residual disease (<3 mm). (*B, C*) False positive case: A second patient who underwent endoscopic resection of attic cholesteatoma in 2013. Follow-up CT-MRI Fusion maps did not show any potential residual until 2017 (*B*). Deemed indeterminate at that stage, a repeat fusion scan was performed in 2019 (*C*). Based on this progressive change the patient underwent a mastoidectomy, at which no cholesteatoma was found. Inflammatory tissue was presumed to have been the cause of the false positive result.

cholesteatoma matrix interface may give a false impression of extent of disease, even in positive cases. Cartilage grafts, often used in reconstruction of the attic or tympanum after endoscopic cholesteatoma removal, can also be a source of a false positive result, leading some authors to propose judicious observation if clinical suspicion for residual disease is low, opting instead for interval imaging.[55] Repeat imaging allows the surgeon to assess change in characteristics over time, which creates more certainty in the suspected positive nature of the findings. If an initial positive finding decreases in dimensions over time, it would likely favor a false positive result. In addition, a positive finding in an area other than the location of the initial cholesteatoma would also point to a likely false positive.[55]

Accurate estimation of the false negative rate for postoperative surveillance is problematic, as most studies do not routinely include operations on every case to confirm recidivism. False negatives may arise due to small-volume residual disease, with the limit of detection generally agreed to be approximately 2 to 3 mm[10,56,57]; however, studies have missed lesions as large as 5 mm.[5] Delay between imaging and second-look surgery can affect this sensitivity due to cholesteatoma growth during the interval.[58] False positives and negatives affect confidence in surveillance imaging such that reliance on a single follow-up scan is problematic and interval imaging over a time course of at least 5 years remains the best way to equilibrate the assurance provided by staged second-look surgery.

PEDIATRIC CONSIDERATIONS
Radiation Dose with Computed Tomography Imaging

CT scanning remains an important part of pediatric cholesteatoma preoperative assessment.[59] Children are, however, more susceptible to the risk of developing cancer from radiation due to the higher dose to organ ratio, developing tissues and longer duration of effect. Life time cancer mortality risks have been estimated at 14% per sievert for a 1-year-old child, 5% per sievert for a middle-aged adult, and 2% per sievert for a person older than 60 years.[60]

"Low-dose" or "Image gently" protocols for imaging the temporal bone, attempt to balance the lowest feasible radiation dose while maintaining a diagnostic image quality[61,62] (ImageGenIty.org). These goals can be balanced at approximately 0.3 mSv for normal anatomy, however, doses as high as 1.2 mSv may be required to delineate pathology with more confidence.[63] CBCT may be used to scan the temporal bone with low radiation (median 0.1 mSv) and acceptable image quality. Caution, however, is warranted when risk counseling parents as individual cone beam machines may vary up to 19-fold in their radiation risk.[64] There are also issues with young children remaining stationary, especially in the sitting or standing position, to avoid movement artifact with CBCT.

When counseling parents, these radiation risk data can be explained by comparing with acceptable risks taken during normal life.[65] For example, a parent could have the amount of radiation compared with the yearly background radiation that their child is exposed to in their home ($\sim$2.28 mSv). Furthermore, cosmic radiation is significantly higher at elevation (sea level 0.28 mSv; city of Denver 0.82 mSv).[66] Ultimately, the clinician and parents balance the risk with what is required to plan for surgery.

MRI for Pediatric Patients

Non-EPI DWI is highly recommended when CT scanning indicates possible intracranial extension[67] but the technique remains most commonly used to examine the

Table 1
Modalities available for imaging of cholesteatoma

Modality	Physical Basis for Diagnosis	Advantages	Limitations	Technical Tips	Future Improvements
Computed tomography (CT)	Bone, soft tissue (including cholesteatoma) and air have distinct CT densities.	Fast, least motion affected Excellent resolution of bony anatomy. Excluding cholesteatoma if mesotympanum aerated. High sensitivity and NPV Excellent spatial resolution (smallest Voxel 0.6–1 mm cube).	Soft tissues (cholesteatoma, effusion, cholesterol granuloma, scar) all have similar CT density lowering specificity. Metallic prostheses can produce artifact. Involves radiation.	Communication between surgeon and radiologist regarding operative findings and reconstruction will improve reporting and image optimization.	Uniform anatomic lexicon between surgeons and radiologists. Lower radiation dose protocols.
MRI T1W, T2W sequences	Soft tissue (including cholesteatoma), effusions and fluid all generate signal of variable degree whereas air generates no signal.	Excellent soft tissue contrast resolution, good delineation of soft tissue, CSF and perilymph. Good spatial resolution (smallest Voxel 1–1.5 mm cube).	Limited bony anatomy. Slow acquisition time. Moderately motion affected. No signal from plastic prostheses. Unreliable differences in signal of cholesteatoma and mimickers. Patient may have contraindication to MRI for example, certain otologic implants, MR nonconditional pacemaker, etc.	Best modality for membranous labyrinth and intracranial extension if suspected.	Increased availability and use of MR conditional implants instead of MR unsafe. Technological advances in MRI hardware and sequences, speeding up scan times, reducing artifacts and improving spatial and contrast resolution.

Diffusion-weighted imaging (DWI MRI)	Cholesteatoma shows high signal on DWI whereas granulation tissue, scar, effusions and simple fluid do not.	High specificity and PPV for cholesteatoma >2–3 mm.	Very motion sensitive. Can be degraded by susceptibility artifact (bone edges) – less evident with non-EPI DWI; Limited anatomic landmarks.	Coronal non-EPI DWI in addition to axial non-EPI DWI can provide valuable additional information.	Newer DWI techniques with less artifact, thinner slices, better spatial resolution, improved reference data for normal ranges, absolute and relative DWI signal and ADC values for different tissue types and magnet strengths.
Fusion MRI-DWI	Localizes DWI abnormality relative to surgically recognisable anatomic landmarks. Overlay of DWI maps on heavily T2W (structural) MRI dataset.	Rigidly identical spatial reference points (assuming no patient motion), achieves excellent co-registration of datasets. Less operator dependent.	Incomplete anatomy demonstration for surgical planning (limited bony anatomy, no signal from prostheses).	Ensure acquisition parameters for DWI and heavily T2W sequences have identical spatial reference points.	

(continued on next page)

Table 1
(continued)

Modality	Physical Basis for Diagnosis	Advantages	Limitations	Technical Tips	Future Improvements
Fusion CT-DWI	Co-registers (fuses) non-EPI DWI dataset with anatomic base dataset from CT.	Current state-of-the-art in attempting to combine high NPV and excellent bony anatomic accuracy of CT with high PPV of DWI sequences. Highest NPV and PPV of all established modalities. Presents a valid alternative to second-look surgery for certain cases (no hearing reconstruction required, low residual risk disease at primary surgery, comorbidity or young age).	Acquiring both CT and MRI has time and cost implications for institutions and patients. Radiation dose of the CT component is a factor when used for surveillance. Time-consuming and operator dependent.	Radiologists should acquire adequate field of view to allow manual fusion on known anatomic landmarks (eg, skull endosteal surface). Acquire at least one whole-of-brain MRI sequence (T1W or FLAIR) in same frame of reference as DWI to fuse with the CT.	Automation of accurate fusion using anatomic landmarks common to both MRI and CT.
Cone Beam CT	Uses the same tissue properties as conventional multidetector CT (MDCT).	Lower radiation dose. Can achieve better spatial resolution than MDCT (75–150 μm). Less distortion from metallic prostheses. Lower cost than MDCT. Size permits installation in office.	Long acquisition times (17–40 s). Subject to movement artifact. Many machines require sitting/standing which is not suited to all patients and makes immobilization problematic.	Variation in both the quality of images and the radiation delivery produced by different machines. Only some machines able to scan temporal bone.	Faster acquisition times to reduce motion artifact. More availability of supine imaging to facilitate patient remaining still for scan.

Dual-energy CT (DECT)	Tissue characterization through different absorptions registered in the same voxel of tissue for 2 spectrally different (but still polychromatic) X-ray beams.	Theoretic aspirational goal of differentiating cholesteatoma from effusion in the same dataset as the structural CT (theoretically achieving the same advantage of a fusion study but in the one modality). Radiation dose can be adjusted to equal that of a standard CT.	Development stage with one study on use in cholesteatoma diagnosis. Clinical application constrained by limited choice of spectral beams and by lack of data pre-processing algorithms specific to cholesteatoma. Time-consuming and operator dependent. Spatial resolution not established.	Requires great caution in interpretation. Use still needs validation.	Requires further study to establish optimal 2-beam spectral settings and optimal data pre-processing algorithms. Further clinical validation of published results.
Optical coherence tomography (OCT)	Uses time-of-flight information from light waves to visualize microstructures.	Very high resolution (5–15 μm). Potential intraoperative application. Use in cholesteatoma surgery may be in ossicular chain assessment.	Development stage. Limited depth of penetration (3 mm). Limited Field of view (15 mm).		Requires further development.
Augmented reality (AR)	Synchronous interaction of computer generated image data with real-world visualization.	Potential intraoperative application providing surgeon with anatomic landmarks beyond their endoscopic vision. May prove useful in pre-surgical rehearsal.	Development stage. Multiple different platforms being trialled. Expensive and at an experimental level.		Requires further development and clinical trials.

Abbreviations: ADC, apparent diffusion coefficient; CSF, cerebrospinal fluid; CT, computed tomography; DECT, dual-energy CT; DWI, diffusion-weighted imaging; EPI, echo-planar imaging; FLAIR, fluid attenuation inversion recovery MRI sequence; MRI, magnetic resonance imaging; non-EPI, non-echo-planar imaging; NPV, negative predictive value; PPV, positive predictive value; T1W, T1-weighted MRI sequence; T2W, T2-weighted MRI sequence.

antrum and mastoid. This guides preoperative discussion with the parent as to the extent of surgery. The great advantage of MRI in this population is a lack of radiation risk. Its limitation is the acquisition time. Most single-shot non-EPI protocols have an acquisition time of 15 minutes. The protocol is frequently achievable without sedation with careful explanation to the child and parent but children under 6 years may require sedation to reduce movement artifact.[68] Movement artifact can lead to false negative results in addition to the other factors seen in adults.[69]

Nonoperative follow-up surveillance is an attractive option in children.[68,70] A recent metanalysis of non-EPI DWI recidivism outcomes examined 10 articles (141 ears)[58] giving a pooled sensitivity and specificity of 89.4% (95% confidence interval [CI] 51.9%–98.5%) and 92.9% (95% CI 81.4%–97.5%), respectively. As with adults, DWI appears limited in its ability to detect lesions smaller than 3 mm. The technique is reproducibly specific but carries uncertain sensitivity in the detection of recidivism in children. False positives, specific to children, can occur from inflammatory causes (proteinaceous fluid, intercurrent infection, tympanosclerosis, cholesterol granuloma, calcified cartilage) or foreign materials (dental appliances, silastic sheet, bone pate, wax and ossicular implants).[68,71]

Fusion CT-DWI holds promise for improving localization accuracy in pediatric primary cholesteatoma. Of relevance to the endoscopic surgeon, specificity in the region of the sinus tympani appears greatly improved (CT 33%, 95% CI 12%–62%; DWI 53%, 95% CI 27%–79%; Fusion 100%, 95% CI 78%–100%). Furthermore, fusion improved assessment of disease medial to the ossicles (Specificity: CT 25%, 95% CI 3%–65%; DWI 75%, 95% CI 35%–97%; Fusion 100%, 95% CI 63%–100%).[19] In the future, these data may aid the endoscopic surgeon to plan ossicular preserving surgery in children.

Postoperative surveillance using fusion in children, although attractive in terms of improved sensitivity and specificity, suffers from the radiation requirement of the CT component. One solution may be to use the preoperative CT scan fused to a postoperative non-EPI DWI follow-up scan, substituting less radiation for a less accurate anatomic layout, but still carrying the fundamental structural aspects of the patient's temporal bone landmarks. In a small study, cholesteatoma was identified with 100% accuracy in 3 of 10 cases using this method.[72]

CONCLUSION

Imaging of cholesteatoma in the preoperative and postoperative setting is fundamental to the endoscopic ear surgeon. Accurate diagnosis of disease is essential to ensure necessary surgery in a timely manner. Prediction of disease extent can better determine surgical strategy. Knowledge of disease interplay with the ossicular chain may help with its preservation and improve hearing outcomes.

In deciding how to use imaging in the postoperative setting, the surgeon must weigh all of the relevant factors, including patient age and comorbidity, availability and expertise of radiology resources, and disease characteristics at the time of surgery, and take into account the limitations in accuracy of the chosen surveillance method (Table 1).

Future research in MRI is needed to establish robust DWI signal and ADC values for different magnet strengths to optimally segregate cholesteatoma from mimickers in order to delineate accurate disease margins. Development of lower-dose techniques and increasing specificity using dual-energy protocols should be the main research focus in CT imaging. Future clinical possibilities include the development of intraoperative real-time imaging, either through end-of-the-scope technologies like OCT and

AR, or perhaps improvements in hybrid operating rooms to ensure complete removal of disease.

Crucial to the success of any imaging is effective collaboration between surgeon and radiologist. Establishing an agreed surgical-radiological anatomic lexicon for the de novo and postsurgical middle ear will allow unambiguous communication. Exchange of information must include from the surgeon the original disease extent, confidence in disease clearance, and what reconstruction was performed (both autologous and prosthetic). This will enable more accurate delineation of future recurrence and essential feedback for what was seen and interpreted in the original preoperative imaging. Equally, the radiologist must appreciate the various approaches to the ear, especially the endoscopic, to report and present useful information of practical benefit to the surgeon.

REFERENCES

1. Williams MT, Ayache D. Imaging of the postoperative middle ear. Eur Radiol 2004; 14(3):482–95.
2. Schwartz KM, Lane JI, Neff BA, et al. Diffusion-weighted imaging for cholesteatoma evaluation. Ear Nose Throat J 2010;89(4):E14–9.
3. Lemmerling MM, De Foer B, VandeVyver V, et al. Imaging of the opacified middle ear. Eur J Radiol 2008;66(3):363–71. https://doi.org/10.1016/j.ejrad.2008.01.020.
4. Chen S, Ikawa F, Kurisu K, et al. Quantitative MR evaluation of intracranial epidermoid tumors by fast fluid-attenuated inversion recovery imaging and echo-planar diffusion-weighted imaging. AJNR Am J Neuroradiol 2001;22(6):1089–96.
5. Aikele P, Kittner T, Offergeld C, et al. Diffusion-weighted MR imaging of cholesteatoma in pediatric and adult patients who have undergone middle ear surgery. Am J Roentgenol 2003;181(1):261–5.
6. Dubrulle F, Souillard R, Chechin D, et al. Diffusion-weighted MR imaging sequence in the detection of postoperative recurrent cholesteatoma. Radiology 2006;238(2):604–10.
7. Cimsit NC, Cimsit C, Baysal B, et al. Diffusion-weighted MR imaging in postoperative follow-up: reliability for detection of recurrent cholesteatoma. Eur J Radiol 2010;74(1):121–3.
8. Vercruysse J-P, De Foer B, Pouillon M, et al. The value of diffusion-weighted MR imaging in the diagnosis of primary acquired and residual cholesteatoma: a surgical verified study of 100 patients. Eur Radiol 2006;16(7):1461–7.
9. Fischer N, Schartinger VH, Dejaco D, et al. Readout-segmented echo-planar DWI for the detection of cholesteatomas: correlation with surgical validation. Am J Neuroradiol 2019;40(6):1055–9.
10. Muzaffar J, Metcalfe C, Colley S, et al. Diffusion-weighted magnetic resonance imaging for residual and recurrent cholesteatoma: a systematic review and meta-analysis. Clin Otolaryngol 2017;42(3):536–43.
11. Lincot J, Veillon F, Riehm S, et al. Middle ear cholesteatoma: compared diagnostic performances of two incremental MRI protocols including non-echo planar diffusion-weighted imaging acquired on 3T and 1.5T scanners. J Neuroradiol J Neuroradiol 2015;42(4):193–201.
12. Lips LMJ, Nelemans PJ, Theunissen FMD, Roele E, van Tongeren J, Hof JR, Postma AA. The diagnostic accuracy of 1.5 T versus 3 T non-echo-planar diffusion-weighted imaging in the detection of residual or recurrent cholesteatoma in the middle ear and mastoid. J Neuroradiol 2019;(18):30332–8. [Epub ahead of print]. https://doi.org/10.1016/j.neurad.2019.02.013.

13. Plouin-Gaudon I, Bossard D, Ayari-Khalfallah S, et al. Fusion of MRIs and CT scans for surgical treatment of cholesteatoma of the middle ear in children. Arch Otolaryngol Neck Surg 2010;136(9):878.

14. Watanabe T, Ito T, Furukawa T, et al. The efficacy of color mapped fusion images in the diagnosis and treatment of cholesteatoma using transcanal endoscopic ear surgery. Otol Neurotol 2015;36(5):763–8.

15. Campos A, Mata F, Reboll R, et al. Computed tomography and magnetic resonance fusion imaging in cholesteatoma preoperative assessment. Eur Arch Otorhinolaryngol 2017;274(3):1405–11.

16. Kanoto M, Sugai Y, Hosoya T, et al. Detectability and anatomical correlation of middle ear cholesteatoma using fused thin slice non-echo planar imaging diffusion-weighted image and magnetic resonance cisternography (FTS-nEPID). Magn Reson Imaging 2015;33(10):1253–7.

17. Kusak A, Rosiak O, Durko M, et al. Diagnostic imaging in chronic otitis media: does CT and MRI fusion aid therapeutic decision making? A pilot study. Otolaryngol Pol Pol Otolaryngol 2018;73(1):1–5.

18. Locketz GD, Li PMMC, Fischbein NJ, et al. Fusion of computed tomography and propeller diffusion-weighted magnetic resonance imaging for the detection and localization of middle ear cholesteatoma. JAMA Otolaryngol Neck Surg 2016; 142(10):947.

19. Sharma SD, Hall A, Bartley AC, et al. Surgical mapping of middle ear cholesteatoma with fusion of computed tomography and diffusion-weighted magnetic resonance images: diagnostic performance and interobserver agreement. Int J Pediatr Otorhinolaryngol 2020;129:109788.

20. Felici F, Scemama U, Bendahan D, et al. Improved assessment of middle ear recurrent cholesteatomas using a fusion of conventional CT and non-EPI-DWI MRI. AJNR Am J Neuroradiol 2019;40(9):1546–51.

21. Casselman JW, Gieraerts K, Volders D, et al. Cone beam CT: non-dental applications. J Belg Soc Radiol 2013;96(6):333.

22. Burd C, Pai I, Connor S. Imaging anatomy of the retrotympanum: variants and their surgical implications. Br J Radiol 2020;93(1105):20190677.

23. Zhang Z, Yin H, Wang Z, et al. Imaging re-evaluation of the tympanic segment of the facial nerve canal using cone-beam computed tomography compared with multi-slice computed tomography. Eur Arch Otorhinolaryngol 2019;276(7): 1933–41.

24. Vaisbuch Y, Hosseini DK, Lanzman B, et al. Temporal bone CT scan for malleal ligaments assessment. Otol Neurotol 2018;39(10):e1054–9.

25. Ikeda R, Kikuchi T, Oshima H, et al. Computed tomography findings of the bony portion of the Eustachian tube with or without patulous Eustachian tube patients. Eur Arch Otorhinolaryngol 2017;274(2):781–6.

26. Güldner C, Diogo I, Bernd E, et al. Visualization of anatomy in normal and pathologic middle ears by cone beam CT. Eur Arch Otorhinolaryngol 2017;274(2): 737–42.

27. Soons JAM, Danckaers F, Keustermans W, et al. 3D morphometric analysis of the human incudomallear complex using clinical cone-beam CT. Hear Res 2016;340: 79–88.

28. Liktor B, Révész P, Csomor P, et al. Diagnostic value of cone-beam CT in histologically confirmed otosclerosis. Eur Arch Otorhinolaryngol 2014;271(8):2131–8.

29. Hashimoto K, Yanagihara N, Hyodo J, et al. Osseous Eustachian tube and peritubal cells in patients with unilateral cholesteatoma comparison between healthy

and diseased sides using high-resolution cone-beam computed tomography. Otol Neurotol 2015;36(5):776–81.

30. Kashiba K, Komori M, Yanagihara N, et al. Lateral orifice of Prussak's space assessed with a high-resolution cone beam 3-dimensional computed tomography. Otol Neurotol 2011;32(1):71–6.

31. Walliczek-Dworschak U, Diogo I, Strack L, et al. Indications of cone beam CT in head and neck imaging in children. Acta Otorhinolaryngol Ital 2017;37(4):270–5.

32. Furlow B. Dual-energy computed tomography. Radiol Technol 2015;86(3): 301ct–21ct, quiz322ct–25ct.

33. Foti G, Beltramello A, Minerva G, et al. Identification of residual–recurrent cholesteatoma in operated ears: diagnostic accuracy of dual-energy CT and MRI. Radiol Med (Torino) 2019;124(6):478–86.

34. MacDougall D, Farrell J, Bance M, et al. Clinical swept-source optical coherence tomography of the middle ear. In: Biomedical optics 2016. Fort Lauderdale, Florida: OSA; 2016. p. JTu3A.47.

35. Tan HEI, Santa Maria PL, Wijesinghe P, et al. Optical coherence tomography of the tympanic membrane and middle ear: a review. Otolaryngol Neck Surg 2018;159(3):424–38.

36. Monroy GL, Pande P, Nolan RM, et al. Noninvasive in vivo optical coherence tomography tracking of chronic otitis media in pediatric subjects after surgical intervention. J Biomed Opt 2017;22(12):1.

37. Park K, Cho NH, Jeon M, et al. Optical assessment of the *in vivo* tympanic membrane status using a handheld optical coherence tomography-based otoscope. Acta Otolaryngol 2018;138(4):367–74.

38. Wong K, Yee HM, Xavier BA, et al. Applications of augmented reality in otolaryngology: a systematic review. Otolaryngol Neck Surg 2018;159(6):956–67.

39. Marroquin R, Lalande A, Hussain R, et al. Augmented reality of the middle ear combining otoendoscopy and temporal bone computed tomography. Otol Neurotol 2018;39(8):931–9.

40. Barber SR, Wong K, Kanumuri V, et al. Augmented reality, surgical navigation, and 3D printing for transcanal endoscopic approach to the petrous apex. OTO Open 2018;2(4). 2473974X1880449.

41. Mills R. Cholesteatoma behind an intact tympanic membrane in adult life: congenital or acquired? J Laryngol Otol 2009;123(5):488–91.

42. Ng JH, Zhang EZ, Soon SR, et al. Pre-operative high resolution computed tomography scans for cholesteatoma: has anything changed? Am J Otolaryngol 2014; 35(4):508–13.

43. Mehanna AM, Baki FA, Eid M, et al. Comparison of different computed tomography post-processing modalities in assessment of various middle ear disorders. Eur Arch Otorhinolaryngol 2015;272(6):1357–70.

44. Himi T, Sakata M, Shintani T, et al. Middle ear imaging using virtual endoscopy and its application in patients with ossicular chain anomaly. ORL J Otorhinolaryngol Relat Spec 2000;62(6):316–20.

45. Morra A, Tirelli G, Rimondini A, et al. Usefulness of virtual endoscopic three-dimensional reconstructions of the middle ear. Acta Otolaryngol 2002;122(4): 382–5.

46. Chung-Wai A, Tiong-Hong M. Is virtual endoscopy of the middle ear useful? Ear Nose Throat J 2011;90(6):256–60.

47. Saxby, AJ., Dawes L, Cheng C, et al. CT vs CT-MRI fusion imaging in preoperative mastoid assessment for cholesteatoma: implications for endoscopic ear surgery. Cholesteatoma Ear Surg – Update 2017. 2017;eBook:255–260.

48. Abdul-Aziz D, Kozin ED, Lin BM, et al. Temporal bone computed tomography findings associated with feasibility of endoscopic ear surgery. Am J Otolaryngol 2017;38(6):698–703.

49. Choi DL, Gupta MK, Rebello R, et al. Cost-comparison analysis of diffusion weighted magnetic resonance imaging (DWMRI) versus second look surgery for the detection of residual and recurrent cholesteatoma. J Otolaryngol Head Neck Surg 2019;48(1):58.

50. Presutti L, Gioacchini FM, Alicandri-Ciufelli M, et al. Results of endoscopic middle ear surgery for cholesteatoma treatment: a systematic review. Acta Otorhinolaryngol Ital 2014;34(3):153–7.

51. Dremmen MHG, Hofman PAM, Hof JR, et al. The diagnostic accuracy of non-echo-planar diffusion-weighted imaging in the detection of residual and/or recurrent cholesteatoma of the temporal bone. Am J Neuroradiol 2012;33(3):439–44.

52. Dhepnorrarat RC, Wood B, Rajan GP. Postoperative non-EchoYPlanar diffusion-weighted magnetic resonance imaging changes after cholesteatoma surgery: implications for cholesteatoma. Screening 2009;30(1):5.

53. Lingam RK, Khatri P, Hughes J, et al. Apparent diffusion coefficients for detection of postoperative middle ear cholesteatoma on non-echo-planar diffusion-weighted images. Radiology 2013;269(2):504–10.

54. Profant M, Sláviková K, Kabátová Z, et al. Predictive validity of MRI in detecting and following cholesteatoma. Eur Arch Otorhinolaryngol 2012;269(3):757–65.

55. Muhonen EG, Mahboubi H, Moshtaghi O, et al. False-positive cholesteatomas on non-echoplanar diffusion-weighted magnetic resonance imaging. Otol Neurotol 2020;41(5):e588–92.

56. Osman NMM, Rahman AA, Ali MTAH. The accuracy and sensitivity of diffusion-weighted magnetic resonance imaging with apparent diffusion coefficients in diagnosis of recurrent cholesteatoma. Eur J Radiol Open 2017;4:27–39.

57. Garcia-Iza L, Guisasola A, Ugarte A, et al. Utility of diffusion-weighted magnetic resonance imaging in the diagnosis of cholesteatoma and the influence of the learning curve. Eur Arch Otorhinolaryngol 2018;275(9):2227–35.

58. Bazzi K, Wong E, Jufas N, et al. Diffusion-weighted magnetic resonance imaging in the detection of residual and recurrent cholesteatoma in children: a systematic review and meta-analysis. Int J Pediatr Otorhinolaryngol 2019;118:90–6.

59. Denoyelle F, Simon F, Chang KW, et al. International Pediatric Otolaryngology Group (IPOG) consensus recommendations: congenital cholesteatoma. Otol Neurotol 2020;41(3):345–51.

60. Brenner DJ, Elliston CD, Hall EJ, et al. Estimated risks of radiation-induced fatal cancer from pediatric CT. Am J Roentgenol 2001;176(2):289–96.

61. Nauer CB, Rieke A, Zubler C, et al. Low-dose temporal bone CT in infants and young children: effective dose and image quality. Am J Neuroradiol 2011;32(8):1375–80.

62. Frush D, Strauss K. Pediatric radiology & imaging | radiation safety – image gently. The image gently alliance. Available at: https://www.imagegently.org/. [Accessed 18 April 2020].

63. Kim SY, Kim H-S, Park MH, et al. Optimal use of CT imaging in pediatric congenital cholesteatoma. Auris Nasus Larynx 2017;44(3):266–71.

64. Stratis A, Zhang G, Jacobs R, et al. The growing concern of radiation dose in paediatric dental and maxillofacial CBCT: an easy guide for daily practice. Eur Radiol 2019;29(12):7009–18.

65. Kasraie N, Jordan D, Keup C, et al. Optimizing communication with parents on benefits and radiation risks in pediatric imaging. J Am Coll Radiol 2018;15(5): 809–17.
66. Aanenson JW, Till JE, Grogan HA. Understanding and communicating radiation dose and risk from cone beam computed tomography in dentistry. J Prosthet Dent 2018;120(3):353–60.
67. Basa K, Levi JR, Field E, et al. A pearl in the ear: intracranial complications of pediatric cholesteatomas. Int J Pediatr Otorhinolaryngol 2017;92:171–5.
68. Nash R, Wong PY, Kalan A, et al. Comparing diffusion weighted MRI in the detection of post-operative middle ear cholesteatoma in children and adults. Int J Pediatr Otorhinolaryngol 2015;79(12):2281–5.
69. Ide S, Ganaha A, Tono T, et al. Value of DW-MRI in the preoperative evaluation of congenital cholesteatoma. Int J Pediatr Otorhinolaryngol 2019;124:34–8.
70. Rajan GP, Ambett R, Wun L, et al. Preliminary outcomes of cholesteatoma screening in children using non-echo-planar diffusion-weighted magnetic resonance imaging. Int J Pediatr Otorhinolaryngol 2010;74(3):297–301.
71. Lingam RK, Bassett P. A meta-analysis on the diagnostic performance of non-echoplanar diffusion-weighted imaging in detecting middle ear cholesteatoma: 10 years on. Otol Neurotol 2017;38(4):521–8.
72. Alzahrani M, Alhazmi R, Bélair M, et al. Postoperative diffusion weighted MRI and preoperative CT scan fusion for residual cholesteatoma localization. Int J Pediatr Otorhinolaryngol 2016;90:259–63.

The Endoscopic Management of Congenital Cholesteatoma

Rachel McCabe, MD[a], Daniel J. Lee, MD[b], Manuela Fina, MD[c],*

KEYWORDS

- Endoscopic ear surgery • Transcanal • Congenital cholesteatoma • Cholesteatoma
- Pediatric otology

KEY POINTS

- Transcanal endoscopic ear surgery is particularly suited for the management of congenital cholesteatoma given the enhanced visualization of protympanic and epitympanic recesses, areas that are more challenging to visualize using a microscopic-assisted transcanal approach.
- Congenital cholesteatoma is primarily a pediatric disease, with an average age of diagnosis of 5 years to 6 years. In adults, congenital cholesteatoma presents at an advanced stage.
- Although the typical presentation of congenital cholesteatoma is a pearly white mass seen behind the anterosuperior aspect of the tympanic membrane, a majority of cases present with extension to multiple quadrants of the middle ear.
- When congenital cholesteatoma is contained within a sac-like structure, it is more likely to be entirely eradicated in a single-stage surgery. Infiltrative disease warrants a second-look procedure, and a transmastoid, endoscopic-assisted approach can be utilized when mastoid extension is seen.
- Overall outcomes of transcanal endoscopic ear surgery for congenital cholesteatoma have been shown to be similar to traditional microscopic ear surgery in terms of risk of residual disease.

INTRODUCTION

As technological advancements and novel applications of endoscopy have proliferated over the past decade, particular interest has been placed in the role of endoscopy

[a] Department of Otolaryngology, University of Minnesota, 420 Delaware Street Southeast, MMC 396, Minneapolis, MN 55455, USA; [b] Pediatric Otology and Neurotology, Department of Otology and Laryngology, Harvard Medical School, Massachusetts Eye and Ear Infirmary, 243 Charles Street, Boston, MA 02114, USA; [c] Department of Otolaryngology, University of Minnesota, HealthPartners Medical Group, 401 Phalen Blvd, St Paul, MN 55130, USA
* Corresponding author.
E-mail address: finax003@umn.edu

Otolaryngol Clin N Am 54 (2021) 111–123
https://doi.org/10.1016/j.otc.2020.09.012
0030-6665/21/© 2020 Elsevier Inc. All rights reserved.

in middle ear surgery. Surgical management of congenital cholesteatoma is especially suited for an endoscopic approach, because congenital cholesteatoma is located within the middle ear space in most cases. This article presents a review of the etiology and clinical aspects of congenital cholesteatoma as well as a surgical guide to the endoscopic management of this primarily pediatric disease.

DEFINITION

Congenital cholesteatoma by definition consists of a sac-like mass of squamous epithelium that has formed in the middle ear space under an intact and normal tympanic membrane with no prior history of middle ear disease or perforation.[1] Previous bouts of otitis media or middle ear effusions do not constitute criteria for exclusion.[2]

Congenital cholesteatoma remains a rare disease, estimated to account for 2% to 5% of all cholesteatomas.[3] In the pediatric population, congenital cholesteatoma has an estimated incidence of 0.12 per 100,000 children. The average age of diagnosis of congenital cholesteatoma is 5 years to 6 years.[4] Increased awareness by pediatricians, implemented preschool screenings, and new clinical tools, such as otoendoscopy, have helped with earlier detection. In a large retrospective series over 24 years, 73% of surgical patients were 15 years old or younger.[5]

Although congenital cholesteatoma is considered a pediatric disease, it can be diagnosed in the adult population. The literature on adult cases of congenital cholesteatoma is limited. Misale and colleagues[6] report on 6 adult cases of congenital cholesteatoma. In their study, most cases had multiple quadrants of tympanic membrane involved secondary to the long duration of symptoms and advanced lesion at presentation. Another study by Doyle and Luxford[7] included patients ranging from 1 years to 59 years of age with congenital cholesteatoma, of whom 13.5% were over the age of 18 at the time of diagnosis.

Congenital cholesteatoma most commonly presents as a pearly white ear mass, most usually in the anterosuperior quadrant of the middle ear and behind an intact and healthy tympanic membrane. The majority of congenital cholesteatoma, however, involves multiple quadrants of the tympanic membrane at presentation due to a delay in diagnosis. One large retrospective study reported disease limited to the anterosuperior quadrant in only 29% of cases; 23% of cases involved the posterosuperior quadrant, and 46% involved both anterior and posterior superior quadrants.[8]

ETIOLOGY

The most widely accepted theory on congenital cholesteatoma formation is the nonresorption of embryonal epithelial rests. This is based on observations of epidermal structures, similar in location and composition, found in the middle ear space of the human fetus.[9] Derivative structures of the first branchial arch are the upper part of the malleus and incus, tensor tympani muscle, and tendon. The second arch derivatives are the facial and chorda tympani nerve, superstructure of the stapes and lower part of the incus and malleus. Clinical observation that congenital cholesteatoma appears at the first and second branchial junction rather than in a random location explains their origin as migration errors of epithelial remnants as well as their location in close proximity of the cochleariform process and tensor tympani tendon.[10]

CLINICAL PRESENTATION

Diagnosis of congenital cholesteatoma often is made after the incidental finding of an asymptomatic small pearly white mass limited to the anterior superior quadrant of the middle ear behind an intact and healthy tympanic membrane. In such cases, the mass does not directly involve the ossicular chain, thus hearing loss is not an initial presenting sign. As congenital cholesteatoma enlarges, the diagnosis may not necessarily become more obvious due to intact drum. Congenital cholesteatoma may be mistaken for a large plaque of myringosclerosis. Although myringosclerosis has sharp, irregular edges, cholesteatoma presents as a white mass with smooth, curved, and well-defined edges. Cholesteatoma also can be mistaken for a mucopurulent effusion if it has grown to involve all quadrants of the tympanic membrane. As congenital cholesteatoma progresses and involves the ossicular chain, then conductive hearing loss can become a more obvious presenting symptom. Other times, congenital cholesteatoma may be present in concomitance with serous otitis media, with images showing a completely opacified middle ear and mastoid. The mass, due to its typical expansion in the anterior superior aspect of the middle ear space, may cause early occlusion of the eustachian tube and obstruction of the tympanic isthmus, resulting in a middle ear and mastoid effusion.[11]

Occasionally, congenital cholesteatoma incidentally is discovered intraoperatively. A white mass may be recognized behind an intact tympanic membrane during myringotomy for recurrent acute otitis media or chronic effusion and in some cases the matrix is violated during the procedure, opening the sac and revealing squamous debris. A myringotomy also could allow epithelial migration to the undersurface of the tympanic membrane. In some cases, a tube may be advantageous in resolving an effusion in a patient with suspected congenital cholesteatoma. On CT imaging, the presence of an effusion in concomitance with a mass may obscure the true extent of disease because of its similar density to soft tissue, hindering surgical planning. In this instance, if the surgeon deems necessary to drain the effusion in preparation for preoperative imaging, it then is advisable to insert a tympanostomy tube, taking care to place it as far as possible from the visible margins of the cholesteatoma.

STAGING

Several staging systems have been proposed for congenital cholesteatoma. The most frequently used is the Potsic staging system that defines the extension of disease, as follows (**Table 1**).

Potsic stage and risk of residual disease are directly correlated, with increasing risk of residual disease with higher stage. In stage I disease, the risk of residual disease is approximately 5%; in stage II, 24%; stage III, approximately 44%; and stage IV, 64%.[3]

More recently, in 2017, the Japan Otological Society (JOS) introduced a new staging system for cholesteatoma, with the goal of more specifically describing borders of division between the middle ear and the mastoid and difficult access sites, including the sinus tympani and the supratubal recess.[11] In addition, a staging system for congenital cholesteatoma was proposed within the JOS staging and classification criteria for middle ear cholesteatoma (**Table 2**).[12]

Table 1	
Potsic staging system for congenital cholesteatoma	
Stage I	Disease confined to a single quadrant
Stage II	Cholesteatoma in multiple quadrants, but without ossicular involvement or mastoid extension
Stage III	Ossicular involvement without mastoid extension
Stage IV	Mastoid disease

Table 2	
Japan Otological Society staging system for congenital cholesteatoma	
Stage I	Cholesteatoma localized in the tympanic cavity
Stage Ia	Cholesteatoma confined to the anterior half of the tympanic cavity
Stage Ib	Cholesteatoma confined to the posterior half of the tympanic cavity
Stage Ic	Cholesteatoma involving both of sides of the tympanic cavity
Stage II	Cholesteatoma involving 2 or more sites
Stage III	Cholesteatoma with infratemporal complications and pathologic conditions
Stage IV	Cholesteatoma with intracranial complications

ANATOMY OF THE PEDIATRIC EAR CANAL

During childhood, the external ear canal undergoes significant structural changes. Although the tympanic membrane, middle ear, and inner ear are almost the same size in infancy as in adulthood, conversely, the pediatric external ear canal is much shorter and narrower compared with its adult size. Although the adult external ear canal usually is described as one-third cartilaginous and two-thirds osseous, the cartilaginous canal of a newborn directly abuts the tympanic ring, with little osseous component. In the first 5 years of life, there is significant lateral extension of the canal, with simultaneous lateral extension of the osseous tympanic ring, forming the osseous portion of the canal. From age 5 years to 18 years, the osseous canal doubles in length, reaching adult proportions.[13] The length of the canal in pediatric patients must be considered carefully in transcanal surgery, especially when raising a tympanomeatal flap. The flap raised is shorter in length and only a few millimeters away from the tympanic annulus. The width and height of the external auditory canal also undergo significant changes during childhood. The neonatal canal is approximately 4.4 mm to 6.3 mm in width and approximately 5.4 mm in height, whereas the canal of the adult is approximately 6.1 mm to 10.4 mm in width and 6.9 mm in height.[14] This is a n important consideration particularly in endoscopic ear surgery, because the bony portion of the canal is a limiting factor in accommodating the endoscope as well as instrumentation. In a young child with a very narrow ear canal, a 3-mm or 2.7-mm endoscope may be required for surgical approach. Larger ear canals in older children may accommodate a 4-mm telescope. Additionally, the angle of the tympanic annulus relative to the bony external ear canal is more acute in children, changing from 34° from horizontal in the infant, to 63° from horizontal in adulthood; this change is due to the growth of the temporal lobe and skull base rather than changes to middle ear morphology.[14] The more acute angle of the tympanic membrane relative to the plane of the bony external ear canal in younger children may make endoscopic or microscope visualization of the epitympanum and retrotympanum more challenging.

PREOPERATIVE EXAMINATION

Depending on the cooperation of the child, the in-office ear examination is performed under microscopy as well as endoscopy. Under microscopy, the ear canal is cleaned from cerumen. Although endoscopy offers a panoramic view of the tympanic membrane with improved visualization of the anterior tympanic rim, microscopic examination offers the possibility of inspecting selected portions of the tympanic membrane under high magnification. In the authors' office, a screen monitor with recording capability (Telepack, Storz, El Segundo, California) is used in order to obtain endoscopic photo documentation that then is uploaded to the medical chart. This allows for the images to be reviewed prior to surgery as well as during follow-up visits. This is useful especially for educational purposes in an academic program. In addition to documenting the appearance of the tympanic membrane, the endoscopic examination is useful to assess the size of the ear canal. In young children with a very narrow ear canal, a 3-mm or a 2.7-mm endoscope may be required for surgical approach.[15] The preoperative endoscopic examination also is important to assess whether there is a prominent anterior canal wall; if the endoscope is unable to capture a view of the entire drum due to a prominent overhang, the surgical team expects greater difficulty with a transcanal approach. An angled scope can help improve visual access, but most dissection instruments do not have a secondary bend to accommodate the curved canal in tight cases.

PREOPERATIVE IMAGING

Temporal bone computed tomography (CT) imaging is obtained to determine extent of the disease in the middle ear, degree of ossicular involvement, and presence of mastoid disease. The authors believe that imaging is important to optimize surgical planning even in smaller congenital cholesteatomas confined to 1 quadrant. Preoperative CT scanning may not be as useful in cases of concomitant effusion, because opacification of the mastoid and middle ear space may mask the extent of disease. In these cases, tympanostomy tube placement may be necessary to resolve the effusion prior to imaging. Although a magnetic resonance image (MRI) with diffusion-weighted imaging may help with differentiating effusion from disease, the authors would not put a child under general anesthesia to obtain a preoperative MRI unless there was a concern for petrous apex disease or intracranial involvement.

SURGICAL MANAGEMENT AND ENDOSCOPIC ADVANTAGES

The primary goals of surgery for cholesteatoma are eradication of disease and preservation of hearing. Despite the fact that congenital cholesteatoma is a benign lesion, prompt surgical intervention is advocated. The disease expands over time, progressively involving multiple compartments of the tympanic cavity, the ossicular chain, with potential to eventually spread to the mastoid. As disease expands and erodes the middle ear anatomy, hearing preservation and disease eradication become more difficult. The introduction of endoscopy in ear surgery has provided improved visualization of previously inaccessible areas in the tympanic cavity and the epitympanic space. Endoscopy also offers advantages in mastoidectomy; after removal of disease, endoscopy grants the ability to inspect areas in the mastoid that are difficult to visualize under microscopy alone.

Without endoscopy, most congenital cholesteatomas can be removed using 2-handed transcanal microscopy with a similarly minimally invasive approach, which brings into question the necessity of endoscopy. Although congenital cholesteatoma of small size can be removed easily under microscopy, full exposure under microscopy becomes difficult when disease is present anterior to the manubrium of the malleus. The manubrium of the malleus, because of its slight tilt toward the promontory, obstructs the visualization of the cochleariform process and tensor tympani tendon. This explains why, under microscopy, surgical maneuvers, such as transection of the tensor tympani tendon to lift the malleus or removal of the malleus, are performed to improve the visualization of the tympanic cavity. Utilization of a 30° angle endoscope and degloving of the manubrium enables a wide-angle view of the anterior mesotympanic and protympanic recesses without any manipulation of the malleus or transection of the tendon.

SURGICAL CONSIDERATIONS

The surgical management of congenital cholesteatoma is different from that of primary acquired cholesteatoma due to the underlying mechanism of disease formation. Patients with congenital cholesteatoma typically have normal middle ear anatomy, an intact tympanic membrane, and normal eustachian tube function. Therefore, when congenital cholesteatoma can be removed while keeping the tympanic membrane intact, the ear is expected to heal uneventfully, with an intact transparent membrane, which also allows for surveillance of residual disease. Because of the normal function of the eustachian tube and middle ear, the occurrence of postoperative tympanic or attic retraction is not expected, which is an unfortunate frequent occurrence after surgery for acquired cholesteatoma. Nevertheless, postoperative atelectasis and attic retraction sometimes are observed after surgery for congenital cholesteatoma, leading to secondary development of acquired cholesteatoma from pars tensa or pars flaccida retraction. This unusual circumstance can be secondary to poorer mastoid ventilation. Studies have shown that the mastoid cells in ears of children with congenital cholesteatoma are poorly pneumatized compared with those of children without middle ear disease, and the degree of pneumatization is significantly poorer than in the opposite side.[16] Decreased gas exchange in a reduced mastoid or sclerotic inflammatory change of the middle ear mucosa after surgery could be responsible for a tendency for delayed tympanic and attic retraction.

The structure of the cholesteatoma is an important determining factor for prognosis and reconstruction. Congenital cholesteatoma, due to its cystic origin from epithelial remnants, is more likely to be collected in a sac-like structure that facilitates complete excision, thus favoring consideration for an immediate ossicular chain reconstruction (OCR) during primary surgery. Conversely, primary acquired cholesteatoma frequently is disorganized in structure with loose or adherent matrix and is more likely to warrant a second-look surgery with staged ossicular reconstruction.

The surgical approach for congenital cholesteatoma is dependent on the extent of the disease. The transcanal approach provides adequate exposure for most congenital cholesteatoma confined to the middle ear, which facilitates the use of endoscopy. When imaging demonstrates mastoid opacification concerning for extent of disease to the mastoid, preoperative discussion about the possible need for a posterior auricular approach with mastoidectomy is discussed with the family.

CHOICE OF ENDOSCOPES

A 3-mm diameter (14-cm length) rigid Hopkins rod telescope is suitable for the majority of pediatric endoscopic cases. Older children with a larger ear canal may accommodate 4-mm endoscopes, with the advantage of providing an enhanced wide-angle view and improved illumination but come at the expense of restricted space with dissection instruments. In very young children or those with especially narrow external canals, a 2.7-mm pediatric rigid sinus endoscope can be utilized. Although this scope may be necessary to access a smaller canal, the 2.7-mm endoscope is disadvantaged by a longer, more fragile shaft (17.5 cm) and a smaller diameter, resulting in reduced wide field view of the surgical area. The authors advocate starting with a 0° 3-mm endoscope. In cases of a prominent anterior canal wall, a 30° 3-mm endoscope may be necessary to improve anterior visualization.

SURGICAL APPROACH
Endoscopic Approach to Congenital Cholesteatoma Limited to the Anterior Superior Quadrant (Stage I)

Endoscopy is particularly advantageous in the approach of a congenital cholesteatoma limited to the anterior superior quadrant. The superior visualization of the anterior rim of the tympanic membrane and protympanic area, compared with microscopy, enables removal of the sac with intact preservation of the ossicular chain. Congenital cholesteatoma limited to the anterosuperior quadrant can be approached in 2 ways: with an anterior tympanomeatal flap designed to expose the anterior portion of the tympanic space and with a posterior tympanomeatal flap that exposes the entire mesotympanum and protympanum after degloving of the manubrium. The latter approach technically is more straightforward and provides improved surgical access to disease.

Anterior tympanomeatal exposure

The anterior tympanomeatal incision is made starting at the anterior rim, anterior to the notch of Rivinus. The incision is made approximately 6 mm away from the tympanic annulus and extended from the 3-o'clock to 9-o'clock position (**Fig. 1**A). The flap is dissected off the anterior tympanic annulus to expose the anterior aspect of the tympanic cavity (**Fig. 1**B). The tympanic membrane is pulled back and detached from the neck and handle of the malleus. Full surgical exposure of the sac is obtained by dissecting the fibrous attachment of the tympanic membrane from the manubrium of the malleus, while maintaining attachment to the umbo (**Fig. 1**C). The reflection of the tympanic membrane exposes the small cholesteatoma and allows retrieval of the sac without exposing the ossicular chain or disrupting the posterior aspect of the tympanic membrane (**Fig. 1**D). This exposure is suitable for small, limited masses, or pearls, that

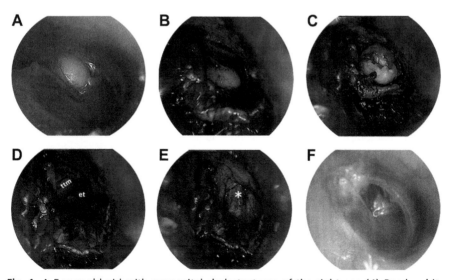

Fig. 1. A 5-year-old girl with congenital cholesteatoma of the right ear. (*A*) Pearly white mass located to the anterior superior quadrant of the tympani muscle. (*B*) Anterior tympanomeatal incision, anterior to the lateral process of the malleus. (*C*) Dissection of the tympanic membrane off the manubrium for surgical exposure of the mass. (*D*) Inspection of the protympanic space after cholesteatoma resection. (*E*) A graft of porcine extracellular mucosa is applied as an underlay. (*F*) Appearance 3.5 years postoperatively. et, eustachian tube orifice; ttm, tensor tympani muscle; *, porcine extracellular mucosal graft.

do not extend past the manubrium of the malleus and do not entirely fill the superior anterior quadrant. One disadvantage of elevating an entirely anteriorly based flap is that dissection may be challenging because the tympanic membrane can be firmly adherent to the tympanic annulus. Other investigators have performed a transtympanic approach with tympanotomy for very small congenital cholesteatoma.[17]

Posterior tympanomeatal exposure
A posterior tympanomeatal incision is made from the 1-o'clock position, anterior to the neck of the malleus, extending posteriorly to the 6-o'clock position, 6 mm to 8 mm in length from the tympanic annulus. Once the tympanic annulus is lifted, the middle ear is entered, and the tympanic membrane is dissected off the manubrium of the malleus to expose the anterior aspect of the tympanic membrane. Endoscopy provides a high degree of magnification, improving visualization of the fibrous attachment of the tympanic membrane over the malleus manubrium. Dissection of this tough fibrous attachment is performed with the sharp edge of a sickle knife or a joint knife to gently dissect the fibrous attachment of the tympanic membrane off the periosteum of the malleus manubrium. The tympanic membrane then is detached from the manubrium, except for a small portion that is left attached to the umbo to avoid postoperative lateralization. Ensuring complete removal of the cholesteatoma from the malleus, tensor tympani tendon, and cochleariform process is crucial because these areas have high risk of harboring residual disease. Curved, angled instruments, such as a Thomassin attic dissector and a Rosen needle, are helpful in removing disease from these structures. Often, the sac appears to be lodged into or protruding over the eustachian tube opening. An endoscopic curved suction is helpful in gently pulling and extracting the sac away from the opening of the eustachian tube.

After sac removal, a 30° or 45° 3-mm scope is used to inspect the protympanic space to assure that no residual disease is left behind. The anatomic structures in this area, the hemicanal of the tensor tympani muscle, the eustachian tube orifice, and the subtensor recess (SR) are inspected for any residual disease (see **Fig. 1**D). The elevated tympanic membrane then is repositioned in place. If any tear occurred during the elevation or the elevated tympanic membrane is particularly thin and fragile, an underlay graft is placed. The authors favor tragal or conchal perichondrium or heterologous porcine extracellular mucosa for its thicker consistency and postoperative transparent appearance (**Fig. 1**E). By keeping the tympanic membrane attached to the umbo, preserving the tympanic rim attachment of the anterior inferior aspect of the tympanic membrane, postoperative blunting is avoided (**Fig. 1**F).

Endoscopic Approach to Congenital Cholesteatoma Involving Multiple Quadrants Without Ossicular Erosion (Stage II)

A congenital cholesteatoma involving multiple quadrants may present as a mass medial to the malleus in a dumbbell shape (**Fig. 2**A). The bulk of the mass extends into the attic and mesotympanic areas, with the narrow portion of the dumbbell medial to the malleus (**Fig. 2**B). This is a challenging situation, because the ossicular chain is in continuity, but the mass is medial in respect to the head of the malleus (**Fig. 2**C). Consequently, it is necessary to disrupt the ossicular chain in order to extract the mass (**Fig. 2**D). In this case, in order to fully expose the attic, the incus is separated from the stapes, and removed, while the head of the malleus is transected at the neck with a malleus nipper and removed (see **Fig. 2**D). Although it may be tempting to remove the entire malleus with the aim of ensuring complete eradication of the disease, the removal of the entire malleus has profound consequences on hearing reconstruction. The tympanic membrane, no longer anchored to the malleus, lateralizes with

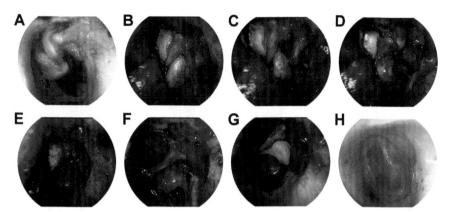

Fig. 2. A 6-year-old boy with congenital cholesteatoma of the left ear. (*A*) Mass involves multiple quadrants of the tympanic membrane. (*B*) Cholesteatoma conformed as a dumbbell-shaped cyst with the narrow portion kinked medial to the malleus. (*C*) Gentle dissection of the mass reveals an intact ossicular chain. (*D*) Incus and malleus head are removed to expose the medial component of the mass. (*E*) Residual mass in protympanic and anterior attic space. (*F*) Attic inspection with 30° endoscopy. (*G*) Autologous incus interposed between stapes capitulum and malleus manubrium. (*H*) Well-healed tympanic membrane 18 months postoperatively.

time. As the tympanic membrane lateralizes, it becomes discontinuous with any form of ossicular reconstruction (prosthesis or autologous incus) with subsequent postoperative conductive hearing loss. To avoid this, the manubrium of the malleus is left attached to the tensor tympani tendon and then lifted to inspect the area of the cochleariform process Endoscopy provides improved visualization of the attic, allowing full inspection for residual disease (**Fig. 2**F). The incus then is sculpted with a 2-mm diamond burr, interposed between the stapes capitulum, and notched under the malleus; this favors a more physiologic OCR than that of a partial ossicular replacement prosthesis (**Fig. 2**G).

Endoscopic Approach to Congenital Cholesteatoma Involving Multiple Quadrants with Ossicular Involvement (Stage III)

When a congenital cholesteatoma occupies a large portion of the middle ear space, the ossicles are enveloped in the large mass, which obscures the degree of erosion (**Fig. 3**A). A posterior incision is made, starting just anterior to the notch of Rivinus, and extending to the inferior aspect of the canal. The tympanic membrane is reflected, and exposure of the middle ear reveals either one large sac or multiple sac-like formations that fill the entire middle ear space. In this particular case, the ossicles are buried under multiple sacs of disease (**Fig. 3**B). At this point, probing or attempting to lift the sac blindly is hazardous, because the degree of involvement with the stapes or facial nerve is unknown. The most prudent course of action is to continue to lift the tympanic membrane and identify the malleus, because this is the ossicle least likely to be eroded (see **Fig. 3**B). Identification of the malleus facilitates palpation of the incus, which can be performed with a blunt instrument, such as a Rosen needle or a short attic dissector. Curetting the scutum with a stapes curette helps to identify the lateral aspect of the body of the incus as well as determine the posterior extension of the cholesteatoma sac. Once the sac of disease is lifted off the mesotympanum and the incus is identified, the stapes and the degree of erosion can be evaluated. If erosion of the

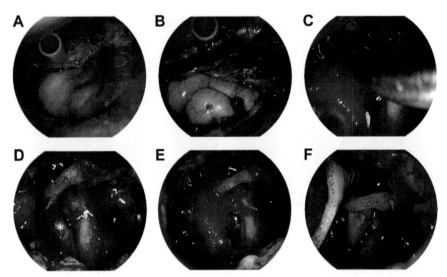

Fig. 3. A 3-year-old boy with congenital cholesteatoma of the left ear. (*A*) Cholesteatoma involves multiple quadrants of the tympanic membrane and a tube had been placed by the referring physician. (*B*) Multiple sacs of cholesteatoma obscure the visualization of incus and stapes. The malleus is identified as first anatomic landmark in the middle ear space. (*C*) A curved suction is utilized to extract a portion of cholesteatoma lodged into the eustachian tube. (*D*) A portion of cholesteatoma deeply lodged over the footplate (*) is removed last. (*E*) After removal of cholesteatoma, the footplate is exposed as stapes superstructure was completely eroded. (*F*) Autologous incus interposition graft from stapes footplate to malleus.

stapes superstructure is present, cholesteatoma matrix can be adherent to the footplate as well as over the tympanic segment of the facial nerve (**Fig. 3**D). The high magnification provided by endoscopy is useful particularly when working delicately in this area. Gentle elevation of matrix from the footplate is performed with a blunt instrument; extreme care is taken to avoid fracturing a thinned footplate or exposing a perilymphatic fistula under an eroded footplate. If necessary, a wider atticotomy is performed with a stapes curette or with a piezoelectric drill, which allows sharp bone curettage with an oscillating blade under a constant flow of saline, providing visualization under water.

Combined Approach for Congenital Cholesteatoma with Mastoid Involvement (Stage IV)

When preoperative imaging shows mastoid opacification, extension of disease to the mastoid should be considered. Congenital cholesteatoma with mastoid extension is present in approximately 13% of all cases.[3] Radiologic signs suggestive of disease extension to the mastoid include loss of air cell trabeculation, blunting of the scutum, and the presence of soft tissue mass with rounded edges in the mastoid. Even when a mastoidectomy appears inevitable, there are several advantages to starting the surgery with a transcanal endoscopic approach. Primarily, a posterior auricular approach or a mastoidectomy would not be committed to until it is evident that the cholesteatoma has extended to the mastoid antrum, beyond the limits of transcanal endoscopy. Additionally, starting the surgery through a transcanal approach allows the prioritization of work time in the middle ear and attic shortly after transcanal injection and delivery of anesthetic and vasoconstrictors.

This brings to question, how far can an atticotomy be extended to retrieve disease that extends into the aditus? The limit of transcanal endoscopy is considered the posterior aspect of the lateral semicircular canal. Although angled endoscopes may visualize the disease, lack of curved instrumentation with grasping capability frequently limits disease removal. The rising popularity of endoscopic ear surgery is inspiring the development of endoscopic ear instruments; curved suctions, angled dissectors, and flexible steering tips are being developed with the goal of improving accessibility of all areas visualized by endoscopy.

When extension of disease to the mastoid is unclear, the decision whether to perseverate with transcanal attempts at removing disease or convert to mastoidectomy may be challenging. If disease still is visualized with angled endoscopy but cannot be removed entirely with curved suctions and angled dissectors, the authors favor avoiding aggressive scutum removal to reduce time and frustration in the operating room and commence with canal-up mastoidectomy. The authors' experience is that cholesteatoma extending past the prominence of the lateral canal can only be removed through an extended atticotomy if it is collected in a well-defined sac. If cholesteatoma is disorganized with loose or infiltrative matrix, it is advisable to move forward with mastoidectomy because small remnants or pedunculated extensions of cholesteatoma may be out of endoscopic view. After completion of a limited canal-up mastoidectomy, 0° and 30° endoscopes are utilized to inspect the recesses of the middle ear and mastoid that are poorly visualized transcanal endoscopically as well as transmastoid microscopically (such as the medial aspect of the posterior auditory canal and the aditus). Using a moist gauze draped over the edge of the mastoid cavity stabilizes the telescope and utilizing a curved suction in the other hand completes débridement of the cholesteatoma.

PRIMARY VERSUS SECONDARY OSSICULAR CHAIN RECONSTRUCTION

It has been shown that resection of an intact sac of congenital cholesteatoma is associated with significantly reduced risk of residual disease.[3] This is due to congenital cholesteatoma's tendency to be collected in a well-defined sac, making it more likely to be completely excised. Therefore, cases in which congenital cholesteatoma is resected are more amenable to primary OCR compared with acquired cholesteatoma. There are certain situations, however, in which primary OCR after congenital cholesteatoma resection is not recommended. Primary OCR is inadvisable when there is concern about possible residual squamous debris in challenging areas, such as the anterior crus, stapes footplate, facial nerve, sinus tympani, and subpyramidal areas. In these circumstances, second-look surgery with secondary OCR should be performed. The incus can be banked in the attic to be used for reconstruction at a later time. In cases of small congenital cholesteatomas resected in entirety, with clear and well-defined borders, primary OCR is advantageous in providing the child with an immediate form of hearing rehabilitation compared with waiting for a planned, staged OCR.

OUTCOMES

Risk of residual disease directly correlates with higher stage. In a review of 82 cases of microscopic surgery for congenital cholesteatoma, cases were stratified according to Potsic staging: 24% of cases were stage I, 21% were stage II, 41% were stage III, and 13% were stage IV. Higher stage also correlated with increased preoperative hearing loss. Residual disease was encountered in 33% of all cases, with rates of residual disease as 5% in stage 1%, 24% in stage 2%, 44% in stage 3%, and 64% in stage 4. In addition to Potsic stage, aspects of disease presentation that were significantly correlated with higher risk of residual disease include congenital cholesteatoma located medial to the malleus or incus, disease abutting the incus or stapes, disease enveloping or eroding the stapes, and disease requiring the removal of ossicles on initial surgery. Having an intact congenital cholesteatoma pearl was associated with greatly reduced rates of residual disease.[3]

Because endoscopic ear surgery is a more recent field, studies on the outcomes of endoscopic ear surgery for congenital cholesteatoma are fewer. These early, encouraging studies, however, have shown similarities in surgical outcomes in the treatment of congenital cholesteatoma using the endoscopic approach compared with using a microscopic technique. In a study of 25 children who underwent endoscopic ear surgery for congenital cholesteatoma of the middle ear, 52% were stage I, 28% were stage II, and 20% were stage III. A majority of the stage I cholesteatomas were located in the anterior superior quadrant (12/13). After an average follow-up period of 24 months ± 8.5 months, 24 of the 25 had no evidence of recurrence.[17] Additionally, James and colleagues[15] reviewed 235 ears in 220 children who had had intact canal wall surgery; 108 underwent microscopic dissection with only endoscopic inspection, and 127 underwent increasing use of endoscopes for dissection. The investigators found a 12% risk reduction in residual disease at 2.5 years when endoscopes were used for dissection, especially in the middle ear (from 22% to 11%).[15]

SUMMARY

Congenital cholesteatoma is a rare disease that comprises approximately 2% to 5% of all cases of cholesteatoma. It primarily is a pediatric disease, with peak age of diagnosis of 5 years to 6 years. Congenital cholesteatoma, as opposed to primary acquired cholesteatoma, often presents in healthy ears with no prior history of disease and with normal eustachian tube function. Transcanal endoscopic ear surgery is particularly suited for congenital cholesteatoma, because this is primarily a disease of the middle ear, and thus the majority of cases can be managed with a transcanal approach. The underlying lack of chronic ear disease in most ears with congenital cholesteatoma, combined with its tendency to be contained in a saclike structure, increases the chances of complete removal during primary surgery. The wide-angled view provided by transcanal endoscopy allows a superior visualization of areas, such as the protympanum and attic, compared with transcanal microscopic-assisted approaches. This further reduces the risk residual disease. In both surgical and clinical practice, the use of endoscopy to document disease and postoperative results is useful not only for surgical planning and family counseling but also as a teaching tool. Initial outcomes on endoscopic management of congenital cholesteatoma show similar residual and recurrent rates compared with microscopic ear surgery. As more surgeons adopt endoscopic-assisted transcanal and transmastoid techniques to manage pediatric ear disease, larger cohort studies can be expected on outcomes of endoscopic ear surgery for congenital cholesteatoma.

DISCLOSURE

Dr M. Fina and Dr R. McCabe have no relevant conflicts of interest or financial ties to disclose.

REFERENCES

1. Derlacki EL, Clemis JD. LX congenital cholesteatoma of the middle ear and mastoid. Ann Otol Rhinol Laryngol 1965;74(3):706–27.
2. Levenson MJ, Michaels L, Parisier SC, et al. Congenital cholesteatomas in children: an embryologic correlation. Laryngoscope 1988;98(9):949–55.
3. Stapleton AL, Egloff AM, Yellon RF. Congenital cholesteatoma: predictors for residual disease and hearing outcomes. Arch Otolaryngol Neck Surg 2012;138(3): 280–5.
4. Nevoux J, Lenoir M, Roger G, et al. Childhood cholesteatoma. Eur Ann Otorhinolaryngol Head Neck Dis 2010;127(4):143–50.
5. Kojima H, Tanaka Y, Shiwa M, et al. Congenital cholesteatoma clinical features and surgical results. Am J Otolaryngol 2006;27(5):299–305.
6. Misale P, Lepcha A. Congenital cholesteatoma in adults-interesting presentations and management. Indian J Otolaryngol Head Neck Surg 2018;70(4):578–82.
7. Doyle KJ, Luxford WM. Congenital aural cholesteatoma: results of surgery in 60 cases. Laryngoscope 1995;105(3):263–7.
8. Lim HW, Yoon TH, Kang WS. Congenital cholesteatoma: clinical features and growth patterns. Am J Otolaryngol 2012;33(5):538–42.
9. Michaels L. Origin of congenital cholestecetoma from a normally occurring epidermoid rest in the developing middle ear. Int J Pediatr Otorhinolaryngol 1988;15(1):51–65.
10. Aimi KMD. Role of the tympanic ring in the pathogenesis of congenital cholesteatoma. Laryngoscope 1983;93(9):1140–6.
11. Yung M, Tono T, Olszewska E, et al. EAONO/JOS joint consensus statements on the definitions, classification and staging of middle ear cholesteatoma. J Int Adv Otol 2017;13(1):1–8.
12. Tono T, Sakagami M, Kojima H, et al. Staging and classification criteria for middle ear cholesteatoma proposed by the Japan Otological Society. Auris Nasus Larynx 2017;44(2):135–40.
13. Isaacson G. Endoscopic anatomy of the pediatric middle ear. Otolaryngol Neck Surg 2014;150(1):6–15.
14. Miller KA, Fina M, Lee DJ. Principles of pediatric endoscopic ear surgery. Otolaryngol Clin North Am 2019;52(5):825–45.
15. James AL. Endoscopic middle ear surgery in children. Otolaryngol Clin North Am 2013;46(2):233–44.
16. Iino Y, Imamura Y, Hiraishi M, et al. Mastoid pneumatization in children with congenital cholesteatoma: an aspect of the formation of open-type and closed-type cholesteatoma. The Laryngoscope 1998;108(7):1071–6.
17. Park JH, Ahn J, Moon IJ. Transcanal endoscopic ear surgery for congenital cholesteatoma. Clin Exp Otorhinolaryngol 2018;11(4):233–41.

Endoscopic Management of Pediatric Chronic Ear Disease

Evette Ronner, BA[a], Michael S. Cohen, MD[b],*

KEYWORDS

- Endoscopic • Chronic ear • Middle ear surgery • Pediatric

KEY POINTS

- Chronic ear disease in children is characterized by Eustachian tube dysfunction and often results in the need for surgical intervention.
- Use of rigid endoscopes provides an alternative approach to the microscope for both in-office examination and surgical procedures.
- The endoscope offers an improved, high-resolution visualization of the middle ear space and adjacent structures.
- Endoscopic ear surgery can reduce the need for postauricular incisions or mastoidectomy, as well as reduce residual disease rates in primary cholesteatoma procedures.

 Video content accompanies this article at http://www.oto.theclinics.com.

INTRODUCTION

Pediatric chronic ear disease is characterized by Eustachian tube dysfunction (ETD) and its sequelae. Common causes of ETD include delayed maturity, heredity, and anomalies of development. Other causes include trauma, adenoid hypertrophy, allergy, reflux, and neoplasm.

Many children with ETD present with otitis media and subsequently will require bilateral myringotomy with tube insertion (BMT) for pressure equalization. Although BMT is the mainstay of treatment for ETD, it is also a leading risk factor for tympanic membrane perforation. ETD can also cause atelectasis of the tympanic membrane, acquired cholesteatoma, and ossicular discontinuity secondary to devascularization and erosion. Congenital cholesteatoma, middle ear tumors, and trauma can also lead to middle ear disease in children in the absence of ETD. Pediatric chronic ear

[a] Geisel School of Medicine at Dartmouth, 1 Rope Ferry Road, Hanover, NH 03755, USA;
[b] Department of Otolaryngology, Massachusetts Eye and Ear and Harvard Medical School, 243 Charles Street, Boston, MA 02114, USA
* Corresponding author.
E-mail address: michael_cohen@meei.harvard.edu

Otolaryngol Clin N Am 54 (2021) 125–128
https://doi.org/10.1016/j.otc.2020.09.013
0030-6665/21/© 2020 Elsevier Inc. All rights reserved.
oto.theclinics.com

disease often results in surgical intervention, such as a myringotomy, tympanoplasty, ossiculoplasty, or removal of cholesteatoma. Endoscopes can enhance both the diagnosis and management of the various sequelae of pediatric middle ear disease. Video 1 demonstrates an endoscopic view of a dehiscent jugular bulb resulting in conductive hearing loss. The visible pulsations and smooth margin help distinguish this from a glomus tympanicum. Office endoscopy helped facilitate this diagnosis, confirmed by MRI.

Traditionally, middle ear surgery in children was performed exclusively using the microscope. Although the microscope provides a stable, highly magnified image and leaves both hands available for dissection, the need for line-of-sight view and long distance from lens to target tissue often necessitates a postauricular incision, canalplasty, and even mastoidectomy just to achieve adequate access and visualization of the middle ear space. The use of a rigid endoscope provides an alternative approach to performing middle ear surgery and affords a broad view of the entire middle ear space without removal of bone in most ears. The endoscope can be used either exclusively through the ear canal to perform transcanal endoscopic ear surgery (TEES) or in a combined approach with the microscope if mastoidectomy is required. Indeed, endoscopes can also augment visualization via a transmastoid approach in cases of a low-hanging dura or difficult to reach posterior epitympanic disease.

There are multiple benefits of performing EES in children. Compared with the microscope, the endoscope allows for a wider viewing angle with an increased depth of field, as well as an improved resolution with magnification, which is particularly helpful when navigating the middle ear space.[1] EES significantly reduces the need for a postauricular incision in all middle ear surgery and for mastoidectomy in cholesteatoma surgery, thus reducing morbidity and surgical risk to the dura, major vascular structures, and the vertical segment of the facial nerve.[2]

DISCUSSION

A high-quality office examination is required to determine the most appropriate management for ear disease. Office-based otoendoscopy delivers a high resolution, panoramic image, thereby enabling the examiner to see the entirety of the tympanic membrane, even in cases of tortuous or narrow ear canals. That said, it is important that the examiner use caution in young children. Use of a shorter, 6-cm endoscope is more suitable for an office examination as it allows the user to stabilize the hands on the patient's head, which provides both support and immediate tactile feedback if the head is turned.

Endoscopes can be helpful for BMT, in particular for children with narrow ear canals. Children with Down syndrome are prone to chronic ETD and often have very narrow ear canals, making it challenging to insert ear tubes in these patients.[3,4] A narrow (1.9 mm) endoscope can facilitate tube insertion, allowing for a more anterior tube placement away from critical middle ear structures. It can increase the likelihood of successful insertion in patients with narrow ear canals because a narrow endoscope can be advanced beyond a bony anterior bulge affording a broad view of the tympanic membrane. These cases are often very challenging with the microscope as it is difficult to manipulate instruments as well as the tube through a very narrow (usually 2 mm or 2.5 mm) speculum. Video 2 demonstrates endoscopic myringotomy with tube insertion in a 3-year-old child with Down syndrome. The drum was not able to be well visualized under the microscope with a 2.5-mm speculum and therefore visualization of the drum was achieved with a 1.9-mm endoscope. This allowed for a clear view of tympanic membrane anatomy and safe incision and tube insertion.

TEES is a feasible and useful method for performing a variety of surgical middle ear procedures. This can be particularly beneficial when performing a tympanoplasty in children as their external auditory canals are narrower than those of adults. Reported tympanoplasty closure rates were similar for both children and adults who underwent endoscopic or microscopic surgeries.[5–7] Use of the endoscope for tympanoplasty is associated with fewer postauricular incisions, and less morbidity, including fewer wound infections, shorter operative time, and decreased length of stay.[5] Outcomes have been similar for children with Down syndrome, who often have narrow ear canals, and endoscopic tympanoplasty enabled many of these children to avoid a postauricular incision.[4] Thus, TEES offers a safe, less morbid, and equally effective approach for pediatric tympanoplasty.

TEES has also proven to be a successful modality for ossiculoplasty. Again, most ossiculoplasty surgery can be successfully completed with TEES, which can potentially reduce postoperative pain and complications associated with a surgical incision. Use of the endoscope for ossiculoplasty has been demonstrated to have similar hearing outcomes compared with those performed with the microscope. Children who underwent endoscopic ossiculoplasty had fewer postauricular incisions and equivalent audiometric outcomes and postoperative complications than those performed microscopically.[2] TEES has also been shown to be an effective approach for performing stapes surgery in children.[8]

There has been an increasing role for use of the endoscope for cholesteatoma removal in children. The success of cholesteatoma surgery depends on the ability to clearly visualize and dissect disease. Therefore, improving visualization of the middle ear cavity is crucial to increase the likelihood of complete cholesteatoma removal and prevent residual disease. The endoscope is well-suited to this task. A meta-analysis of 11 studies involving 915 patients demonstrated that TEES was associated with lower rates of residual cholesteatoma than those surgeries performed with some or total use of the microscope.[9] EES also significantly reduces the frequency of mastoidectomy and postauricular incisions required compared with cases performed with the microscope alone.[1,10,11]

Because TEES can reduce the need for a postauricular approach, use of the endoscope may also reduce postoperative pain for pediatric ear surgery patients. Reported postoperative pain and analgesic use was significantly lower in patients who underwent TEES that in those who underwent microscopic surgery.[12] This is particularly relevant to national efforts to reduce opioid prescription in response to the current opioid crisis.

SUMMARY

- In summary, EES for chronic ear disease in children provides multiple advantages to the traditional microscopic approach, such as the following:
- Augments visualization and diagnosis in the office setting;
- Allows for safer and more effective ear tube insertion in narrow ear canals, particularly in children with Down syndrome;
- Reduces the need for postauricular incision in tympanoplasty, with equivalent closure rates;
- Reduces the need for postauricular incisions in ossiculoplasty, with equivalent hearing outcomes;
- Reduces mastoidectomy rates in primary cholesteatoma procedures;
- Reduces residual disease rates in primary cholesteatoma procedures;
- Allows for improved visualization via the mastoidectomy approach;

PATHOGENESIS OF CHOLESTEATOMA

Cholesteatoma is a disease of the middle ear and mastoid characterized by the accumulation of keratinizing stratified squamous epithelium that results in local inflammation and destruction. The estimated annual incidence of cholesteatoma is 6 to 15 cases per 100,000 people.[2–4] There are 2 types of aural cholesteatoma: congenital and acquired. Congenital cholesteatoma originates from ectopic rests of squamous epithelium that form in the middle ear under an intact tympanic membrane. Acquired cholesteatoma originates from migration of the epithelium in the middle ear from a retraction or a perforation of the tympanic membrane. Acquired cholesteatoma comprises the vast majority of cholesteatoma cases and is further divided into primary and secondary acquired.[5] Primary acquired cholesteatoma results from tympanic membrane retraction. The retraction may involve the pars flaccida, the pars tensa, or both. Secondary acquired cholesteatoma results from a direct injury or perforation of the tympanic membrane due to infection or iatrogenic causes.

There are several theories on the pathogenesis of primary acquired cholesteatoma. These include (1) invagination, (2) basal cell hyperplasia, (3) metaplasia, and (4) epithelial invasion.[6] More recently, 2 new theories have been proposed: mucosal traction and selective epitympanic dysventilation theory. In the theory of mucosal traction, adhesions of opposing mucosal surfaces exert traction on the tympanic membrane, stimulating cytokine production and keratinocyte proliferation.[7] The theory of selective epitympanic dysventilation postulates that retraction of the pars flaccida occurs secondary to a block of ventilation pathways between the mesotympanic space and the epitympanic compartment. This results from a complete tensor fold that obstructs the epitympanic compartment while the remaining mesotympanic space is ventilated by the eustachian tube. The selective epitympanic dysventilation theory attempts to explain how epitympanic cholesteatoma can be associated with a well-ventilated and normal appearing pars tensa.[8]

Primary acquired cholesteatoma can occur at any age. Within the pediatric population, the estimated incidence of cholesteatoma is 3 cases per 100,000 individuals, with the majority of these attributed to acquired cholesteatoma.[9,10] In the pediatric acquired cholesteatoma population, the average age of presentation is approximately 10 years.[11,12] Pediatric primary acquired cholesteatoma typically has a more aggressive growth pattern compared to its adult counterpart.[13,14] This is attributed to more active keratinocyte proliferation and more rapid spread in widely pneumatized pediatric mastoids compared to a slower spread in adult osteitic mastoids with dense bone.[15]

ADVANTAGES OF THE ENDOSCOPIC APPROACH

Endoscopy provides superior visualization of portions of the middle ear that are not well-visualized with a microscope; these regions include the attic, sinus tympani, anterior epitympanic rim, protympanum, and hypotympanum.[1] Initially, endoscopes were used as an adjunct tool to inspect the middle ear and mastoid following microscopic work.[16] With improvements in optics and instrumentation, more surgeons have adopted endoscopes as the primary tool for repair of tympanic perforations and management of cholesteatoma with limited attic extension.[16,17] Outcomes for microscopic and endoscopic tympanoplasty show equivalent closure rates of 85% to 97%, while endoscopy obviates the need for a postauricular incision, resulting in less postoperative pain and morbidity.[18,19] Endoscopy is uniquely suited for management of attic cholesteatoma as it confers improved visualization of the attic and sinus tympani areas, the 2 most common sites of residual disease.[20,21] The improved endoscopic view allows the surgeon to follow the pathway of the disease from the middle ear into the attic. This creates a tailored, less invasive approach that extends up to the limits of the disease and may preserve the ossicular chain and the mastoid.

IN-OFFICE ENDOSCOPIC EXAMINATION

Surgical planning for cholesteatoma begins in the office with a combined microscopic and endoscopic ear examination. Microscopy is used first to clean the ear and inspect the tympanic membrane under high magnification. The ear is then examined with a rigid endoscope. In the clinic we use 4-mm rigid sinus endoscopes that are readily available. Pediatric 2.7-mm sinus endoscopes are an alternative for pediatric and narrow ear canals. The endoscopic examination supplies a panoramic view of the entire tympanic membrane with improved visualization of the anterior tympanic rim and pars flaccida. Photo documentation is obtained and uploaded to the medical chart to help with surgical planning. Endoscopic assessment of the size of the ear canal, prominence of the anterior and/or posterior canal wall are all important details that are documented for preoperative surgical planning.

PREOPERATIVE IMAGING

We routinely order a computed tomography (CT) scan for surgical planning. In certain circumstances, such as cholesteatoma with significant tegmen erosion and a poorly defined dural plane, an MRI of the brain with gadolinium and diffusion-weighted images (DWI) is ordered to rule out a meningocele or encephalocele. Another indication for an MRI is concern for petrous apex extension. Some investigators have reported on the utility of obtaining a routine preoperative non–echo planar DWI MRI to differentiate cholesteatoma from mastoid fluid or granulation tissue to predict the feasibility of an exclusive transcanal endoscopic approach.[22]

IMAGING CONSIDERATIONS FOR ENDOSCOPIC MANAGEMENT OF CHOLESTEATOMA
Ear Canal

Although the size of the ear canal is assessed by physical examination, the CT scan supplies details on the size of the ear canal, tortuosity, possible exostosis or prominent scutum. Depending on these findings, the surgeon may anticipate drilling the canal to enlarge transcanal access or removing an exostosis before proceeding with a transcanal endoscopic approach. Tortuous or narrow ear canals may require smaller and angled endoscopes for access. In ears with pronounced exostosis, an exclusive transcanal endoscopic approach may not be feasible and the surgeon must discuss with the patient that a posterior auricular or an endaural incision may be required to remove the prominent exostosis and gain access to the middle ear.

   Blunting of the scutum is a characteristic radiologic finding consistent with attic erosion and is pathognomonic for epitympanic cholesteatoma. However, a mesotympanic cholesteatoma may not present with scutal blunting as the pars flaccida is frequently spared.

Middle Ear Involvement

A high-resolution temporal bone CT provides detailed images of middle ear anatomy. Poorly defined ossicles, ossicular erosion, and soft tissue located medial to the ossicular chain suggest that cholesteatoma has involved the ossicles or is lodged medial to the ossicular chain. In addition, the CT scan offers details on the depth and involvement of the sinus tympani, which is often the limiting factor in a transcanal microscopic approach. Shallower sinus tympani conformations are often amenable to an exclusive transcanal endoscopic approach, while a deeper sinus tympani may require a mastoidectomy with a retrofacial approach.[23] However, angled endoscopes may increase visualization and access to a deep sinus tympani.

Mastoid Involvement

It is essential to evaluate the extent of mastoid involvement, as most surgeons agree that cholesteatoma is endoscopically accessible as long as it does not extend beyond the dome of the horizontal semicircular canal. Mastoid opacification on CT imaging may represent cholesteatoma or trapped mucus from a blocked tympanic isthmus. Cholesteatoma is suspected if there is erosion of the mastoid trabeculae or other bony structures, or if the opacification has a discrete, rounded shape. However, the surgeon should be prepared for both possibilities, as the sensitivity and specificity of CT scan in detecting mastoid cholesteatoma when compared to intraoperative assessment has been reported to be as low as 65% and 87%, respectively.[24]

When cholesteatoma is present in a small, contracted mastoid, the entire mastoid may only extend a few millimeters past the horizontal semicircular canal. In such cases an exclusive transcanal atticotomy may be adequate to remove the disease (**Fig. 1**A). In other circumstances the mastoid is small, but with greater antral extension past the horizontal canal. The endoscopic approach cannot reach this space despite an extensive atticotomy and utilization of curved instruments; thus, a mastoidectomy is necessary (see **Fig 1**B).

Occasionally, cholesteatoma with involvement beyond the dome of the horizontal semicircular canal can be removed from the antrum if it possesses a well-defined sac structure. Conversely, a cholesteatoma with lesser involvement of the antrum but with a loose matrix quality may not be amenable to transcanal removal and may require a mastoidectomy.

Mastoid Pneumatization

The extent of mastoid development is an important factor in surgical planning. The degree of mastoid pneumatization is an important predictor of middle ear ventilation.[25] When a widely pneumatized mastoid is partially drilled, residual mastoid air cells

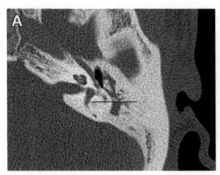 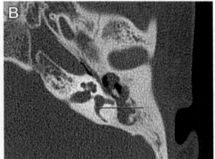

Fig. 1. CT temporal bone axial cross-sections of two left contracted mastoids with cholesteatoma. (*A*) In this case with limited mastoid extension beyond the horizontal semicircular canal, a transcanal endoscopic atticotomy was possible. (*B*) In this case with greater mastoid extension beyond the dome of the horizontal semicircular canal, a canal wall down mastoidectomy was necessary.

continue to produce nitrous gas and contribute to middle ear homeostasis. In these circumstances, it is favorable to perform a canal wall up mastoidectomy, as the mastoid is partially functional. Conversely, a small sclerotic mastoid cavity has poor gas exchange and does not significantly contribute to middle ear pressure homeostasis, especially once it has been opened and drilled. This small mastoid is more likely to self-obliterate with fibrous tissue postoperatively. We have a lower threshold to perform a canal wall down in smaller mastoids as these small drilled mastoids essentially represent a dead space without gas exchange.

Tegmen Condition and Orientation

The tegmen is evaluated for bony dehiscence or disease eroding into the tegmen. In addition, there are few intraoperative landmarks for the tegmen when performing a transcanal atticotomy. Thus, the height and thickness of the tegmen tympani must be evaluated preoperatively to prevent an iatrogenic tegmen defect.

The orientation of the tegmen plane is also assessed. If cholesteatoma extends into the antrum and the tegmen lies in a horizontal plane, the anterior aspect of the attic and aditus ad antrum are easily accessible through a mastoidectomy (**Fig. 2**A). Conversely, a low-lying or sloping tegmen obstructs transmastoid access to the attic. In this circumstance a transcanal endoscopic extended atticotomy is preferred to access the anterior epitympanic space (see **Fig. 2**B).

SURGICAL GUIDE
Prepping the Ear for Endoscopic Approach

The ear is first anesthetized by injecting local anesthetic with a diluted epinephrine solution in the cartilaginous portion of the ear canal, tragus, and posterior auricular sulcus prior to prepping. This allows the anesthetic to infiltrate in the ear canal while prepping and draping is performed. Monitored hypotension and reverse Trendelenburg positioning may help reduce bleeding. The bed is turned 180° and the screen monitor is positioned at eye level approximately 6 feet away from the surgeon. Sitting or standing while performing endoscopic ear surgery is per surgeon preference. The senior author prefers a standing position as it is ergonomically favorable with respect to the arm and shoulder girdle, avoiding neck and shoulder strain. The ear canal hair is trimmed with scissors and the canal is injected just beyond the hair-bearing skin, making sure the entire canal skin blanches and hydrodissects off the canal bone.

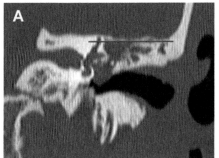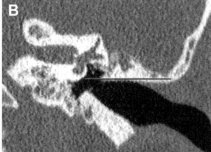

Fig. 2. CT temporal bone coronal cross-sections of 2 left ears with different tegmen conformations. (*A*) The tegmen lies in a horizontal plane allowing transmastoid access to the attic. (*B*) The tegmen is low-lying and overhanging, obstructing transmastoid access to the attic.

We always start with a transcanal endoscopic approach, even when a mastoidectomy is contemplated. This has several advantages. The initial endoscopic inspection of the tympanic membrane may reveal details about the pathophysiology of the disease that may affect the surgical approach. Additionally, starting in the middle ear not only maximizes the vasoconstrictive effects of the local anesthetic, but more importantly, allows removal of disease beginning at its origin and continuing along the pathway of spread.

Endoscopic Management of Epitympanic Cholesteatoma with Limited Attic Extension

Epitympanic cholesteatoma limited to the attic represents the ideal indication for a transcanal endoscopic approach. In epitympanic cholesteatoma, the most common pattern of disease spread is posterior and medial to the ossicular chain. Less frequently, cholesteatoma can migrate posteriorly in the attic and remain lateral to the ossicular chain. Rarely, cholesteatoma spreads toward the anterior attic without direct ossicular chain involvement. Under microscopy, the transcanal view of the attic is limited by the narrow segment of the ear canal. In contrast, endoscopes provide a wide visual field and an angled view of the posterior aspect of the attic.

The tympanomeatal incision is started anterior to the neck of the malleus to facilitate exposure of the entire attic. The flap should be 8 to 10 mm long, as significant curettage of the scutum is often necessary to gain adequate exposure and a longer tympanomeatal flap is required to cover the resultant defect (**Fig. 3**B).

It is safest to elevate the tympanic annulus in an area that is uninvolved by disease. In epitympanic cholesteatoma, this is most often the posteroinferior aspect. The sac frequently extends into the middle ear space and obscures the ossicles. Curettage

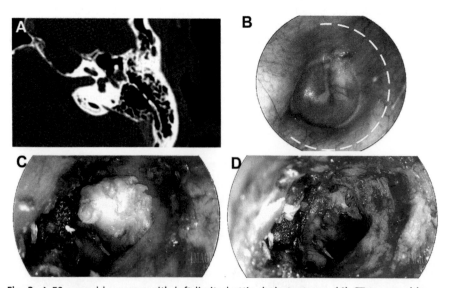

Fig. 3. A 59-year-old woman with left limited attic cholesteatoma. (*A*) CT temporal bone, axial cross-section shows the most common growth pattern of cholesteatoma, posterior and medial to the ossicular chain. (*B*) Endoscopic examination with planned incision marked by the dashed line. (*C*) Surgical exposure after curetting of the scutum to reach the lateral extent of the cholesteatoma sac. (*D*) Endoscopic inspection following removal of disease and incus.

of the posterior ear canal may facilitate identification of the lateral borders of the cholesteatoma sac as well as the bodies of the incus and malleus.

Once the middle ear is entered and the ossicular chain is identified, the surgeon must decide if the ossicular chain must be disrupted in order to eradicate the disease. We advocate removing enough of the scutum to expose the lateral edge of the cholesteatoma. This enables identification of whether the cholesteatoma lies lateral or medial to the ossicular chain.

If the cholesteatoma involves the medial aspect of the ossicular chain, it is necessary to remove the body of the incus, and depending on extension, the head of the malleus. If the malleus is transected, it is best to do so at the neck so that the manubrium remains attached to the tensor tympani tendon. This provides better stability for tympanic membrane reconstruction.

After disease removal, the posterior wall of the epitympanic space is inspected with 30-degree and 45-degree angled endoscopes. Special endoscopic instruments such as curved suctions, curved microcurettes and attic dissectors are used to remove residual squamous debris adherent to the bone. The attic defect is then reconstructed with a cartilage graft (**Fig. 4**). One of the most challenging steps of the surgery is shaping a cartilage graft to match the size of the attic defect and to lay it as a smooth surface adjacent to the tympanic membrane remnant. If the graft is too small, it will fall medially into the attic defect and allow a postoperative retraction to develop. If the graft is too large, it will obstruct visualization and postoperative monitoring of the anterior epitympanic rim. Inadequate juxtaposition of the graft with the native tympanic membrane will allow epithelium to infiltrate medial to the graft, resulting in cholesteatoma formation. It is helpful to fashion a template made of pressed Gelfoam or sterile suture metal packaging to approximate the atticotomy defect prior to shaping the cartilage graft.

Combined Endoscopic and Microscopic Management of Primary Acquired Cholesteatoma with Mastoid Extension

When cholesteatoma extends into the antrum, the crucial question is whether or not an endoscopic transcanal atticotomy is sufficient to reach the antral disease or if a mastoidectomy is required. A limited endoscopic atticotomy can be easily performed with a stapes curette. However, a wider endoscopic atticotomy requires a small diamond otologic burr or a piezoelectric drill for more expedient bone removal. The piezoelectric drill differs from a traditional otologic drill because it uses a blade that oscillates at ultrasonic frequency. Piezoelectric drilling is performed under a constant flow of saline, which reduces heat transmission. In addition, the ultrasonic frequency reduces

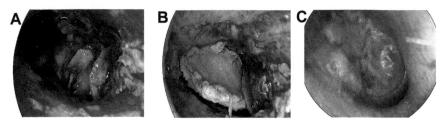

Fig. 4. Right ear cartilage graft placement after cholesteatoma resection. (*A*) Atticotomy defect and autologous incus interposed between the stapes capitulum and malleus manubrium. (*B*) The cartilage graft is sized and positioned to cover the atticotomy defect. (*C*) Well-healed attic cartilage graft.

potential for soft tissue injury. Results of revision mastoidectomy for chronic otitis media and cholesteatoma using the piezoelectric drill have reported no injury to the facial nerve, lateral sinus, or dura.[26]

If the disease is beyond the reach of a transcanal atticotomy, a mastoidectomy is performed to gain full access. Once a mastoidectomy is completed, we inspect the mastoidectomy defect with 0-degree and 30-degree endoscopes to visualize potential blind areas of disease under microscopy such as the medial surface of the skeletonized external auditory canal and the anterior and lateral attic wall.

Endoscopic Management of Mesotympanic Cholesteatoma

Whereas epitympanic cholesteatoma originates from a pars flaccida retraction, mesotympanic cholesteatoma originates from a pars tensa retraction. Tos[27] characterized mesotympanic cholesteatoma into 2 subtypes: (1) sinus cholesteatoma, which involves only the posterior mesotympanum with a normal anterior tympanic membrane (**Fig. 5**A), and (2) tensa retraction cholesteatoma which involves the entirety of the tympanic cavity. At times cholesteatoma may involve both the pars tensa and pars flaccida, making classification challenging. Rosito and colleagues[28] noted in a cohort of 356 patients that 14% of cases of cholesteatoma involved both the pars flaccida and pars tensa, and in 16% of cases no pattern of growth could be identified on otoscopy.

Of note, mesotympanic cholesteatoma occurs more frequently than epitympanic cholesteatoma in children.[28] Eustachian tube function is not fully matured in the pediatric population, predisposing them to otitis media and tympanic membrane retraction, leading to mesotympanic cholesteatoma formation.

The tympanic segment of the facial nerve, the stapes, and retrotympanic space are involved more often in mesotympanic cholesteatoma than in epitympanic

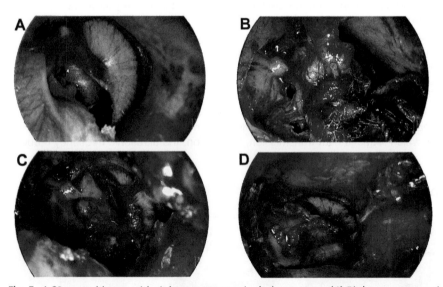

Fig. 5. A 22-year-old man with right mesotympanic cholesteatoma. (*A*) Right mesotympanic cholesteatoma with normal anterior portion of tympanic membrane. (*B*) A cottonoid pledget is used to dissect the atrophic tympanic membrane off the retrotympanic space. (*C*) After disease removal, only a small portion of the anterior tympanic membrane remains. (*D*) A cartilage graft is placed lateral to the manubrium of the malleus.

cholesteatoma.[28] These structures are difficult to reach with transcanal microscopy and often require a transmastoid facial recess approach. Endoscopy affords improved visualization which facilitates an exclusive transcanal approach.

A critical point in the approach to mesotympanic cholesteatoma is to gain wide exposure of the posterior tympanic cavity. A wide semi-circumferential incision is made to create a long tympanomeatal flap as there is often scutal erosion. To accomplish this, the incision is started anterior to the notch of Rivinus and extended 180°, taking care to preserve an 8-mm to 10-mm-wide flap. Elevation of the tympanomeatal flap may be challenging, as the tympanic membrane is often atrophic and adherent to the floor of the middle ear space. The epithelium is also often adherent to the capitulum of the stapes or the tympanic segment of the facial nerve, which may have bony dehiscence. Cottonoids soaked in epinephrine solution (1:1000) are used to dissect the flap anteriorly and away from its adhesions to the promontory (see **Fig. 5**B). Once the middle ear is opened, the anatomy may be distorted because of scutal erosion or granulation tissue in the location of the facial nerve and stapes. Elevation of the tympanomeatal flap continues inferiorly to identify the round window. This may be the only landmark when the rest of the middle ear is filled with disease.

When the incus and stapes are not readily identifiable, curetting the posterior superior aspect of the scutum can allow identification of the neck of the malleus, ensuring a safe anatomic landmark to start the middle ear dissection. If cholesteatoma occupies the retrotympanic space, there may be erosion of the posterior canal bone and pyramidal eminence, distorting the landmarks for the second genu of the facial nerve. The stapes may have partial or total erosion of its suprastructure and matrix may cover the footplate. Squamous debris extending into the sinus tympani and retrotympanic space can be removed under endoscopy with curved endoscopic instruments or attic dissectors, avoiding the need for a mastoidectomy with a posterior tympanotomy. Access to the retrotympanic space may be improved by standing on the opposite side of the patient, rotating the patient away from the operative ear, and using a 30-degree endoscope. This direct endoscopic retrotympanic approach requires experience in endoscopy to maintain orientation (**Fig. 6**).

After removing disease from the mesotympanum and retrotympanic space, often only a small portion of the anterior half of the tympanic membrane is preserved (see **Fig. 5**C). A cartilage graft is preferred for tympanic membrane reconstruction as it is stiffer and resists postoperative retraction. Placement of the underlay cartilage graft lateral to the malleus helps prevent postoperative retraction, a frequent sequela observed when placing the cartilage graft medial to the manubrium of the malleus (see **Fig. 5**D).[29]

Endoscopic Management of Mesotympanic Cholesteatoma with Infracochlear Extension

When there is extensive retrotympanic involvement, disease can extend into the petrous apex via the infracochlear and infracarotid air cell tracts (**Fig. 7**). If the preoperative CT shows indistinct opacification between the middle ear and the infracochlear air cell tract, a non–echo planar DWI MRI can differentiate cholesteatoma from effusion, cholesterol granuloma, or normal bone marrow. Microscopic access to the infracochlear region requires significant removal of the inferior rim of the external ear canal which places the mastoid segment of the facial nerve at risk of injury. Endoscopic approaches to this area may offer better visualization without significant removal of the inferior canal wall. When cholesteatoma has involved the infracochlear air cell tract, the anatomy can be significantly distorted. The round window niche may be eroded and the bony boundaries widened (**Fig. 8**). Matrix in the hypotympanic region must

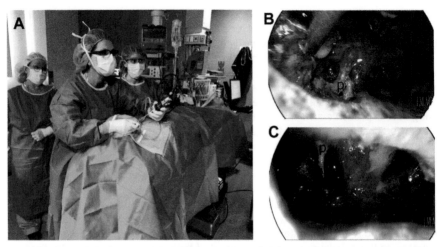

Fig. 6. Direct endoscopic retrotympanic inspection of right ear. (*A*) The surgeon stands on the opposite side of the operative ear using a 30-degree endoscope. (*B*) Right ear. Traditional endoscopic view of sinus tympani. Cholesteatoma is present along the stapedial tendon and pyramidal eminence. (*C*) Direct retrotympanic inspection of the same ear illustrates an upside-down view of the retrotympanic space after cholesteatoma removal. p, pyramidal eminence.

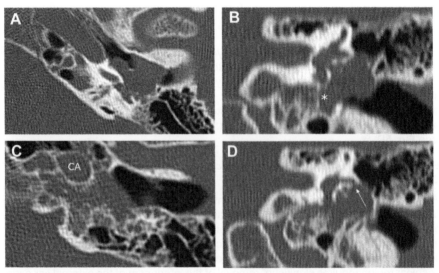

Fig. 7. CT scan of a 47-year-old man with left mesotympanic cholesteatoma. (*A*) Axial cross-section showing opacification of the entire middle ear and sinus tympani. (*B*) Coronal cross-section showing opacification extending in the infracochlear air cell tract. (*C*) Axial cross-section showing opacification in the infracarotid air cell tract. (*D*) Coronal cross-section showing possible lateral semicircular canal fistula. arrow, labyrinthine fistula; *, infracochlear air cell tract; CA, carotid artery.

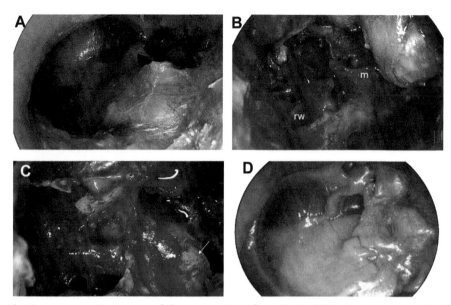

Fig. 8. Intraoperative images of the same patient from **Fig. 7**. (*A*) Endoscopic exam of left ear. (*B*) Cholesteatoma has eroded a significant portion of the posterior scutum with distorted anatomy. The malleus manubrium is the sole landmark to help with orientation. The round window anatomy is distorted due to niche erosion and enlargement of the bony boundaries. (*C*) After cholesteatoma removal, there is a blue lining of the dome of the horizontal semicircular canal. (*D*) Postoperative examination at 6 months. m, malleus manubrium; rw, round window; arrow, blue lining of horizontal semicircular canal.

be carefully lifted and structures palpated to assess for bony dehiscence over the jugular bulb and carotid region (**Fig. 9**).

Endoscopic Management of Cholesteatoma with Labyrinthine Fistula

Perilymphatic fistulas due to invasion by cholesteatoma is not an uncommon occurrence. Labyrinthine fistulas are classified according to degree of erosion. In type I,

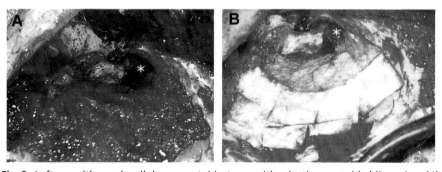

Fig. 9. Left ear with canal wall down mastoidectomy with selective mastoid obliteration. (*A*) The mastoid defect is obliterated with DBX and bone pate. (*B*) The mastoid cavity is lined with Biodesign graft as there was insufficient temporalis fascia to line the defect secondary to multiple prior surgeries. *, exteriorized attic.

the perilymphatic membrane is still covered with bone (blue lining); type II occurs when the perilymphatic membrane is exposed; and type III occurs when cholesteatoma has eroded the perilymphatic membrane or invaded into the labyrinth.[30] The estimated incidence of labyrinthine fistula is 6% to 8% in all cholesteatoma cases, with 90% or more occurring at the lateral semicircular canal.[31,32] Portier and colleagues[31] further reported a 9% incidence of a second fistula identified intraoperatively. Schmidt Rosito and colleagues[33] identified 9 labyrinthine fistulas in their cohort of 333 patients with cholesteatoma, all of which were in the setting of a posterior epitympanic cholesteatoma.

The surgical management of labyrinthine fistulas depends on several factors, including size and depth of the fistula, location, hearing status of the operative and contralateral ear, as well as the surgeon's level of comfort. A fistula can be managed conservatively by leaving cholesteatoma matrix over the fistula and performing a canal wall down mastoidectomy to exteriorize the disease. However, this approach leaves the patient with persistent symptoms as the labyrinthine fistula is not repaired but simply exteriorized into a large mastoid cavity.

More advanced techniques include complete removal of cholesteatoma matrix from perilymphatic fistulas while preserving labyrinthine function and enabling a canal wall up approach.[34] Removal of cholesteatoma matrix from the fistula is performed by carefully lifting the matrix and avoiding direct suction over the fistula. Continuous irrigation allows removal of the debris without using suction; however, the irrigation stream may obscure the field of view. Yamauchi and colleagues[35] described underwater endoscopic repair of labyrinthine fistulas. The mastoid is filled with saline and the endoscope is submerged to perform the repair, thus avoiding the refractive effects of the traditional stream of irrigation. Once the matrix is completely removed, the fistula can be repaired with temporalis fascia, perichondrium, and bone pate.

Indications for Canal Wall Down Mastoidectomy

The utilization of endoscopy as an adjunct tool in cases of cholesteatoma with mastoid involvement can facilitate the choice of a canal wall up mastoidectomy.[16] However, there are still circumstances when a canal wall down mastoidectomy is unavoidable. A canal wall down mastoidectomy is often performed to eradicate recidivistic disease after multiple canal wall up procedures have failed. There are however, situations in which a canal wall down mastoidectomy is discussed with the patient at the time of primary surgery for cholesteatoma.

Indications for a primary canal wall down mastoidectomy in the contemporary era of endoscopic ear surgery can be divided into patient characteristics, disease extent, and anatomic factors. Patient characteristics include patients with multiple comorbidities who are poor candidates for multiple ear surgeries or if the cholesteatoma is present in the patient's only hearing ear. A single, canal wall down procedure may also be optimal if there is concern for follow-up.

Disease-related indications for a canal wall down mastoidectomy can be further divided by disease extent and patient anatomy. Cholesteatoma with more than 50% bony erosion of the posterior canal wall, extensive labyrinthine fistula, or presence of a large tegmen defect with dural attachment to cholesteatoma is an indication for a canal wall down mastoidectomy. The surgeon should also take into consideration their own experience, comfort level and likelihood of completely eradicating disease.

Anatomic factors that may require canal wall down mastoidectomy as a primary surgery include cholesteatoma in a small mastoid with a low-lying tegmen. When the tegmen is low-lying, it may obstruct visualization of the anterior epitympanum via the microscopic transmastoid route. This frequently leads to the decision to take the canal wall down to achieve an unobstructed view of the attic. In selected cases of cholesteatoma present in a small mastoid antrum and a low-lying tegmen, it is possible to perform an exclusive endoscopic transcanal retrograde inside-out mastoidectomy. This is achieved by extending the transcanal atticotomy to fully expose the mastoid antrum. In this case, a small meatoplasty may be sufficient to access the small mastoid cavity, which will require less maintenance than a traditional large mastoid cavity.

However, if a low-lying tegmen is associated with a prominent anterior canal wall, even endoscopic techniques are challenging. In this situation the prominence of the anterior canal wall precludes a satisfactory transcanal approach to the attic. In addition, when there is a prominent canal wall, reconstructive efforts to cover the attic defect with a cartilage graft may fail. The acute angle between the anterior canal wall and the anterior tympanic rim impedes good control of graft placement. Epithelium can grow under the graft at the junction between the anterior tympanic rim and the graft. In this situation a canal wall down mastoidectomy with the attic space left exteriorized and lined by fascia is a safer option for long-term disease control.

Innovations in Mastoid Obliteration Techniques

When cholesteatoma has extended in a widely pneumatized mastoid and a canal wall down mastoidectomy is performed, patients are left with a large mastoid cavity that requires long-term maintenance. One option to reduce the cavity size and minimize postoperative chronic granulations is to selectively obliterate the mastoid cavity.

Techniques for selective mastoid obliteration differ from the traditional tympanomastoid obliteration of a radical cavity, in which the entire mastoid and middle ear space, voided of ossicles, are obliterated with a large pedicled Palva flap and the canal oversewn.[36] Recently, mastoid obliteration techniques have been applied to both canal wall down mastoidectomy and canal wall up mastoidectomy with the goal of selectively obliterating the mastoid while preserving the middle ear space. Obliteration of the mastoid alone creates a small mastoid cavity that is, more manageable in terms of cleaning and debridement. In addition, a smaller mastoid cavity requires a smaller meatoplasty, avoiding the cosmetic disfigurement of a large meatoplasty. When the mastoid is selectively obliterated in a canal wall up mastoidectomy, the purpose of obliteration is to occlude the dead space and prevent cholesteatoma formation.

A recent systematic review of patients who underwent mastoid obliteration with canal wall up and canal wall down mastoidectomy found better rates of residual and recurrent cholesteatoma than the published rates for those who did not undergo obliteration. Overall rates of recurrent and residual disease were low, at 4.6% and 5.4%, respectively.[37] If the decision is made to obliterate the cavity, there are several commercially available materials. Demineralized Bone Matrix (DBX; DePuy Synthes, West Chester, PA) combined with bone dust collected during drilling has been used with stable long-term results.[38] Other materials include bioactive glass polymers,[39] titanium micromesh, hydroxyapatite, and silicone.[40] When performing mastoid obliteration techniques, postoperative monitoring with a non–echo planar DWI MRI is required to rule out occult cholesteatoma within the obliteration. A modified technique for mastoid obliteration is a partial obliteration with the epitympanum left exteriorized and lined by fascia. In this case the area at most risk for residual disease is left exposed and exteriorized.

MRI AS AN ALTERNATIVE TO SECOND-LOOK SURGERY FOR POSTOPERATIVE SURVEILLANCE

The paradigm of a second-look surgery following cholesteatoma removal has shifted with the advent of non–echo-planar DWI MRI, which was first described in identifying cholesteatoma in 2006.[41] Multiple systematic reviews comparing non–echo planar DWI MRI to intraoperative identification of cholesteatoma have reported sensitivity and specificity over 90%.[42,43] The decision to select non–echo planar DWI MRI versus a second-look surgery depends on patient factors, extent of cholesteatoma, and surgeon confidence in the resection of the cholesteatoma. MRI is appropriate for surveillance in adults with low risk of residual or recurrent disease. A second-look surgery is preferred in children, as cholesteatoma tends to be more aggressive. In addition, MRIs may require sedation for the child to participate.[42] A second-look surgery may also be preferable if there is concern for patient compliance with long-term surveillance. Finally, the surgeon must keep in consideration that MRI does not routinely detect cholesteatoma less than 3 mm in size.

Our practice has shifted from a routine second-look surgery in all cholesteatoma cases to a more tailored protocol specific for each case. In general, in cases with low concern for residual disease, a non–echo planar DWI MRI is ordered 12 to 18 months following primary surgery. In cases with increased concern for residual disease a second-look surgery is scheduled 9 to 12 months after the primary surgery.

OUTCOMES

Outcome data regarding endoscopic approaches to surgery, while limited, are promising. The endoscopic approach to cholesteatoma removal has at least equivalent outcomes with regard to residual and recurrent disease, similar rates of postoperative complications, and decreased pain and shorter healing time compared to microscopic surgery.[44–46] Hearing outcomes are also comparable. Further investigation is needed to compare operative time as well as long-term outcomes.

A primary concern following cholesteatoma resection is recidivism, which includes residual and recurrent disease. These rates are widely variable in traditional microscope otologic surgeries, with meta-analysis data reporting recurrence rates of cholesteatoma of 9% to 70% following a canal wall up procedure and lower rates of 5% to 17% after a canal wall down procedure.[47] Endoscopic ear surgery has demonstrated noninferior outcomes with regards to residual and recurrent disease rates. Presutti and colleagues[16] reported in their meta-analysis that 6.2% of patients had residual disease and 3.1% of patients had recurrence after endoscopic middle ear surgery for cholesteatoma; however, this was limited by a small number of studies and short mean follow-up period (23.4 months). Subsequent studies that compared endoscopic surgery to a microscopic control group for cholesteatoma showed equivalent rates of residual and recurrent disease, of up to 17% and 20%, respectively.[44,45] Long-term data regarding outcomes and need for revision surgery for other indications, such as perforation or graft failure, are future areas of investigation.

Differences in operative time are widely variable. One randomized controlled trial reported a mean decrease in operating time of 20 minutes with endoscopic approaches for limited attic cholesteatoma compared with microscopic approaches.[46] Other studies reported equivalent or increased time for endoscopic approaches, but with a decrease in operative time with experience.[44,45] Acute postoperative complications are rare and do not differ significantly between those undergoing microscopic versus endoscopic ear surgery. Most studies do not report facial nerve injury following either approach[17,44,46]; Killeen and colleagues[45] reported one patient with a facial nerve palsy following endoscopic ear surgery that resolved during follow-up. Incidence of dizziness and dysgeusia following surgery did not differ by surgical approach.[44] Of note, endoscopic ear surgery appears to offer a distinct benefit in decreased pain and recovery time.[18,44]

Studies comparing endoscopic surgery with a microscopic surgery control group have not shown significant differences in hearing outcomes as measured by changes in air-bone gap closure, air conduction thresholds, median pure tone averages, and word recognition scores.[44–46]

SUMMARY

Endoscopic ear surgery is increasingly accepted as a primary modality for cholesteatoma surgery. One of its major advantages is the superior visualization of the attic and sinus tympani, the 2 sites at highest risk for residual disease in cholesteatoma surgery. Transcanal endoscopic ear surgery is particularly suited for management of limited epitympanic and mesotympanic cholesteatoma. When cholesteatoma extends in the mastoid beyond the dome of the horizontal semicircular canal, a combined approach with mastoidectomy is often necessary. Even with endoscopic assistance, certain anatomic constraints such as a low-lying tegmen associated with a prominent anterior canal wall may preclude full access to the anterior attic and complete disease removal, necessitating a canal wall down mastoidectomy. When a canal wall down mastoidectomy is necessary, partial mastoid obliteration techniques allow a selective obliteration of the mastoid cavity with preservation of the middle ear space. This has reduced the long-term sequelae of large mastoid cavities. Data comparing outcomes in endoscopic ear surgery show at least equivalent outcomes compared to microscopic ear surgery in rates of residual and recurrent disease, and are associated with decreased postoperative morbidity and shorter recovery times.

DISCLOSURE

The authors have nothing to disclose.

REFERENCES

1. Marchioni D, Alicandri-Ciufelli M, Piccinini A, et al. Inferior retrotympanum revisited: an endoscopic anatomic study. Laryngoscope 2010;120(9):1880–6.
2. Kemppainen HO, Puhakka HJ, Laippala PJ, et al. Epidemiology and aetiology of middle ear cholesteatoma. Acta Otolaryngol 1999;119(5):568–72.
3. Tos M. Incidence, etiology and pathogenesis of cholesteatoma in children. Adv Otorhinolaryngol 1988;40:110–7.
4. Harker L. Cholesteatoma - an incidence study. In: McCabe BF, Sade J, Abramson M, editors. First International Conference on Cholesteatoma. Birmingham: Aesculapius Publishing Co; 1977. p. 308–12.
5. Tos M. A new pathogenesis of mesotympanic (congenital) cholesteatoma. Laryngoscope 2000;110(11):1890–7.
6. Semaan MT, Megerian CA. The pathophysiology of cholesteatoma. Otolaryngol Clin North Am 2006;39(6):1143–59.
7. Jackler RK, Santa Maria PL, Varsak YK, et al. A new theory on the pathogenesis of acquired cholesteatoma: mucosal traction. Laryngoscope 2015;125(Suppl 4): S1–14.
8. Marchioni D, Alicandri-Ciufelli M, Molteni G, et al. Selective epitympanic dysventilation syndrome. Laryngoscope 2010;120(5):1028–33.

9. Dornelles CeC, da Costa SS, Meurer L, et al. Comparison of acquired cholesteatoma between pediatric and adult patients. Eur Arch Otorhinolaryngol 2009; 266(10):1553–61.

10. Dornhoffer JL, Friedman AB, Gluth MB. Management of acquired cholesteatoma in the pediatric population. Curr Opin Otolaryngol Head Neck Surg 2013;21(5): 440–5.

11. Morita Y, Yamamoto Y, Oshima S, et al. Pediatric middle ear cholesteatoma: the comparative study of congenital cholesteatoma and acquired cholesteatoma. Eur Arch Otorhinolaryngol 2016;273(5):1155–60.

12. Ghadersohi S, Carter JM, Hoff SR. Endoscopic transcanal approach to the middle ear for management of pediatric cholesteatoma. Laryngoscope 2017; 127(11):2653–8.

13. Glasscock ME, Dickins JR, Wiet R. Cholesteatoma in children. Laryngoscope 1981;91(10):1743–53.

14. Palva A, Karma P, Kärjä J. Cholesteatoma in children. Arch Otolaryngol 1977; 103(2):74–7.

15. Hildmann H, Sudhoff H. Cholesteatoma in children. Int J Pediatr Otorhinolaryngol 1999;49(Suppl 1):S81–6.

16. Presutti L, Gioacchini FM, Alicandri-Ciufelli M, et al. Results of endoscopic middle ear surgery for cholesteatoma treatment: a systematic review. Acta Otorhinolaryngol Ital 2014;34(3):153–7.

17. Tarabichi M. Transcanal endoscopic management of cholesteatoma. Otol Neurotol 2010;31(4):580–8.

18. Plodpai Y. Endoscopic vs microscopic overlay tympanoplasty for correcting large tympanic membrane perforations: a randomized clinical trial. Otolaryngol Head Neck Surg 2018;159(5):879–86.

19. Tseng CC, Lai MT, Wu CC, et al. Comparison of the efficacy of endoscopic tympanoplasty and microscopic tympanoplasty: a systematic review and meta-analysis. Laryngoscope 2017;127(8):1890–6.

20. Hulka GF, McElveen JT. A randomized, blinded study of canal wall up versus canal wall down mastoidectomy determining the differences in viewing middle ear anatomy and pathology. Am J Otol 1998;19(5):574–8.

21. Palva T. Surgical treatment of chronic middle ear disease. II. Canal wall up and canal wall down procedures. Acta Otolaryngol 1987;104(5–6):487–94.

22. Migirov L, Wolf M, Greenberg G, et al. Non-EPI DW MRI in planning the surgical approach to primary and recurrent cholesteatoma. Otol Neurotol 2014;35(1): 121–5.

23. Marchioni D, Valerini S, Mattioli F, et al. Radiological assessment of the sinus tympani: temporal bone HRCT analyses and surgically related findings. Surg Radiol Anat 2015;37(4):385–92.

24. Gerami H, Naghavi E, Wahabi-Moghadam M, et al. Comparison of preoperative computerized tomography scan imaging of temporal bone with the intraoperative findings in patients undergoing mastoidectomy. Saudi Med J 2009; 30(1):104–8.

25. Sadé J, Fuchs C. Secretory otitis media in adults: II. The role of mastoid pneumatization as a prognostic factor. Ann Otol Rhinol Laryngol 1997;106(1):37–40.

26. Salami A, Mora R, Dellepiane M, et al. Results of revision mastoidectomy with Piezosurgery(®). Acta Otolaryngol 2010;130(10):1119–24.

27. Tos M. Upon the relationship between secretory otitis in childhood and chronic otitis and its sequelae in adults. J Laryngol Otol 1981;95(10):1011–22.

28. Rosito LS, Netto LF, Teixeira AR, et al. Classification of cholesteatoma according to growth patterns. JAMA Otolaryngol Head Neck Surg 2016;142(2):168–72.
29. Yawn RJ, Carlson ML, Haynes DS, et al. Lateral-to-malleus underlay tympanoplasty: surgical technique and outcomes. Otol Neurotol 2014;35(10):1809–12.
30. Dornhoffer JL, Milewski C. Management of the open labyrinth. Otolaryngol Head Neck Surg 1995;112(3):410–4.
31. Portier F, Lescanne E, Racy E, et al. Studies of labyrinthine cholesteatoma-related fistulas: report of 22 cases. J Otolaryngol 2005;34(1):1–6.
32. Soda-Merhy A, Betancourt-Suárez MA. Surgical treatment of labyrinthine fistula caused by cholesteatoma. Otolaryngol Head Neck Surg 2000;122(5):739–42.
33. Rosito LPS, Canali I, Teixeira A, et al. Cholesteatoma labyrinthine fistula: prevalence and impact. Braz J Otorhinolaryngol 2019;85(2):222–7.
34. Quaranta N, Liuzzi C, Zizzi S, et al. Surgical treatment of labyrinthine fistula in cholesteatoma surgery. Otolaryngol Head Neck Surg 2009;140(3):406–11.
35. Yamauchi D, Yamazaki M, Ohta J, et al. Closure technique for labyrinthine fistula by "underwater" endoscopic ear surgery. Laryngoscope 2014;124(11):2616–8.
36. Saunders JE, Shoemaker DL, McElveen JT. Reconstruction of the radical mastoid. Am J Otol 1992;13(5):465–9.
37. van der Toom HFE, van der Schroeff MP, Pauw RJ. Single-stage mastoid obliteration in cholesteatoma surgery and recurrent and residual disease rates: a systematic review. JAMA Otolaryngol Head Neck Surg 2018;144(5):440–6.
38. Leatherman BD, Dornhoffer JL. The use of demineralized bone matrix for mastoid cavity obliteration. Otol Neurotol 2004;25(1):22–5, discussion 25–26.
39. Bernardeschi D, Pyatigorskaya N, Russo FY, et al. Anatomical, functional and quality-of-life results for mastoid and epitympanic obliteration with bioactive glass s53p4: a prospective clinical study. Clin Otolaryngol 2017;42(2):387–96.
40. Skoulakis C, Koltsidopoulos P, Iyer A, et al. Mastoid obliteration with synthetic materials: a review of the literature. J Int Adv Otol 2019;15(3):400–4.
41. Dubrulle F, Souillard R, Chechin D, et al. Diffusion-weighted MR imaging sequence in the detection of postoperative recurrent cholesteatoma. Radiology 2006;238(2):604–10.
42. Lingam RK, Bassett P. A meta-analysis on the diagnostic performance of non-echoplanar diffusion-weighted imaging in detecting middle ear cholesteatoma: 10 years on. Otol Neurotol 2017;38(4):521–8.
43. Li PM, Linos E, Gurgel RK, et al. Evaluating the utility of non-echo-planar diffusion-weighted imaging in the preoperative evaluation of cholesteatoma: a meta-analysis. Laryngoscope 2013;123(5):1247–50.
44. Magliulo G, Iannella G. Endoscopic versus microscopic approach in attic cholesteatoma surgery. Am J Otol 2018;39(1):25–30.
45. Killeen DE, Tolisano AM, Kou YF, et al. Recidivism after endoscopic treatment of cholesteatoma. Otol Neurotol 2019;40(10):1313–21.
46. Das A, Mitra S, Ghosh D, et al. Endoscopic versus microscopic management of attic cholesteatoma: a randomized controlled trial. Laryngoscope 2020;130(10): 2461–6.
47. Tomlin J, Chang D, McCutcheon B, et al. Surgical technique and recurrence in cholesteatoma: a meta-analysis. Audiol Neurootol 2013;18(3):135–42.

Endoscopic Stapes Surgery
Pearls and Pitfalls

Kristen L. Yancey, MD[a],*, Nauman F. Manzoor, MD[b],
Alejandro Rivas, MD[b]

KEYWORDS

- Endoscopic ear surgery • Surgical techniques • Stapedotomy • Middle ear disease

KEY POINTS

- Although an investment in time is required to master transcanal endoscopic stapes surgery, this approach offers an expanded view of the middle ear, as it allows visualization beyond the shaft of surgical instruments and increased illumination.
- Evidence suggests endoscopic techniques result in similar audiologic outcomes as traditional microscopic stapes surgery.
- Establishing a relatively bloodless field is key. Strategies to optimize intraoperative visibility include instrument and camera choice, anesthetic and hemodynamic considerations, and patient positioning.

 Videos on the endoscopic stapes surgery cases described in this article can be found at http://www.ototheclinics.com/.

INTRODUCTION

The first reported stapes surgery is often credited to Johannes Kessel in 1876 and the first stapes mobilization for otosclerosis to Samuel Rosen in 1953.[1] Further advances include the incorporation of the laser in stapedotomy by Rodney Perkins in 1978 and the use of endoscopic approaches.[2] Endoscopic techniques for visualization of the middle ear was initially described in 1967 by Mer and colleagues, and the use of transcanal endoscopic ear surgery (TEES) has since expanded to a wider range of otologic applications including tympanoplasty, excision of cholesteatomas, and other middle ear lesions, as well as ossiculoplasty and stapes surgery.[3–8]

[a] Department of Otolaryngology–Head and Neck Surgery, The Bill Wilkerson Center for Otolaryngology & Communication Sciences, 7209 Medical Center East South Tower, 1215 21st Avenue South, Nashville, TN 37232-8605, USA; [b] Department of Otolaryngology–Head and Neck Surgery, University Hospitals, ENT Institute, Case Western Reserve University, 11100 Euclid Avenue, Stop Mail: LKSD 5045, Cleveland, OH 44106, USA
* Corresponding author.
E-mail address: kristen.yancey@vumc.org
Twitter: @KLYancey (K.L.Y.)

Otolaryngol Clin N Am 54 (2021) 147–162
https://doi.org/10.1016/j.otc.2020.09.015
0030-6665/21/© 2020 Elsevier Inc. All rights reserved.
oto.theclinics.com

The main advantages of TEES include increased visibility of the operative field and its minimally invasive approach. Enhanced visibility is especially advantageous in the setting of patients with abnormal middle ear anatomy, whether from prior surgeries, congenital anomalies, or other pathology. Proponents of endoscopic techniques also cite a lower incidence of complications from chorda tympani manipulation and injury.[9–13] Drawbacks include the learning curve, single-handed operative techniques, loss of stereopsis, and the potential risk for thermal injury.[14,15] Specifically during endoscopic stapes surgery, the lack of depth perception can make the maneuvers centered on the stapedial footplate (ie, creation of a fenestra) more challenging, especially in the setting of deep oval window niches.[9]

Outcomes in Endoscopic Stapes Surgery

Literature to date supports endoscopic approaches as safe and effective in the management of stapes fixation[16] (**Table 1**). Surgical success in stapes surgery is often defined as air-bone gap closure to within 10 dB.[17] With TEES, reported rates of air-bone gap (ABG) closure less than or equal to 10 dB range between 56% and 88% of patients,[18,19] with pooled analysis rates ranging between 72% and 77%.[16,20] Furthermore, audiologic outcomes are comparable to the microscopic approach, with recent systematic reviews reporting no significant difference between the two techniques.[11,20,21]

Regarding complications, published data indicate endoscopic stapes surgery has a comparable risk profile as microscopic techniques, with similar rates of tympanic membrane perforation,[21,22] dizziness,[11,21,23–25] and facial nerve dysfunction.[22] Facial nerve injuries are rare, with temporary nerve palsies occurring in 0.95% (N = 3) in a pooled analysis of 314 patients undergoing endoscopic stapes surgery.[16] Of note, 2 of these cases were attributed to local anesthetic. Postoperative sensorineural hearing loss (SNHL) is also rare following stapes surgery. Hall and colleagues performed a pooled analysis of 313 endoscopic stapes cases, identifying 2 patients (0.6%) who developed moderate SNHL (bone conduction pure tone averages of 43- and 46-dB HL) in a single series, but no severe cases or cophosis have been reported.[16]

In contrast, recent systematic reviews have found chorda tympani nerve injury is up to 3 times more likely in microscopic stapes surgery.[11,21,22] Similarly, reported rates of dysgeusia are lower with TEES (5.9% vs 16.9%), representing an approximately 69% lower chance of incurring postoperative taste disturbance (odds ratio = 0.31, 95% confidence interval 0.14, 0.69).[20]

Few studies have directly compared mean operating times between endoscopic and microscopic approaches, and there is no consensus regarding superiority of a given approach. Koukkoullis and colleagues and Manna and colleagues did not find a significant difference in their recent meta-analyses.[11,21] However, the limited number of existing studies precludes drawing definitive conclusions. Not surprisingly, operating time is influenced by surgeon experience. Iannella and Magliulo found endoscopic stapes surgery initially took longer than microscope approaches. However, this difference disappeared by the last third of their year-long study as surgeons gained more experience.

EQUIPMENT AND INSTRUMENTS

Success in endoscopic stapes surgery is supported by having access to the appropriate equipment and instruments (**Box 1**). For the novice TEES surgeon, this includes a draped microscope should significant bleeding occur or if the surgeon needs to verify the footplate depth with the microscope's binocular view. With the exception

Table 1
Review of published outcomes on endoscopic stapes surgery. Ranges and standard deviations are provided when available

Author, Year	Country	Endoscopic Procedure (Footplate Management)	N	Mean Follow-up (Months)	ABG (%) <10 dB	ABG (%) <20 dB	Mean ABG Improvement (dB)	Chorda Tympani Preservation	Chorda Tympani Dysgeusia	Mean Operative Time (min)
Tarabichi,[5] 1999	UAB	Stapedectomy (NR)	13	NR	86	NR	NR	NR	NR	NR
Poe,[56] 2000	USA	Stapedioplasty (L)	5	≥6	NR	NR	NR	100%	NR	NR
Nogueira et al,[12] 2011	Brazil	Stapedotomy (P)	15	1	NR	NR	NR	100% (manipulated in 20%)	7%	NR
Migirov & Wolf,[57] 2013	Israel	Stapedotomy (D)	8	≥6 (6–11)	75	100	NR	100%	NR	NR
Sarkar et al,[58] 2013	India	Stapedotomy (P)	30	3	56	100	NR	NR	NR	NR
Kojima et al,[24] 2014	Japan	Stapedotomy (P)	15	8.6	87	93	17.9 ± 9.06	100%	0%	53[a]
Naik & Nemade,[18] 2015	India	Stapedotomy (P)	20	1.5	55	85	NR	100% (manipulated in 25%)	0%	31 (20–48)
Özdek et al,[59] 2016	Turkey	Stapedotomy (L)	29	13 (4–27)	79	93	NR	NR	NR	NR
Daneshi & Jahandideh,[25] 2016	Iran	Stapedotomy (P)	19	7.4 (1–15)	58	95	NR	100%	NR	31.8[b]
Hunter et al,[60] 2016	USA, Columbia, Brazil	Stapedectomy, stapedotomy (D, L)	51	13.4 (0.8–57.4)	NR	90	NR	88%	10%	77.4 (35–170)

(continued on next page)

Table 1
(continued)

Author, Year	Country	Endoscopic Procedure (Footplate Management)	N	Mean Follow-up (Months)	ABG (%)		Mean ABG Improvement (dB)	Chorda Tympani		Mean Operative Time (min)
					<10 dB	<20 dB		Preservation	Dysgeusia	
Iannella & Magliulo,[23] 2016	Italy	Stapedotomy (P)	20	10.3 (6–15)	85	95[a]	NR	100% (manipulated in 85%)	20%[a] (transient)	45[c]
Marchioni et al,[44] 2016	Italy	Stapedectomy (83%, NR), stapedotomy (17%, NR)	6	NR	83	100	28.5 ± 18.2	NR	NR	NR
Surmelioglu et al,[61] 2017	Turkey	Stapedotomy (D)	22	15.8 (12–28)	NR	NR	27.6 ± 8.7[b]	NR	5%	65.1[b]
Sproat et al,[62] 2017	Scotland	Stapedotomy (D)	34	5 (1–26)	79[a]	100[a]	21 ± 10[b]	94%	6%	NR
Harikumar & Kumar,[63] 2017	India	Stapedotomy (P)	30	NR	57	90	NR	100% (manipulated in 7%)	0%	54.1[a]
Moneir et al,[64] 2018	Egypt	Stapedotomy (P)	14	4.5 (1–8.5)	71	93	22.5	NR	7%	39.1[b]
Kuo & Wu,[19] 2018	Taiwan	Stapedotomy (L)	14	NR	88	100	22.0[a]	100%	0%	107 (40–160)[c]
Nassiri et al,[65] 2018	USA	Stapedectomy (52%; L), stapedotomy (48%; D, L)	81	Median 5.3 (1.2–50.4)	84	100	NR	93%	8%	Median 86 (43–151)
Bianconi et al,[66] 2020	Italy	Stapedotomy (D)	150	≥6	78	93	20 ± 22	99%	1%	34 (18–76)

Abbreviations: ABG, air-bone gap; D, drill; L, laser; NR, not reported; P, perforator.
[a] Indicates outcomes were not significantly different from microscopic stapes surgery. Statistical significance was set at $P<.05$.
[b] Outcomes were better in the patients undergoing endoscopic stapes surgery compared with a microscopic approach ($P<.05$).
[c] Outcomes were superior for the microscopic group ($P<.05$).
Data from Refs[5,12,18,19,23,24,44,56–65]

Box 1
Basic equipment required for endoscopic stapes surgery

- High-definition, 3CCD camera
- High-definition monitor
- Rigid endoscopes: 0°, 30°, 45°; 14 cm long, 3 mm in diameter
- Standard otologic instrument set that includes a measuring rod
- Suction elevator
- Laser, micro drill, or hand drill

---

of a micro-ear suction elevator, a standard set of otologic instruments is sufficient for stapes surgery and most TEES procedures. A 3-chip (3CCD) camera is preferred to avoid the red-dominant hue associated with single-CCD cameras that can skew the optics within the narrow confines of the middle ear cavity.

Although acknowledging endoscope selection is subject to individual surgeon preference, the senior author recommends the 3-mm diameter, 14-cm long endoscopes as balancing an optimal working length with maneuverability within the ear canal. Image stabilization and operator fatigue can be compromised with longer working lengths, and instrument crowding can occur with shorter scope lengths. In addition, greater temperature elevations have been associated with larger diameter scopes and xenon light sources.[26] Dundar and colleagues measured oval window temperature changes during endoscopic stapedectomy in a Guinea pig model and found the least temperature change was associated with a 3-mm endoscope and LED light source.[27] The senior author also prefers to keep the light intensity less than or equal to 40 to help mitigate the risk for thermal injury (**Box 2**). The 0° and 30° scopes are most often used, with rare need for the 45° scope. Larger angulations have not been found to aid visualization and may inadvertently pose risk to the ossicular chain or tympanic membrane from the disoriented view.

PERIOPERATIVE CONSIDERATIONS AND SURGICAL TECHNIQUE

Although the procedural steps are essentially the same in endoscopic stapes surgery as the traditional microscopic approach, the surgeon should be aware of particular nuances specific to TEES. Optimizing visualization by minimizing blood in the operative field is crucial to support the one-handed surgeon's ability to efficiently progress through the case without having to continually pause and suction. Total intravenous anesthesia (TIVA) is a useful mechanism for decreasing intraoperative blood loss and improve visualization, as it produces comparatively less vasodilation than inhalational agents.[28,29]

Box 2
Strategies to mitigate risk of potential thermal injury

- LED light source and light intensity $\leq$ 40
- Smaller diameter endoscopes
- Limiting the middle ear to prolonged, uninterrupted endoscope exposure
- Frequent suctioning
- Intermittent irrigation

After induction with TIVA, the patient is positioned into a modified "beach chair" (**Fig. 1**B). The back of the bed is raised between 15° and 30° to increase venous return, and the head is extended to improve exposure of the stapes footplate and oval window. Two-channel, bipolar facial nerve electrodes are placed into the orbicularis oris and oculi muscles for continuous electromyography monitoring. Local anesthesia (1% lidocaine 1:100,000 epinephrine) is injected into the tragus. The patient is then prepped and draped in the usual fashion. An example room and Mayo instrument set-up is shown in **Figs. 1A and 2**.

Using a zero-degree endoscope, standard, 4-quadrant canal injections are made just lateral to the osseocartilaginous junction with approximately 1 mL of 2% lidocaine 1:50,000 epinephrine. A cotton ball soaked in 1:1000 epinephrine is placed into the external auditory canal (EAC) for additional vasoconstriction, and the canal hair is trimmed to further aid visibility in preventing smearing of the scope lens. Standard stapes tympanomeatal flap incisions are made at 6 and 12 o'clock, connected with a

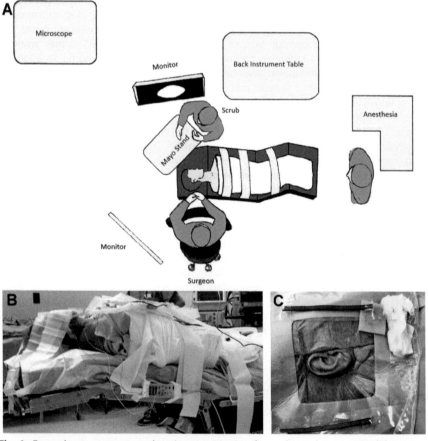

Fig. 1. Example room set-up and patient positioning for endoscopic ear cases. (*A*) Perspective shown from above. (*B*) Patient positioning for standard endoscopic middle ear procedures. The back of the bed is raised between 15° and 30° to increase venous return. Head extension also improves exposure of the stapes footplate and oval window. (*C*) Ear is draped with placement of defogging pad and wet sponge to facilitate efficient cleaning of scope.

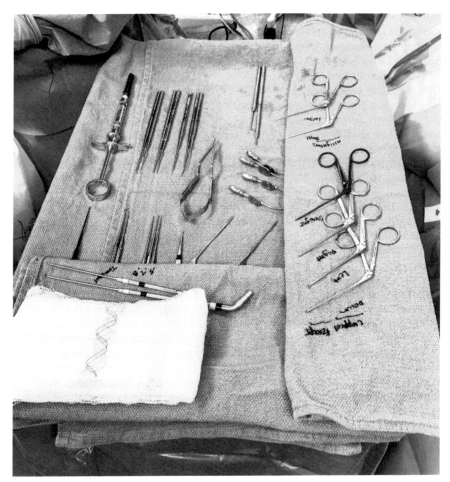

Fig. 2. Example layout for Mayo stand with various microear instruments. The senior author prefers to use dental carpules for canal injections to guarantee correct dosing of local anesthetic and the ease of administering injection under controlled pressure.

lateral incision parallel to and 5 to 8 mm from the annulus (Video 1). In cases where substantial scutum removal is anticipated, a wider flap is designed in order to accommodate redraping at closing.

The tympanomeatal flap is raised down to the annulus and elevated from the annular sulcus. A cotton ball or pledget soaked in 1:1000 epinephrine is used to provide hemostasis and can aid in flap elevation along with a suction elevator. The middle ear is entered preferentially along the posteroinferior annulus to facilitate identification of the chorda tympani nerve and thereby avoid traction injury or avulsion. The ear drum is then reflected anteriorly to the level of the malleus neck and lateral process.

Although excellent visualization of the oval window niche is generally feasible without scutum removal, an ear curette is used to partially take down its posterior aspect to allow sufficient access for the endoscope and instruments (**Fig. 3**). To gain stability during curetting, the anterior EAC can serve as a fulcrum for the instrument shaft to help direct the vector of force inferiorly and laterally. The lateral chain and stapes are then palpated to identify the location and degree of fixation. If stapes pathology is not encountered, and instead ossicular fixation is due to lateral chain pathology such as a fixed and immobile anterior malleolar ligament, the tympanomeatal flap should be elevated further anteriorly, beyond the malleus (**Fig. 4**). If necessary, malleus or incus fixation can be addressed endoscopically with a limited atticotomy and malleostapedotomy (**Fig. 5**).

The stapedius tendon is first cut with a microscissor or laser, and the posterior crus of the stapes is divided with a carbon dioxide (CO_2) laser. The incudostapedial joint is then separated with a joint knife or small, right-angled micro pick. Next, the stapes suprastructure is downfractured and removed. Of note, the anterior crus can also be divided if needed, a distinct advantage of the endoscopic approach. Subsequently, the distance between the footplate and the incudal lenticular process is measured with a measuring rod.

If a stapedectomy is being performed, the mucosa adjacent to the oval window niche can be removed or laser ablated. A tissue graft (perichondrium, fascia, vein or fat) is placed on the promontory, inferior to the oval window before addressing the footplate. After partial or total stapedectomy, the tissue graft on the promontory is then positioned over the oval window to seal the vestibule. The prosthesis is placed between this graft and long process of the incus.

The senior author typically performs stapedotomies and uses a CO_2 laser at 3 W to create the fenestra. When footplate disease is excessive and cannot be effectively addressed with the laser, a stapedotomy can be made with a 7 mm burr to drill at 7000 rpm. Using serial perforators from 0.5 to 0.7 mm, the hole is measured. Sizing is confirmed, and a piston-type prosthesis is placed into the stapedotomy hole and hooked around the long process of the incus. The laser is then used to crimp the prosthesis securely onto the lenticular process. Next, the promontory is scratched in order to create a blood patch to help secure the prosthesis to the footplate (**Fig. 6**).

The round window reflex is assessed with the endoscope to confirm appropriate coupling of the prosthesis. The endoscope also enables a detailed examination of the round window to readily determine its potential involvement by disease, estimated in up to 13% of cases.[30] Furthermore, a pulsating round window can be easily identified with an endoscope (Case example 3). This finding can indicate an underlying gusher, and responsible consideration should be given to abort the procedure before manipulating the stapes to decrease the risk of sensorineural hearing loss.

At the end of the procedure, the tympanomeatal flap is laid back into position, covering the exposed osseous canal. The ear canal is packed with Gelfoam anteriorly and then filled with antibiotic ointment, followed by a cotton ball and a band-aid.

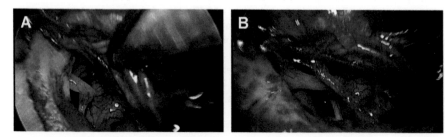

Fig. 3. View with a 0° endoscope after tympanomeatal flap elevation (*A*) and following limited curettage of posterior scutum (*B*).

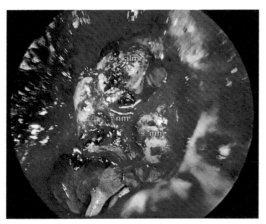

Fig. 4. Congenital abnormalities of the ossicular chain with prominent anterior malleolar ligament fixation. i, malformed incus; mh, malleolar head; nm, neck of malleus; alm, anterior malleolar ligament; s, malformed stapes.

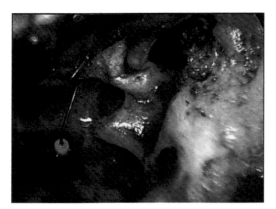

Fig. 5. A curved pick is used to position a piston prosthesis from the malleus to the fenestra following a malleostapedotomy.

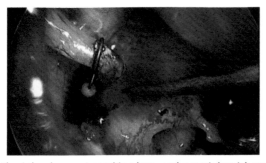

Fig. 6. Piston prosthesis has been crimped in place, and a straight pick was used to create a blood patch.

HIGHLIGHTED SCENARIOS IN ENDOSCOPIC STAPES SURGERY
Revision Stapedotomy

TEES offers a viable option for revision cases and affords excellent visualization of the middle ear space to determine the cause of prior surgical failure.[31,32] Lack of diagnosis has been associated with poorer outcomes.[33] In general, however, revision cases are associated with worse hearing outcomes compared with primary stapes surgeries for otosclerosis.[34–36]

Failure following stapes surgery can be temporally divided into 2 categories—immediate and delayed. When patients deny hearing improvement immediately after surgery, causes include an incorrect diagnosis that led to an unaddressed lateral chain fixation, excess tissue graft, or reparative granuloma.[34,37,38] In contrast, patients may report initial improvement only to experience a decline in hearing later. Delayed hearing loss may indicate a progression of otosclerosis within the middle ear and recurrence of oval window pathology, tympanosclerosis, and ossicular chain discontinuity from incus erosion or displaced prosthesis.[36,38] Overall, a misaligned prosthesis with or without ossicular erosion is the most common cause detected at revision cases.[38]

Video 2 demonstrates a revision stapes surgery performed in a 46-year-old woman who presented to clinic 9 years after undergoing a previous stapedotomy. She denied improvement in hearing following the initial surgery and wished to undergo revision to address her left conductive hearing loss. On otoscopy, there was retraction at the scutum, and the prosthesis could be seen contacting the tympanic membrane.

Intraoperatively, once the flap was elevated and adhesions were cleared, the prosthesis was found to be malpositioned. The old prosthesis was removed, and a new prosthesis was sized. A laser was used to make a new stapedotomy fenestra, and the piston prosthesis was then lowered into place. Care is taken to crimp the prosthesis proximal to the prior prosthesis-incudal attachment where there is often some degree of bony erosion (**Fig. 7**). A tragal cartilage graft was used to reconstruct the scutum. Her postoperative audiogram showed closure of the ABG within 10 dB.

Perilymphatic Leak Gusher

Robust perilymphatic leaks or gushers are an uncommon complication encountered during stapes surgery for otosclerosis, with an estimated rate of 0.3%.[39] Video 3 demonstrates a case in a 16-year-old female patient with a history of osteogenesis imperfecta, left greater than right conductive hearing loss, and a normal examination on otoscopy. Intraoperatively, round window pulsations were noted, and perilymph could be visualized leaking through the fenestra following stapedotomy. After placing the

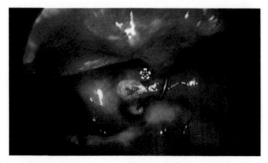

Fig. 7. When revising a prior stapedotomy, there is often ossicular erosion. The new prosthesis is placed proximal to area of focal bone loss (*) on the incus long process.

prosthesis, a perichondrium graft was tucked around its base to seal the vestibule. The patient did well postoperatively with ABG closure less than 5 dB, representing a 20 dB improvement. She endorsed disequilibrium on the first postoperative day, which subsequently spontaneously resolved. Of note, her preoperative computed tomography did not demonstrate any radiologic abnormality.[40]

The most common cause for stapes gushers is thought to be secondary to an abnormal connection with the subarachnoid space via defects in the internal auditory canal or a patent cochlear aqueduct.[41,42] As others have reported, the senior author has found most cases of perilymphatic leaks can be managed with tissue grafts, and a prosthesis can often be placed.[39] However, poorer outcomes may be expected in the setting of perilymphatic leaks with more than half of patients reporting postoperative hearing that is either unchanged (28%) or worse (31%).[39,43]

Narrow Oval Window Niche

The most prominent advantage of TEES is the wider intraoperative field of view. This can be particularly useful in the setting of particular anatomic variants including narrow oval window niches. In this case example, a 57-year-old man with a history of otosclerosis presented for left-sided endoscopic stapes surgery after a prior microscopic approach was aborted in the setting of a narrow oval window niche (Video 4). His preoperative audiogram demonstrated bilateral conductive hearing loss, maximal on the left. Intraoperatively, a view of the stapes was obtained with the 0° endoscope and demonstrated bony overgrowth of the promontory and a low lying, prolapsed facial nerve. Limited amount of promontory drilling was performed to enlarge the niche to accommodate a prosthesis (**Fig. 8**). There was also a slow perilymph leak that was managed with a perichondrium graft tucked around a piston prosthesis. The patient did well postoperatively, with closure of his ABG to within 5 dB.

Congenital Stapes Fixation

An otherwise healthy 52-year-old woman presented with several years of progressive right-sided conductive hearing loss (Video 5). Her history was consistent with

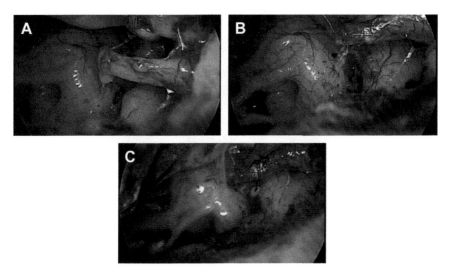

Fig. 8. A narrow oval window niche before (*A*) and after (*B*) limited drilling of the promontory. The prosthesis is crimped into place with a laser (*C*).

otosclerosis, but intraoperatively, the stapes was noted to be malformed. On inspection, the stapes was fixed posteriorly but mobile anteriorly. The stapedius tendon and pyramidal process were absent, but the tympanic segment of the facial nerve followed a traditional course. The lateral chain was mobile, and an ossicular chain reconstruction was performed following stapedotomy. There were no complications, and her postoperative course was uneventful. Follow-up audiometry demonstrated closure of her ABG to less than or equal to 10 dB.

Endoscopic techniques are often ideally suited to address congenital fixations due to the improved visibility that facilitates identification of anatomic variations.[44] In addition, concomitant middle ear structural abnormalities have been reported,[45–51] including an anomalous facial nerve in up to 11.2% of cases.[46,47,52] When the tympanic course of the facial nerve is dehiscent and overlaps the oval window niche, prosthesis placement can be challenging (**Fig. 9**) and in some cases impossible (**Fig. 10**). In addition, several investigators have reported lateral chain pathology (37%–100%) or involvement of the stapes superstructure coexistent with a congenital fixed stapes footplate, underscoring the importance of examining the entirety of the ossicular chain.[44,46,49–51] Thomeer and colleagues found no significant difference in hearing outcomes between patients who underwent malleostapedotomy versus incudostapedotomy ($P = .09$).[50]

In general, reported hearing results are worse following surgery for congenital stapes footplate fixation (CSFF), indicating the need for appropriate preoperative counseling regarding expectations.[46,48,53] Published rates of postoperative ABG closure less than 10 dB vary, ranging between 44% and 77%.[48,50,53–55] Massey and colleagues compared outcomes between isolated congenital fixation and otosclerosis, noting poorer performance for CSFF patients.[53] Nearly half (48%) of the cases with congenital stapes fixation achieved ABG closure within 10 dB, compared with 86%

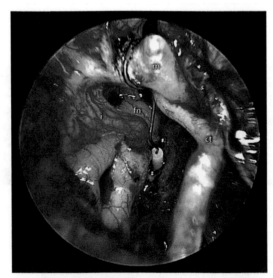

Fig. 9. Right ear during malleostapedotomy in a patient with congenital stapes fixation. The stapes superstructure was partially eroded in the setting of a prominent dehiscent tympanic segment of the facial nerve, and the crura were malformed. Only a small portion of the anterior footplate was visible and accessible for the malleostapedotomy. ct, chorda tympani; fn, facial nerve; i, incus; m, malleus.

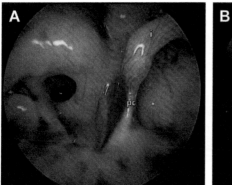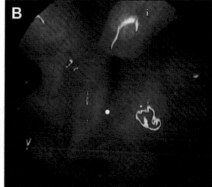

Fig. 10. (*A*) An endoscopic view of left ear. The stapes is malformed with an absent foot-plate, foreshortened anterior crura, and posterior crura lacking distal attachment. (*B*) After the malformed stapes was removed, the entirety of the footplate recess resulted in facial nerve stimulation secondary to a bifid facial nerve obliterating the oval window. This re-vented ossiculoplasty, and the procedure was concluded. i, incus; pc, posterior crura.

of otosclerosis cases, respectively (*P* = .001). However, the mean postoperative ABG was 12.2 dB, and no complications occurred, supporting the role of surgery in appropriate candidates.[53]

SUMMARY

Over the last 20 years, an endoscopic approach to stapes surgery has been increasingly pursued, with favorable results. Similar audiologic and safety outcomes have been reported in TEES compared with traditional, microscopic approaches. The endoscope increases visibility in stapes surgery with a wider, magnified field of view. Its use is particularly advantageous in the setting of variant anatomy including revision cases and congenital abnormalities. Limitations include the lack of depth perception and single-handed instrumentation, yet TEES can still be a useful tool in challenging cases as the above examples demonstrate.

DISCLOSURE

The senior author (A.R) is a consultant for Cook Medical, Stryker, Grace Medical, Cochlear Corporation, Med-EL, Advanced Bionics. K.L.Y. and N.F.M. have nothing to disclose.

SUPPLEMENTARY DATA

Supplementary data related to this article can be found online at https://doi.org/10.1016/j.otc.2020.09.015.

REFERENCES

1. Nazarian R, McElveen JT Jr, Eshraghi AA. History of otosclerosis and stapes surgery. Otolaryngol Clin North Am 2018;51(2):275–90.
2. Perkins RC. Laser stapedotomy for otosclerosis. Laryngoscope 1980;90(2):228–40.
3. Mer SB, Derbyshire AJ, Brushenko A, et al. Fiberoptic endotoscopes for examining the middle ear. Arch Otolaryngol 1967;85(4):387–93.

4. Ayache S, Tramier B, Strunski V. Otoendoscopy in cholesteatoma surgery of the middle ear: what benefits can be expected? Otol Neurotol 2008;29(8):1085–90.
5. Tarabichi M. Endoscopic middle ear surgery. Ann Otol Rhinol Laryngol 1999; 108(1):39–46.
6. Rosenberg SI, Silverstein H, Willcox TO, et al. Endoscopy in otology and neurotology. Am J Otol 1994;15(2):168–72.
7. Isaacson B, Nogueira JF. Endoscopic management of middle ear and temporal bone lesions. Otolaryngol Clin North Am 2016;49(5):1205–14.
8. Kapadiya M, Tarabichi M. An overview of endoscopic ear surgery in 2018. Laryngoscope Investig Otolaryngol 2019;4(3):365–73.
9. Isaacson B, Hunter JB, Rivas A. Endoscopic stapes surgery. Otolaryngol Clin North Am 2018;51(2):415–28.
10. Lee SY, Lee DY, Seo Y, et al. Can endoscopic tympanoplasty be a good alternative to microscopic tympanoplasty? A systematic review and meta-analysis. Clin Exp Otorhinolaryngol 2019;12(2):145–55.
11. Manna S, Kaul VF, Gray ML, et al. Endoscopic versus microscopic middle ear surgery: a meta-analysis of outcomes following tympanoplasty and stapes surgery. Otol Neurotol 2019;40(8):983–93.
12. Nogueira Junior JF, Martins MJ, Aguiar CV, et al. Fully endoscopic stapes surgery (stapedotomy): technique and preliminary results. Braz J Otorhinolaryngol 2011; 77(6):721–7.
13. James AL. Endoscope or microscope-guided pediatric tympanoplasty? Comparison of grafting technique and outcome. Laryngoscope 2017;127(11):2659–64.
14. Kozin ED, Kiringoda R, Lee DJ. Incorporating endoscopic ear surgery into your clinical practice. Otolaryngol Clin North Am 2016;49(5):1237–51.
15. Kozin ED, Lehmann A, Carter M, et al. Thermal effects of endoscopy in a human temporal bone model: implications for endoscopic ear surgery. Laryngoscope 2014;124(8):E332–9.
16. Hall AC, Mandavia R, Selvadurai D. Total endoscopic stapes surgery: systematic review and pooled analysis of audiological outcomes. Laryngoscope 2020; 130(5):1282–6.
17. Bittermann AJ, Rovers MM, Tange RA, et al. Primary stapes surgery in patients with otosclerosis: prediction of postoperative outcome. Arch Otolaryngol Head Neck Surg 2011;137(8):780–4.
18. Naik C, Nemade S. Endoscopic stapedotomy: our view point. Eur Arch Otorhinolaryngol 2016;273(1):37–41.
19. Kuo CW, Wu HM. Fully endoscopic laser stapedotomy: is it comparable with microscopic surgery? Acta Otolaryngol 2018;138(10):871–6.
20. Nikolaos T, Aikaterini T, Dimitrios D, et al. Does endoscopic stapedotomy increase hearing restoration rates comparing to microscopic? A systematic review and meta-analysis. Eur Arch Otorhinolaryngol 2018;275(12):2905–13.
21. Koukkoullis A, Toth I, Gede N, et al. Endoscopic versus microscopic stapes surgery outcomes: a meta-analysis and systematic review. Laryngoscope 2020; 130(8):2019–27.
22. Pauna HF, Pereira RC, Monsanto RC, et al. A comparison between endoscopic and microscopic approaches for stapes surgery: A systematic review. J Laryngol Otol 2020;134(5):398–403.
23. Iannella G, Magliulo G. Endoscopic versus microscopic approach in stapes surgery: are operative times and learning curve important for making the choice? Otol Neurotol 2016;37(9):1350–7.

24. Kojima H, Komori M, Chikazawa S, et al. Comparison between endoscopic and microscopic stapes surgery. Laryngoscope 2014;124(1):266–71.

25. Daneshi A, Jahandideh H. Totally endoscopic stapes surgery without packing: novel technique bringing most comfort to the patients. Eur Arch Otorhinolaryngol 2016;273(3):631–4.

26. Ito T, Kubota T, Takagi A, et al. Safety of heat generated by endoscope light sources in simulated transcanal endoscopic ear surgery. Auris Nasus Larynx 2016; 43(5):501–6.

27. Dundar R, Bulut H, Guler OK, et al. Oval window temperature changes in an endoscopic stapedectomy. J Craniofac Surg 2015;26(5):1704–8.

28. Kelly EA, Gollapudy S, Riess ML, et al. Quality of surgical field during endoscopic sinus surgery: a systematic literature review of the effect of total intravenous compared to inhalational anesthesia. Int Forum Allergy Rhinol 2013;3(6):474–81.

29. Little M, Tran V, Chiarella A, et al. Total intravenous anesthesia vs inhaled anesthetic for intraoperative visualization during endoscopic sinus surgery: a double blind randomized controlled trial. Int Forum Allergy Rhinol 2018;8(10):1123–6.

30. Mansour S, Magnan J, Nicolas K, et al. Otosclerosis. In: Middle ear diseases: advances in diagnosis and management. Cham: Springer International Publishing; 2018. p. 1–83.

31. Fernandez IJ, Villari D, Botti C, et al. Endoscopic revision stapes surgery: surgical findings and outcomes. Eur Arch Otorhinolaryngol 2019;276(3):703–10.

32. Nassiri AM, Yawn RJ, Dedmon MM, et al. Audiologic and surgical outcomes in endoscopic revision stapes surgery. Laryngoscope 2019;129(10):2366–70.

33. Wegner I, Vincent R, Derks LSM, et al. An internally validated prognostic model for success in revision stapes surgery for otosclerosis. Laryngoscope 2018; 128(10):2390–6.

34. Ramaswamy AT, Lustig LR. Revision surgery for otosclerosis. Otolaryngol Clin North Am 2018;51(2):463–74.

35. Gros A, Vatovec J, Zargi M, et al. Success rate in revision stapes surgery for otosclerosis. Otol Neurotol 2005;26(6):1143–8.

36. Blijleven EE, Wegner I, Tange RA, et al. Revision stapes surgery in a tertiary referral center: surgical and audiometric outcomes. Ann Otol Rhinol Laryngol 2019;128(11):997–1005.

37. Huber A, Koike T, Wada H, et al. Fixation of the anterior mallear ligament: diagnosis and consequences for hearing results in stapes surgery. Ann Otol Rhinol Laryngol 2003;112(4):348–55.

38. Fisch U, Acar GO, Huber AM. Malleostapedotomy in revision surgery for otosclerosis. Otol Neurotol 2001;22(6):776–85.

39. Alicandri-Ciufelli M, Molinari G, Rosa MS, et al. Gusher in stapes surgery: a systematic review. Eur Arch Otorhinolaryngol 2019;276(9):2363–76.

40. Krouchi L, Callonnec F, Bouchetemble P, et al. Preoperative computed tomography scan may fail to predict perilymphatic gusher. Ann Otol Rhinol Laryngol 2013; 122(6):374–7.

41. Glasscock ME 3rd. The stapes gusher. Arch Otolaryngol 1973;98(2):82–91.

42. Wiet RJ, Harvey SA, Bauer GP. Complications in stapes surgery. Options for prevention and management. Otolaryngol Clin North Am 1993;26(3):471–90.

43. Antonelli PJ. Prevention and management of complications in otosclerosis surgery. Otolaryngol Clin North Am 2018;51(2):453–62.

44. Marchioni D, Soloperto D, Villari D, et al. Stapes malformations: the contribute of the endoscopy for diagnosis and surgery. Eur Arch Otorhinolaryngol 2016;273(7): 1723–9.

45. McRackan TR, Carlson ML, Reda FA, et al. Bifid facial nerve in congenital stapes footplate fixation. Otol Neurotol 2014;35(5):e199–201.

46. Carlson ML, Van Abel KM, Pelosi S, et al. Outcomes comparing primary pediatric stapedectomy for congenital stapes footplate fixation and juvenile otosclerosis. Otol Neurotol 2013;34(5):816–20.

47. An YS, Lee JH, Lee KS. Anomalous facial nerve in congenital stapes fixation. Otol Neurotol 2014;35(4):662–6.

48. De la Cruz A, Angeli S, Slattery WH. Stapedectomy in children. Otolaryngol Head Neck Surg 1999;120(4):487–92.

49. Teunissen B, Cremers CW. Surgery for congenital stapes ankylosis with an associated congenital ossicular chain anomaly. Int J Pediatr Otorhinolaryngol 1991; 21(3):217–26.

50. Thomeer HG, Kunst HP, Cremers CW. Congenital stapes ankylosis associated with another ossicular chain anomaly: surgical results in 30 ears. Arch Otolaryngol Head Neck Surg 2011;137(9):935–41.

51. Albert S, Roger G, Rouillon I, et al. Congenital stapes ankylosis: study of 28 cases and surgical results. Laryngoscope 2006;116(7):1153–7.

52. Visvanathan A, Rinaldi V, Visvanathan PG. Fallopian canal stapedotomy in congenital stapes fixation with aberrant facial nerve. Ann Otol Rhinol Laryngol 2011;120(6):377–80.

53. Massey BL, Hillman TA, Shelton C. Stapedectomy in congenital stapes fixation: are hearing outcomes poorer? Otolaryngol Head Neck Surg 2006;134(5):816–8.

54. Kisilevsky VE, Bailie NA, Dutt SN, et al. Hearing results of stapedotomy and malleo-vestibulopexy in congenital hearing loss. Int J Pediatr Otorhinolaryngol 2009;73(12):1712–7.

55. House HP, House WF, Hildyard VH. Congenital stapes footplate fixation; a preliminary report of twenty-three operated cases. Laryngoscope 1958;68(8):1389–402.

56. Poe DS. Laser-assisted endoscopic stapedectomy: a prospective study. Laryngoscope 2000;110(5 Pt 2 Suppl 95):1–37.

57. Migirov L, Wolf M. Endoscopic transcanal stapedotomy: how i do it. Eur Arch Otorhinolaryngol 2013;270(4):1547–9.

58. Sarkar S, Banerjee S, Chakravarty S, et al. Endoscopic stapes surgery: our experience in thirty two patients. Clin Otolaryngol 2013;38(2):157–60.

59. Özdek A, Ö Bayır, Tatar EÇ, et al. Fully endoscopic stapes surgery: preliminary results. Ann Otolaryngol Rhinol 2016;3:1085.

60. Hunter JB, Rivas A. Outcomes following endoscopic stapes surgery. Otolaryngol Clin North Am 2016;49(5):1215–25.

61. Surmelioglu O, Ozdemir S, Tarkan O, et al. Endoscopic versus microscopic stapes surgery. Auris Nasus Larynx 2017;44(3):253–7.

62. Sproat R, Yiannakis C, Iyer A. Endoscopic stapes surgery: a comparison with microscopic surgery. Otol Neurotol 2017;38(5):662–6.

63. Harikumar BAKK. Comparative study between microscopic and endoscopic stapes surgery. Int J Otorhinolaryngol Head Neck Surg 2017;3(2):285–9.

64. Moneir W, Abd El-Fattah AM, Mahmoud E, et al. Endoscopic stapedotomy: merits and demerits. J Otol 2018;13(3):97–100.

65. Nassiri MA, Yawn JR, Dedmon MM, et al. Primary endoscopic stapes surgery: audiologic and surgical outcomes. Otol Neurotol 2018;39(9):1095–101.

66. Bianconi L, Gazzini L, Laura E, et al. Endoscopic stapedotomy: safety and audiological results in 150 patients. Eur Arch Otorhinolaryngol 2020;277(1):85–92.

Endoscopic Assisted Lateral Skull Base Surgery

Brandon Isaacson, MD[a],*, Daniel E. Killeen, MD[a], Luca Bianconi, MD[b],
Daniele Marchioni, MD[b]

KEYWORDS

- Endoscopic ear surgery • Acoustic neuroma • Vestibular schwannoma
- Cholesterin granuloma • Cholesteatoma • Paraganglioma • Cerebrospinal fluid
- Facial nerve tumor

KEY POINTS

- There are 3 transcanal approaches to access the lateral skull base, including the supra-geniculate fossa, transpromontorial, and infracochlear.
- The indictions for the transpromontorial approach to the internal auditory canal and cerebellopontine angle include a progressively enlarging acoustic neuroma, confined to the internal auditory canal, and with nonserviceable hearing.
- The transcanal suprageniculate and infracochlear approaches provide access to the superior and inferior petrous apex while preserving the integrity of the otic capsule.

INTRODUCTION

The complex anatomy of the lateral skull base poses a significant challenge for the management of the various pathologies that occur in this area. Traditional approaches are well established for the management of lateral skull base pathology, but they require extensive bone removal, and in some cases, still provide poor access to hidden recesses within the temporal bone.[1] The endoscope was introduced for otologic surgery in the 1990s as an adjunct, but in the past 10 years the role of the endoscope has expanded as a primary visualization tool.[2–4] The concept of using a minimally invasive approach to the skull base is now routine for anterior skull base surgeons.[5] In the past 30 years, endoscopic sinus surgery has become the gold standard visualization tool for addressing various pathologic processes. The management of nasal pathologies with the endoscope has been shown to have similar outcomes to the classic open craniofacial approaches with reduced morbidity and improved cosmesis.[6]

[a] Department of Otolaryngology, UT Southwestern Medical Center, 2001 Inwood Road, Dallas, TX 75390-9035, USA; [b] ENT Department, University Hospital of Verona, Piazzale Aristide Stefani, 1, Verona 37126, Italy
* Corresponding author.
E-mail address: brandon.isaacson@utsouthwestern.edu

Otolaryngol Clin N Am 54 (2021) 163–173
https://doi.org/10.1016/j.otc.2020.09.020
0030-6665/21/© 2020 Elsevier Inc. All rights reserved.

Technological improvements in camera, endoscope, and light source design have further enhanced intraoperative visualization and magnification. These technological advancements in endoscopy have enhanced the surgeon's ability to identify landmarks with confidence and precision within the temporal bone.[7,8] The external auditory canal is a natural access point for addressing temporal bone pathology that has been traditionally performed with a microscope either through a retro-auricular incision or via a per-meatal approach.[9,10] The curvilinear shape of the external auditory canal limits more medial visualization and illumination of the middle ear and petrous apex when the microscope is used, but this issue is readily mitigated with the endoscope.[11] Endoscopic ear surgery has been increasingly used for the management of middle ear pathology, but has only recently been described to address pathology of the internal auditory canal and petrous apex.[7,8,12–15] Marchioni and colleagues[9] described 3 novel transcanal endoscopic approaches to the lateral skull base and demonstrated lower morbidity as well as reduced length of hospitalization. In addition to using the endoscope as the primary visualization tool for the management of lateral skull base pathology, it also has been used as an adjunct for traditional microscopic approaches to confirm completeness of tumor removal especially in areas out of the line of sight.[16,17]

Transcanal Approaches

Marchioni and colleagues[9] categorized endoscopic lateral skull base approaches per their relationship with the otic capsule. The 3 transcanal endoscopic approaches include the *transcanal transpromontorial approach* passing through the otic capsule, the *transcanal suprageniculate approach* passing superior to the otic capsule, and the *transcanal infracochlear approach* passing inferior to the otic capsule.[9]

TRANSCANAL SUPRAGENICULATE CORRIDOR

In all transcanal endoscopic approaches, the external auditory canal (EAC) is used as a natural corridor to access the inner ear and petrous apex via the tympanic cavity.[9] The suprageniculate approach permits access the superior petrous apex as defined by the petrous bone superior to the internal auditory canal (IAC).[18,19] The suprageniculate fossa (SGF) is a pyramidal-shaped anatomic area bounded inferiorly by geniculate ganglion and tympanic facial nerve, superiorly by the dura of the middle cranial fossa, and posteriorly by the ampullated end of the lateral semicircular canal, and medially consists of the petrous apex cells superior to the IAC.[9,18]

Indications

- Neoplasms (ie, facial nerve hemangiomas, schwannomas) involving the suprageniculate fossa, with limited extension into the petrous apex cells lying superiorly to the geniculate ganglion and the labyrinthine facial nerve, with significant facial paresis (House-Brackmann III-VI).
- Cholesteatoma of the superior petrous apex.
- Traumatic injury to the geniculate ganglion and distal labyrinthine facial nerve requiring decompression or removal of bone spicules.

Surgical Technique

The patient is positioned supine with the operative ear facing laterally, as per traditional otologic surgery. Facial nerve function is monitored throughout the procedure with electrophysiological monitoring (NIM; Medtronic, Dublin, Ireland). A 0-degree endoscope (3 or 4 mm diameter, 0°, 14 cm length; Storz, Tuttlingen, Germany) is inserted through the EAC. An inferiorly based tympano-meatal flap is elevated by making canal incisions along the anterior superior canal (2 o'clock) and the posterior inferior canal (7 o'clock). The flap is raised off the bone of the posterior-superior EAC and the annulus is elevated from the sulcus. The chorda tympani nerve is identified and preserved and the retrotympanic area is exposed. The eardrum is partially dissected from the malleus neck and handle and the flap is positioned along the anterior inferior portion of the EAC. An extensive atticotomy is performed exposing the entire malleus head and incus body. The incus is carefully separated from the stapes capitulum and is removed along with the head of the malleus. The neck and manubrium of the malleus and the tensor tympani tendon are preserved to perform an ossiculoplasty with a prosthesis or an autograft (incus interposition) after the primary pathology has been managed. The boundaries of the approach are limited posteriorly by the ampullated end of the lateral semicircular canal, superiorly by the dura of the middle fossa, inferiorly by the tympanic facial nerve and geniculate ganglion. Identification of the tympanic facial nerve and geniculate ganglion between the cog and the cochleariform process is warranted in the management of facial nerve neoplasms (schwannoma, hemangioma). In select facial nerve tumor cases, it may be possible to preserve a portion of the nerve, but a reconstruction with an interposition graft is also feasible using the endoscope.[19] In cases of long-standing complete facial paralysis, a muscle free tissue transfer with an alternate nerve source graft (masseter or hypoglossal nerve) may be performed. A static procedure is also an option. Extension of epitympanic cholesteatoma into the superior petrous apex can also be managed using the suprageniculate fossa approach depending on the extent of temporal bone pneumatization. The last steps of this approach are reconstruction of the ossicular chain followed by tympanic membrane grafting if necessary, and tympanomeatal flap repositioning.[9,18]

Advantages

- Facilitates identification of landmarks and nonline of sight structures.
- Otic capsule and subsequent hearing preservation with a possibility of middle ear reconstruction with an autograft or prosthesis.
- Eliminates the need for dura and temporal lobe retraction with reduced morbidity by avoiding an intensive care unit (ICU) admission.

Disadvantages

- Unsuitable for extensive lesions.
- Mandatory incus body and malleus head removal, necessitating ossiculoplasty with the potential for postoperative conductive hearing loss.
- Substantial dural or intradural involvement will likely necessitate a more extended approach with the microscope.
- In cases in which excision of the facial nerve becomes necessary, an end to end reconstruction is rarely possible, but an interposition cable nerve graft is possible but challenging.

TRANSCANAL INFRACOCHLEAR CORRIDOR

The infracochlear approach provides access to the petrous apex cells located inferior to the cochlea and IAC. The boundaries of this approach are the cochlea superiorly, the vertical segment of the petrous internal carotid artery anteriorly and the jugular bulb posterior-inferiorly. The ossicular chain and the cochlea are preserved.[9,11,20]

Indications

- Pathology localized to the inferior petrous apex with limited extent.
- Cholesterol granuloma of the petrous apex.
- Cholesteatoma with subcochlear canaliculi and petrous apex involvement.

Surgical Technique

The patient is positioned in the same fashion as the suprageniculate approach. A superiorly based tympanomeatal flap is used to access the meso, hypo, and retrotympanum. Canal incisions are made at 3 o'clock and 9 o'clock and are connected along the inferior canal wall. The inferior canal skin is elevated down to the tympanic annulus, which is then elevated out of the osseous sulcus exposing the middle ear mucosa. In most cases the tympanic membrane is left attached to the malleus handle and umbo. The ossicular chain is preserved and the landmarks identified including the round window, the fustis, the subiculum, and the funiculus. In some patients, there is a tunnel between the fustis and the funiculus, that connects the middle ear with the cells of the petrous apex known as the subcochlear canaliculus. The subcochlear canaliculus varies between patients and may extend medial and inferior to the cochlea between jugular bulb and internal carotid artery ending in the petrous apex. In some cases of extensive middle ear cholesteatoma, the subcochlear canaliculus can be a pathway by which disease can extend into the petrous apex. The variable pneumatization and dimensions of the infracochlear approach dictates which pathologies can be appropriately managed using the infracochlear approach. Once the pathology has been treated, an angled or 0° endoscope can be used to visualize the petrous apex through the infracochlear corridor. The tympanomeatal flap is replaced back onto the osseous EAC at the end of the procedure.[9,11]

Advantages

- Facilitates identification of landmarks and exploration of hidden areas.
- Ossicular chain and hearing function preservation.
- Minimally invasive approach with lower morbidity and reduced hospitalization.

Disadvantages

- Not suitable for extensive infralabyrinthine, or infralabyrinthine-apical cholesteatoma.
- Not feasible in patients with a high jugular bulb or when the jugular bulb and petrous carotid artery are in close proximity to each other.

TRANSCANAL TRANSPROMONTORIAL CORRIDOR

The transpromontorial approach differs from the previously described transcanal procedures in that it requires a partial or complete removal of the cochlea to expose the IAC and cerebello-pontine angle (CPA).[8,12,21,22] Opening the otic capsule, as expected, results in profound sensorineural hearing loss that rarely can be restored via a cochlear implantation provided some of the cochlea and the cochlear nerve are preserved. Further, opening the subarachnoid space necessitates obliteration of the Eustachian tube, and middle ear and typically requires overclosure of the ear canal to mitigate the risk of a cerebrospinal fluid (CSF) leak. This approach differs from the traditional transcochlear/transotic approaches because it preserves the mastoid and the vestibular portion of the otic capsule. The transpromontorial approach also does not require a significant amount of bone removal and thus is a minimally invasive and bone sparing alternative.[12]

There are 2 variants of the transpromontorial approach:

- *Exclusive endoscopic transcanal transpromontorial approach.*
- Expanded transcanal transpromontorial approach.

Exclusive Endoscopic Transcanal Transpromontorial Approach

Indications

- Intralabyrinthine schwannomas with or without extension to the fundus of the IAC with the following characteristics: profound hearing loss, progressive growth and/or intractable vestibular symptoms.
- Symptomatic or growing intracanalicular vestibular schwannomas with profound hearing loss.
- Cholesteatoma, or middle ear neoplasms with extension of the pathology into the cochlea.

Advantages

- Direct approach to intra-otic capsule and IAC pathology.
- Minimally invasive approach obviating the need for brain and meningeal retraction.
- Potential for standard postsurgical unit admission as opposed to the ICU.
- Potentially reduced morbidity.

Disadvantages

- Limited to (Koos I-II) IAC lesions with limited CPA extension.
- Resultant anacusis.
- Poor control of the vascular structures in the CPA.[8,23]

Expanded Transcanal Transpromontorial Approach

Indications

- Internal auditory canal and CPA neoplasms with limited CPA expansion outside of the line of site of the IAC in patients with nonserviceable hearing.
- Lesions with petrous apex extension or involvement in patients with nonserviceable hearing (eg, cholesteatoma, cholesterol granuloma, chondroid series tumors).

Advantages

- Two-handed technique with the possibility to merge the advantages of the microscope and the endoscope.
- Direct surgical approach to the inner ear, IAC and CPA up to the brainstem.
- Minimally invasive approach without brain or dural retraction with possible reduced morbidity.
- Improved control of the CPA vascular structures compared with the more limited transpromontorial approach.

Disadvantages

- Not suitable for tumor extending to the level of the lower cranial nerves and or trigeminal nerve.
- Resultant anacusis.

Surgical technique

The facial nerve is monitored per standard protocol for temporal bone surgery. The transpromontorial approach typically necessitates closure of the EAC to prevent a CSF leak. There are 2 techniques for EAC overclosure either by the blind sac closure, or by the modified Rambo approach.[10,21,23] The Rambo technique begins by making incisions in the cartilaginous ear canal at 6 and 12 o'clock with an anterior medial incision at the bony cartilaginous junction. The anterior tragal skin is then elevated off of the tragal cartilage in a medial to lateral direction, creating an anteriolaterally based skin flap. This skin flap is then extended over to the concha to identify the location of final tension-free closure. A curvilinear incision is then made in the conchal bowl connecting up to the apices of the prior membranous canal incisions. The conchal and posterior membranous ear canal skin are then dissected away from the underlying cartilage down to the osseo-cartilaginous junction, and removed. A monopolar cautery is then used to remove all of the remaining membranous canal skin down to the osseous canal. At this point, surgical hooks are used to retract the anterior skin flap and posterior conchal skin to provide an unobstructed view of the osseous EAC.[16,21]

Under endoscopic visualization, the remaining medial EAC skin is then dissected away from the bone until the tympanic annulus is visualized. The fibrous annulus is then elevated away from the osseous annulus circumferentially and the middle ear is entered. The incudostapedial joint is visualized and divided.[2] The incus is then removed.[2] At this point, the medial ear canal skin, tympanic membrane, and malleus are then completely removed. The chorda tympani nerve is also sacrificed[2] (**Fig. 1**). A wide canaloplasty is performed with an otologic drill. The limits of dissection are the vertical petrous carotid artery anteriorly, the jugular bulb inferiorly, the tympanic segment of the facial nerve superiorly, and the mastoid segment of the facial nerve posteriorly.[2] The stapes is then removed and the oval window is connected to the

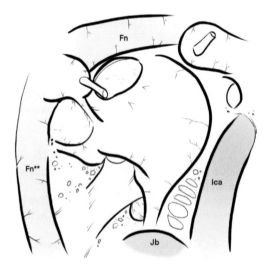

Fig. 1. This illustration demonstrates the boundaries of the transpromontorial approach after the lateral chain and stapes have been removed. The superior boundary is the tympanic facial nerve (Fn), the posterior boundary is the mastoid facial nerve (Fn**), the anterior boundary is the vertical petrous carotid artery (Ica), and the inferior boundary is the jugular bulb (Jb).

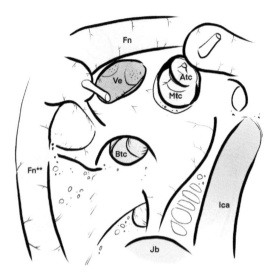

Fig. 2. This illustration demonstrates the basal (Btc), middle (Mtc), and apical turns (Atc) of the cochlea and the vestibule (Ve) after opening the round window, promontory, and oval window.

round window niche exposing the hook region of the basal cochlear turn using the otologic drill. The promontory is then opened to define the basal, middle, and apical turns of the cochlea (**Fig. 2**). The fundus of the IAC is opened and allows the surgeon to remove smaller fundal or intravestibular tumors (**Figs. 3** and **4**). On completion of tumor removal, some temporalis muscle or abdominal fat is used to plug the fundus, the Eustachian tube. This more limited approach facilitates reduced operative times and

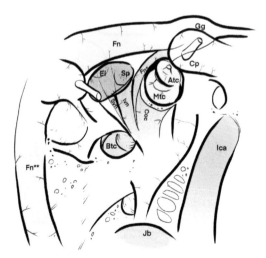

Fig. 3. This illustration shows the position of neural elements within the IAC after it has been opened and their position relative to the cochlear turns (Btc, Mtc, Atc), cochleariform process (Cp), and geniculate ganglion (Gg). Coc, cochlear nerve; Ivn, inferior vestibular nerve; Svn, superior vestibular nerve; Fn*, labyrinthine facial nerve.

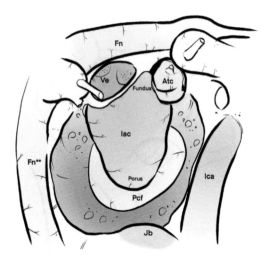

Fig. 4. For more extensive tumors extending to the porus and into the posterior cranial fossa, more extensive bone removal is necessary up to the previously described boundaries of the transpromontorial approach. Iac, internal auditory canal; Pcf, posterior cranial fossa.

possible the risk of a CSF leak. A more extensive approach is often necessary for tumors that extend to or involve the porus acusticus or with limited involvement of the CPA. In the extended approach, the infracochlear tract is opened to expose the IAC porus, as well as the posterior cranial fossa dura. The internal auditory canal is skeletonized creating anterior and posterior troughs, which may allow for 270° of IAC exposure (**Fig. 4**; **Figs. 5** and **6**). The cochlear aqueduct is usually encountered and allows for the release of CSF. The internal auditory is then opened and the tumor is

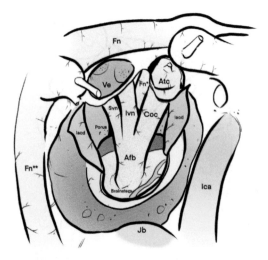

Fig. 5. This illustration demonstrates the extended transpromontorial approach. The internal auditory canal dura (Iacd) has been opened from the fundus to the porus exposing the brainstem, 8-nerve complex (Afb), distal meatal and labyrinthine facial nerve (Fn*).

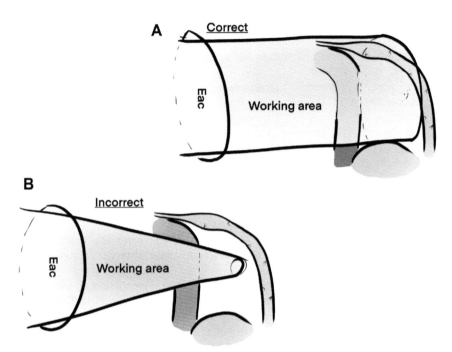

Fig. 6. This illustration depicts the transpromontorial surgical corridor. (*A*) Demonstrated is the correct approach, which uses the full extent of the surgical corridor outlined by the tympanic and mastoid facial nerve, jugular bulb, and petrous carotid artery. (*B*) Demonstrated is a very limited exposure of the IAC as a result of not removing all of the bone up to the previously described boundaries. External auditory canal (Eac).

removed.[2] After completion of tumor removal the Eustachian tube is then obliterated with fat or temporalis muscle. The tensor tympani muscle can also facilitate Eustachian tube obliteration by elevating the muscle out of its osseous canal to create a pedicled flap. An abdominal fat graft is further used to fill the middle ear and EAC. The previously created anterior tragal skin flap is then sutured to the posterior conchal skin to complete the Rambo ear closure.[9,21,22]

Postoperative care and follow-up
The patients usually are discharged between 3 and 5 days after surgery. A head computed tomography scan is obtained in all patients after surgery and antibiotics are administered for 24 to 48 hours. Weight lifting and exercise restrictions are recommended for 4 to 6 weeks after surgery to reduce the risk of a CSF leak. An MRI is obtained 1, 5, and 10 years after the surgery to monitor for recurrent disease. Contralateral routing of sound hearing rehabilitation options are discussed with the patient before and after surgery.

DISCLOSURE

The authors have nothing to disclose.

REFERENCES

1. Zanoletti E, Martini A, Emanuelli E, et al. Lateral approaches to the skull base. Acta Otorhinolaryngol Ital 2012;32:281–7.

2. Thomassin JM, Korchia D, Doris JM. Endoscopic-guided otosurgery in the prevention of residual cholesteatomas. Laryngoscope 1993;103:939–43.

3. Tarabichi M. Endoscopic middle ear surgery. Ann Otol Rhinol Laryngol 1999;108: 39–46.

4. Tarabichi M. Endoscopic management of limited attic cholesteatoma. Laryngoscope 2004;114:1157–62.

5. Ketcham AS, Wilkins RH, Vanburen JM, et al. A combined intracranial facial approach to the paranasal sinuses. Am J Surg 1963;106:698–703.

6. Albonette-Felicio T, Rangel GG, Martinez-Perez R, et al. Surgical management of anterior skull-base malignancies (endoscopic vs. craniofacial resection). J Neurooncol 2020. https://doi.org/10.1007/s11060-020-03413-y.

7. Marchioni D, Gazzini L, De Rossi S, et al. The management of tympanic membrane perforation with endoscopic type I tympanoplasty. Otol Neurotol 2020; 41:214–21.

8. Marchioni D, Alicandri-Ciufelli M, Mattioli F, et al. From external to internal auditory canal: surgical anatomy by an exclusive endoscopic approach. Eur Arch Otorhinolaryngol 2013;270:1267–75.

9. Marchioni D, Alicandri-Ciufelli M, Rubini A, et al. Endoscopic transcanal corridors to the lateral skull base: initial experiences. Laryngoscope 2015;125(Suppl 5): S1–13.

10. Wick CC, Arnaoutakis D, Barnett SL, et al. Endoscopic transcanal transpromontorial approach for vestibular schwannoma resection: a case series. Otol Neurotol 2017;38:e490–4.

11. Wick CC, Hansen AR, Kutz JW Jr, et al. Endoscopic infracochlear approach for drainage of petrous apex cholesterol granulomas: a case series. Otol Neurotol 2017;38:876–81.

12. Marchioni D, Alicandri-Ciufelli M, Rubini A, et al. Exclusive endoscopic transcanal transpromontorial approach: a new perspective for internal auditory canal vestibular schwannoma treatment. J Neurosurg 2017;126:98–105.

13. Yawn RJ, Hunter JB, O'Connell BP, et al. Audiometric outcomes following endoscopic ossicular chain reconstruction. Otol Neurotol 2017;38:1296–300.

14. Nikolaos T, Aikaterini T, Dimitrios D, et al. Does endoscopic stapedotomy increase hearing restoration rates comparing to microscopic? A systematic review and meta-analysis. Eur Arch Otorhinolaryngol 2018;275:2905–13.

15. Presutti L, Marchioni D, Mattioli F, et al. Endoscopic management of acquired cholesteatoma: our experience. J Otolaryngol Head Neck Surg 2008;37:481–7.

16. Presutti L, Alicandri-Ciufelli M, Bonali M, et al. Expanded transcanal transpromontorial approach to the internal auditory canal: pilot clinical experience. Laryngoscope 2017;127:2608–14.

17. Presutti L, Alicandri-Ciufelli M, Rubini A, et al. Combined lateral microscopic/ endoscopic approaches to petrous apex lesions: pilot clinical experiences. Ann Otol Rhinol Laryngol 2014;123:550–9.

18. Marchioni D, Rubini A, Nogueira JF, et al. Transcanal endoscopic approach to lesions of the suprageniculate ganglion fossa. Auris Nasus Larynx 2018;45:57–65.

19. Wick CC, Sakai M, Richardson TE, et al. Transcanal endoscopic ear surgery for excision of a facial nerve venous malformation with interposition nerve grafting: a case report. Otol Neurotol 2017;38:895–9.

20. Rihani J, Kutz JW Jr, Isaacson B. Hearing outcomes after surgical drainage of petrous apex cholesterol granuloma. J Neurol Surg B Skull Base 2015;76:171–5.

21. Isaacson B, Tolisano AM, Patel AR, et al. Transcanal microscopic transpromonto-rial approach for vestibular schwannoma. J Neurol Surg B Skull Base 2019;80: S279–80.
22. Komune N, Matsuo S, Miki K, et al. The endoscopic anatomy of the middle ear approach to the fundus of the internal acoustic canal. J Neurosurg 2017;126: 1974–83.
23. Marchioni D, Carner M, Rubini A, et al. The fully endoscopic acoustic neuroma surgery. Otolaryngol Clin North Am 2016;49:1227–36.

New Navigation Approaches for Endoscopic Lateral Skull Base Surgery

Samuel R. Barber, MD

KEYWORDS

- Image-guided surgery • IGS • Navigation • Lateral skull base
- Endoscopic ear surgery

KEY POINTS

- Endoscopic lateral skull base surgery requires a mastery knowledge of 3-dimensional anatomy to operate in narrow spaces while preserving critical structures.
- Image-guided navigation has existed since the start of endoscopic ear surgery, yet accuracy was not adequate for the lateral skull base until recent years.
- Modern navigation systems are safe and feasible in the lateral skull base using optical or magnetic tracking and fiducial markers for registration.
- Novel transcanal-exclusive approaches with image-guided navigation can access the internal auditory canal, posterior cranial fossa, or petrous apex without a craniotomy.

INTRODUCTION

Innovations in image-guided navigation technology have changed the way surgery of the lateral skull base (LSB) is performed. The use of endoscopes in ear surgery was described 25 years ago,[1,2] but early techniques identified risks of complications with dissection in areas, including the internal auditory canal (IAC) and posterior cranial fossa.[3] Transcanal-exclusive approaches for endoscopic ear surgery (EES) rely on intimate knowledge of middle ear anatomy while offering many advantages in return. Outcomes of these minimally invasive procedures have shown a decreased need for craniotomy or larger surgery, shorter hospital stays, and reduced postoperative pain.[4–7] EES already has a steep learning curve, yet complexity only increases when operating in the LSB. Whether in the mastoid, the labyrinth, or the petrous apex, there are many structures at risk during dissection.[8–10] The internal carotid artery (ICA), jugular bulb (JB), and basal turn of the cochlea all may be within 1 mm to 2 mm of an infracochlear corridor.[11] Accordingly, some experts in the field regard endoscopic LSB surgery as the last step in comprehensive EES training.[12]

Department of Otolaryngology–Head and Neck Surgery, University of Arizona College of Medicine, 1501 North Campbell Avenue, Tucson, AZ 85724, USA
E-mail address: sambarber@oto.arizona.edu

Otolaryngol Clin N Am 54 (2021) 175–187
https://doi.org/10.1016/j.otc.2020.09.021
0030-6665/21/© 2020 Elsevier Inc. All rights reserved.
oto.theclinics.com

Image-guided Navigation

Image-guided navigation, also known as surgical navigation, image-guided surgery (IGS), stereotactic navigation, and neuronavigation, all describe the same adjunctive intraoperative technology. In the broad field of IGS, this application specifically refers to stereotactic surgery with imaging studies, such as computed tomography (CT) or structural magnetic resonance imaging (MRI), being registered to the surgical field using common anatomic reference markers.[13] Intraoperatively, displayed imaging data correspond to specific coordinates of positionally tracked instruments relative to patient-specific anatomy.[14–16] Multiplanar reformatted views of imaging in navigation serve an important role in computer-assisted surgery, because they confirm critical landmarks in the surgical field with real-time visual data. Endoscopic LSB surgery requires submillimeter accuracy of tracking hardware, which has been achieved over multiple decades.[13,17,18] Historically, the choice for LSB approach has been determined by the size and location of the tumor, necessary exposure for the region of interest, and the degree of morbidity deemed acceptable by both the patient and care team.[10] It is important to emphasize that image-guided navigation revolutionizes patient selection and the surgical plan: a greater preservation of structures reduces lifelong morbidity for patients, and patients with previously inoperable disease may become surgical candidates.[19,20] This article reviews advancements in image-guided navigation over time, presents examples of new image-guided navigation approaches in endoscopic LSB surgery, and discusses developing technologies for next-generation navigation systems.

NAVIGATION TECHNOLOGY FOR THE LATERAL SKULL BASE
Medical Imaging Modalities for Lateral Skull Base Navigation

Stereotactic surgery using cartesian coordinates originally began with frame-based systems fixed to the head for neurosurgery, dating back to 1906.[21] With the advent of CT and MRI, imaging was registered with frame-based systems in the 1970s and 1980s.[13,14] Over time, frameless systems transitioned from mechanically linked to fully wireless components that were the foundation of modern-day workstations. These comprised electromagnetic (EM), ultrasound, and light emitting-based systems.

Although accuracy always has been a limiting factor for feasibility of navigation in endoscopic LSB surgery, image guidance is only as good as the image series utilized.

Computed Tomography Imaging

Resolution of CT imaging has increased significantly over 4 decades. Early image-guided navigation systems utilized step-and-shoot CT scanners that acquired 1 direct axial image at a time with 1-mm slice thickness.[22] Thin-slice axial reconstructions with submillimeter resolution became possible with the advent of single-detector row helical (spiral) CT; however, image quality was improved markedly with multidetector row CT (MDCT).[23] MDCT series with at least 4 channels can have isotropic voxels,[24,25] meaning that spatial resolution for the in-plane axis (x-y) is equal to the long axis (z). As a result, images are acquired as volume data rather than individual slices, offering the ability to reformat a series in any desired plane without degrading quality.[23,26] In-plane spatial resolution must have a field of view and pixel size adequate to resolve microanatomic structures in the middle and inner ear.[27]

Two other CT modalities include cone beam (CBCT) and flat-panel volume CT. These both have potential advantages when visualizing the ossicular chain or cochlear implant electrodes but at the expense of lower signal-to-noise ratio and contrast resolution.[28–32] Overall, all CT techniques are adequate for image-guided navigation with acceptable spatial resolution in both axes.

The long axis is represented by slice thickness, which is arguably the greatest determinant of feasibility for navigation.[24] Anisotropic voxels have inadequate spatial resolution for multiplanar and 3-dimensional (3-D) reconstructions, because details are severely degraded with increased slice thickness.[22,26] If a temporal bone CT has a slice thickness of 3 mm, and a semicircular canal falls between slices, no interpolation algorithm can visually represent that structure if a tracked instrument encounters it[33] (**Fig. 1**). If the Nyquist theorem is applied to spatial resolution, a sample twice that of the desired value is necessary.[27] This corresponds to the recommended 0.5-mm slice thickness reported for both diagnostic radiology and image navigation literature,[16,22,34,35] although voxel size of 0.625 mm also is common.[26,36,37]

Magnetic Resonance Imaging

MRI has an adjunctive role in navigation given that registration is based on fixed, bony landmarks best seen on CT. Soft tissue regions of interest, however, can be represented with great specificity when strategic MRI sequences are chosen. MRI can be registered with CT data on navigation workstations to superimpose both imaging modalities. In general, T1-weighted and T2-weighted sequences should have small, isotropic voxels to delineate boundaries of soft tissue structures. T2-weighted sequences for the IAC can reveal neurovascular structures within the cerebrospinal fluid, whereas postcontrast enhanced T1-weighted sequences reveal tumors with varying patterns of intensity based on the pathology.[38] Lastly, some diffusion-weighted imaging sequences may highlight cholesteatoma,[39,40] whereas diffusion tensor imaging tractography can represent white matter tracts.[41] Currently, navigation with diffusion imaging is used predominantly by neurosurgeons.[41,42] There are potential applications for endoscopic LSB surgery; however, it is important to understand fundamental differences compared to traditional structural MRI sequences. Diffusion-weighted signal intensity represents calculated values based on the diffusion of water molecules. These sequences are susceptible to geometric distortion and require additional postprocessing and distortion correction for reliable registration with structural image series.[43]

Positional Tracking and Registration Strategies

Modern image-guided navigation workstations are frameless, non–mechanically linked systems. The 2 main methods for positionally tracking registered anatomy and surgical instruments are optical and EM tracking (**Fig. 2**). Capabilities increased

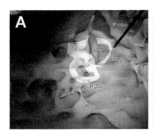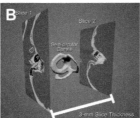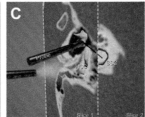

Fig. 1. CT slice thickness matters. (A) Virtual transmastoid endoscopic view of a left ear shows a probe lateral to the position of the superior semicircular canal (*yellow outline*). (B) Slices are too far apart to capture the region of interest. (C) Oblique superior-lateral 3-D view shows the probe tip is between slices. HSC, horizontal semicircular canal; PSC, posterior semicircular canal; SSC, superior semicircular canal.

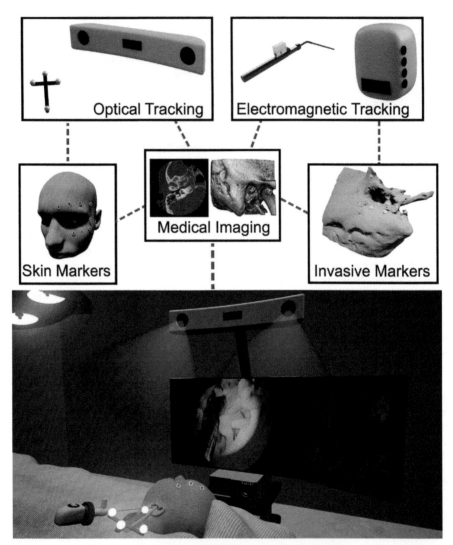

Fig. 2. Image navigation components. Tracking equipment uses optical or electromagnetic systems to register medical imaging with patient anatomy and surgical instruments (top). A schematic of optical tracking equipment for transcanal endoscopic approaches (bottom). Concept tracking equipment rendered with computer-aided design.

for both tracking strategies over decades to become adequate for endoscopic LSB. Just as spatial resolution has increased in imaging modalities, multiple key parameters determine feasibility to achieve submillimeter accuracy. Emphasis on accuracy is defined broadly, yet both components of tracking and registration factor into resultant accuracy for a navigation system.

Pioneering work by Maurer, West, Fitzpatrick, and others established standard metrics to assess clinical accuracy.[44–48] Markers that defined points for registration were named, *fiducials*. The first measurement of the error in determining positions of markers was named, *fiducial localization error (FLE)*.[48] There are separate FLE for image markers and physical markers.[16] Second, a measurement of distance between these respective fiducials after registration was named the *fiducial registration error* (*FRE*). This value reflects how well imaging and physical markers are aligned. Third, a measurement of distance between respective points after registration anywhere else in the coordinate system was named, *target registration error* (*TRE*).[49] These measurements typically are reported as scalar values that represent lengths of respective component vectors.[45]

Most importantly, TRE values are not uniform within a surgical field.[16,45,46,49] TRE decreases with increasing number of fiducials, even as FRE goes up.[45] Additionally, TRE is most accurate at the central point of all fiducials and least accurate on the periphery. Hence, the TRE represents an average accuracy, and the largest outlier value (sometimes referred to as maximum error or maximum accuracy) may be unacceptable for safe navigation.[50]

Registration of imaging with patient anatomy can be achieved via multiple strategies. One strategy is paired-point registration, in which corresponding points between multiple fiducials are aligned using transform functions.[51] These include anatomic landmarks and artificial markers either applied to skin or invasively anchored in bone.[16,50,52] A second strategy is surface registration, in which the external border of soft tissue of the head is measured with a pointer or laser surface scanner.[53] A third, less common strategy, involves intraoperative image acquisition with concurrent registration with the scanner equipment.[52,54] Accuracy is highest for invasive markers with reports of mean accuracy for bone-anchored titanium as low as 0.66 mm.[36,55] Hybrid registration strategies combining markers with surface registration have varying results but do not outperform invasive markers alone.[50,55] Traditional surface scanning overall has had the highest TRE,[51,52,55] and current commercially available systems may not be adequate in LSB approaches.

Optical tracking is the most utilized tracking system for otologic and LSB surgery.[13,14,16,36,56–58] The oldest systems used active tracking via infrared light-emitting diodes and a dedicated camera.[14] These probes had the drawback of requiring active power, which led to an alternate design solution using reflective spheres for passive tracking.[59] Optical tracking consistently has the lowest recorded TRE and outlier values, but the main limitation for this system is that direct line of sight is required. Studies have shown decreased accuracy away from the center of a tracking area and with increased distance between instrument tips and reference frames.[49]

EM tracking is the other most common strategy in image-guided navigation. The need for line-of-sight tracking is eliminated through the use of an EM field generator and small sensor coils.[17,37,60] Positional tracking errors are caused by magnetic field distortion from a variety of devices in the operating room and can include displays, drills, and even surgical lights.[37,60,61] Field generators must be placed close to the patient's head, and troubleshooting may be required to reduce static and dynamic sources of error. Older comparison studies found optical tracking to be more accurate, whereas EM tracking had larger variance in TRE.[17] Recent systems have significant improvements, however, in algorithms to filter random noise and compensate for field distortion.[37,59]

Accuracy of Navigation Systems in Lateral Skull Base Surgery

Given that TRE is different based on fiducial marker arrangements and relative position of targets, navigation systems must be evaluated specifically for feasibility in LSB. For registration, some hybrid registration techniques may achieve submillimeter accuracy; however, invasive markers remain the gold standard.[50,55] Modern systems using either optical or EM tracking strategies have demonstrated overall accuracy less than 1 mm[13,18,37] (see **Fig. 2**).

NEW NAVIGATION APPROACHES FOR ENDOSCOPIC LATERAL SKULL BASE SURGERY

Novel approaches for endoscopic LSB surgery achieve minimally invasive access to regions, including the posterior cranial fossa and IAC. The risks identified by early pioneers of EES were addressed through advancements in surgical technique and technology. Approaches described by Marchioni,[62,63] Presutti,[8] and others involve transcanal-exclusive approaches beyond the middle ear as well as endoscope-assisted translabyrinthine, infralabyrinthine, transpetrosal, and middle fossa approaches. Although not explicit, it is noted in their reports that navigation has useful utility during various steps.[8] These approaches have well-established risks to major structures, such as the ICA, JB, facial nerve along multiple segments, and even the anterior inferior cerebellar artery.[62]

Cadaver Studies

Earlier research by neurosurgeons investigated the use of navigation with endoscopes in the retrosigmoid approach to the IAC for vestibular schwannoma. In a cadaver study with 10 fresh heads, TRE measurements ranged from 0.28 mm to 0.82 mm, and the entire IAC was drilled out without violating the labyrinth.[64] Since then, cadaver studies investigating transcanal-exclusive procedures of the middle ear have been performed. Although not using navigation, a study by Master and colleagues[65] sought out to quantify the transpromontory surgical corridor required to reach the IAC endoscopically. Although creation of the fundostomy preserved critical structures in all 17 cadaver specimens, mean distance from fundostomy to the ICA was approximately 4 mm, with 2 specimens measuring less than 2 mm from the ICA. Some specimens had additional hypotympanic bone for removal depending on the height of the JB.

When an infracochlear approach is utilized to preserve hearing, image-guided navigation is helpful with such anatomic constraints (**Fig. 3**). In 1 study by Kempfle and colleagues,[66] endoscopic infracochlear dissection to the IAC with navigation was performed on 7 heads. Registration was achieved with 7 bone-anchored fiducials, and EM tracking was used. TRE ranged between 0.2 mm and 0.6 mm. No critical

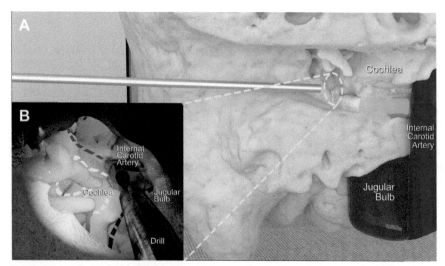

Fig. 3. (*A*) Virtual 3-D coronal view shows location of transcanal infracochlear surgical corridor (*highlighted in green*). (*B*) Virtual endoscopic view emphasizes proximity of critical structures.

structures were encountered. A similar pilot study was performed by Trakimas and colleagues[67] investigating a vestibular neurectomy using the same approach. The endoscopic, transcanal infracochlear approach was performed with EM tracking, with successful exposure of the IAC and selective neurectomy of the inferior vestibular nerve in 3 cadaver specimens. Postprocedure imaging was performed to confirm that the ICA, JB, and facial nerve all were intact without exposure. This work and others both identified feasibility for safe access through a transcanal, endoscopic approach, while also identifying anatomic variations of ICA and JB that may preclude patients from being surgical candidates.[68]

Another application of endoscopic LSB with image-guided navigation is for keyhole middle fossa craniotomy approaches. A cadaver study investigated feasibility of this approach for superior semicircular canal repair.[69] Bone-anchored fiducials were placed for registration, and EM tracking was utilized for navigation. Accuracy was reported to be less than 1 mm. In this study, navigation was helpful for a keyhole craniotomy to optimally position the bone window as well as confirm the arcuate eminence after identifying it endoscopically. These results were repeatable for 6 temporal bones. Benefits to this procedure in vivo theoretically would decrease operative time, minimize temporal lobe retraction, and minimize morbidity with a minimally invasive approach.

The Komune and colleagues[37] study investigating accuracy of EM tracking for LSB recreated the keyhole middle fossa craniotomy study and achieved access to the petrous apex using an endoscopic infralabyrinthine approach. Overall, TRE was 0.5 mm using bone-anchored fiducials, and no critical structures were encountered in cadaver dissections.

Clinical Studies

Transpromontory approaches without navigation for vestibular schwannoma have been described in multiple case series, requiring sacrifice of the cochlea.[63,70] For surgery with preservation of other structures, there are a few examples where image-guided navigation has benefit. One unique example is for endoscopic transmastoid repair of superior canal dehiscence. Creighton and colleagues[71] described a method of underwater ESS using balanced salt solution in the mastoid so that the endoscope lens and drill are both submerged. Navigation with optical tracking and fiducial skin markers facilitated a targeted mastoidotomy to rapidly expose the superior semicircular canal for repair.

A second example is a case report of a diagnostic petrous apicotomy. In this report by Plontke and colleagues,[72] an endoscopic infracochlear approach using navigation safely exposed a petrous apex lesion for biopsy without complications. The pathology demonstrated chondrosarcoma, and the patient underwent radiation therapy.

A third example is another transcanal, infracochlear approach to the petrous apex in a patient with a cystic lesion abutting the ICA and a high riding JB. In this novel report by the senior author, image-guided navigation was used for the surgical procedure but also was combined with 3-D printing and virtual surgical planning for preoperative simulation[73] (**Fig. 4**). First, segmentation of CT imaging generated a 3-D model with surface meshes. The model was used to build a mobile augmented reality (AR) application that allowed virtual evaluation of 3-D patient-specific anatomy. This model was also 3-D printed via stereolithography using 25-μm resolution. A CT scan of the model then was performed, and the series was registered with the original scan in navigation software. Registration accuracy of scans was 0.7 mm, validating the printing methodology. The 3-D printed model was set up with navigation equipment using anchored fiducials and the original CT imaging, and surgical simulation with the planned

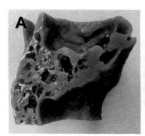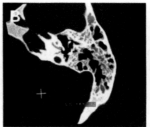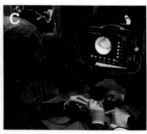

Fig. 4. (*A*) A 3-D print of temporal bone used for preoperative simulation. (*B*) CT scan of 3-D print was a 1:1 match with the original and able to be registered for navigation. (*C*) Transcanal approach to petrous apex was simulated on 3-D print with navigation. *From* Barber SR, Wong K, Kanumuri V, et al. Augmented Reality, Surgical Navigation, and 3D Printing for Transcanal Endoscopic Approach to the Petrous Apex. OTO Open. October 2018. https://doi.org/10.1177/2473974X18804492.

approach was performed (see **Fig. 3**). During simulation, the carotid canal was encountered anteriorly by a 1-mm burr and confirmed with navigation. This finding optimized the trajectory for the surgical corridor in live surgery the following day, and the procedure was completed without any complications. The patient had successful drainage of the cyst and was symptom free at 1 year follow-up. For this difficult case, virtual 3-D anatomy predicted the location of structures at risk, and 3-D printing with navigation allowed simulation to optimize decision making in the operating room for a successful outcome.

FUTURE TECHNOLOGY FOR SURGICAL NAVIGATION IN THE LATERAL SKULL BASE

Selesnick and colleagues'[14] description of an ideal image-guided navigation system at the turn of the century has stood the test of time. Ongoing research is developing systems with accuracy less than 1 mm, small equipment, and wireless, real-time image display. A recent publication by Zhou and colleagues[74] have made strides in noninvasive registration accuracy. A novel registration algorithm combines surface matching using imaging data with point-paired fiducial matching from a physical tracking tool to achieve mean errors ranging 0.16 mm to 0.23 mm and maximum error of 0.44 mm. Various registration strategies were incorporated into a custom image-guided navigation system comprising a portable tablet and optical tracking system linked wirelessly via Bluetooth.[34] TRE in a technical phantom study using fiducial screws was 0.20 mm,[34] whereas a study investigating noninvasive registration strategies reported TRE of approximately 0.5 mm.[58]

Additionally, AR likely will have a large role in image-guided navigation this decade. Recently, some microscopes allow AR projection of medical imaging into the digital eyepiece to view regions of interest superimposed in the surgical field.[75] One AR study for EES described a novel algorithm for navigation without physical trackers using computer vision algorithms to register CT data.[76] The proof of concept demonstrated mean error ranging from 0.2 mm to 0.38 mm based on employed algorithms. These findings show promise for next-generation image-guided navigation systems in endoscopic LSB surgery.

SUMMARY

Image-guided navigation continues to push the boundaries of endoscopic LSB surgery. Over multiple decades, navigation technology has improved performance enough to meet the demands of intricate anatomy in the temporal bone and surrounding regions. Modern commercial workstations have adequate accuracy below 1 mm, and each has its advantages and limitations. To date, invasive markers are the most reliable for accurate registration in the LSB. Ongoing research may improve noninvasive strategies.

As endoscopic techniques and other surgical technology continue to develop, image-guided navigation will need to follow suit. Once reliable accuracy is achieved for endoscopic approaches to LSB, there is a need for improvement in how data can be optimally utilized in computer-assisted surgery. Future research may investigate the use of augmented surgical displays with processed imaging data or surgical guides to decrease operative time and the risk for complications.

CLINICS CARE POINTS

Steps to successful navigation in endoscopic LSB surgery

- CT imaging should have slice thickness of 0.625 mm or less. MDCT, CBCT, and flat panel CT all are adequate to obtain high spatial resolution.
- MRI sequences should have slice thickness of 1 mm or less. These can highlight regions of interest superimposed with CT, such as tumors or cysts.
- Invasive bone-anchored fiducial markers provide the most reliable tracking accuracy. Some hybrid systems achieve accuracy less than 1 mm, but results in the LSB are highly variable.
- TRE decreases with an increase in the number of fiducials used. TRE is lowest in the center of a tracking sphere, so fiducial markers should be arranged appropriately based on the surgical approach. A smaller tracking area defined by fiducials is associated with a smaller mean TRE.
- Optical and EM tracking both are capable of accuracy less than 1 mm. Optical systems require direct line of sight, and accuracy is improved with proximity of components. EM systems are prone to errors from many sources in the operating room and may need frequent troubleshooting during setup.
- Some systems offer instrument tracking of the endoscope in addition to surgical tools.
- Preoperative planning can identify anatomic constraints in different anatomic regions, such as the location of the ICA and JB for a transcanal, infracochlear approach. Pneumatization of the hypotympanum and petrous apex makes surgical access easier with less dissection.
- Real-time image navigation does not replace fund of knowledge for complex, 3-D anatomic relationships. Images in navigation only confirm what landmarks are suspected by the surgeon. Visual feedback optimizes surgical approaches and efficiency.

DISCLOSURE

The authors have nothing to disclose.

REFERENCES

1. Bowdler DA, Walsh RM. Comparison of the otoendoscopic and microscopic anatomy of the middle ear cleft in canal wall-up and canal wall-down temporal bone dissections. Clin Otolaryngol Allied Sci 1995;20:418–22.
2. Bottrill ID, Poe DS. Endoscope-assisted ear surgery. Am J Otol 1995;16:158–63.

3. Rosenberg SI, Silverstein H, Willcox TO, et al. Endoscopy in otology and neuro-tology. Am J Otol 1994;15:168–72.
4. Cohen MS, Landegger LD, Kozin ED, et al. Pediatric endoscopic ear surgery in clinical practice: lessons learned and early outcomes. Laryngoscope 2016;126: 732–8.
5. Kapadiya M, Tarabichi M. An overview of endoscopic ear surgery in 2018. Laryn-goscope Investig Otolaryngol 2019;4:365–73.
6. Kozin ED, Gulati S, Kaplan AB, et al. Systematic review of outcomes following observational and operative endoscopic middle ear surgery. Laryngoscope 2015;125:1205–14.
7. Pollak N. Endoscopic and minimally-invasive ear surgery: a path to better out-comes. World J Otorhinolaryngol Head Neck Surg 2017;3:129–35.
8. Presutti L, Nogueira JF, Alicandri-Ciufelli M, et al. Beyond the middle ear: endo-scopic surgical anatomy and approaches to inner ear and lateral skull base. Oto-laryngol Clin North Am 2013;46:189–200.
9. Tarabichi M, Marchioni D, Presutti L, et al. Endoscopic transcanal ear anatomy and dissection. Otolaryngol Clin North Am 2013;46:131–54.
10. Zanoletti E, Martini A, Emanuelli E, et al. Lateral approaches to the skull base. Acta Otorhinolaryngol Ital 2012;32:281–7.
11. Anschuetz L, Alicandri-Ciufelli M, Wimmer W, et al. The endoscopic anatomy of the cochlear hook region and fustis: surgical implications. Acta Otorhinolaryngol Ital 2019;39:353–7.
12. Alicandri-Ciufelli M, Marchioni D, Pavesi G, et al. Acquisition of surgical skills for endoscopic ear and lateral skull base surgery: a staged training programme. Acta Otorhinolaryngol Ital 2018;38:151–9.
13. Azagury DE, Dua MM, Barrese JC, et al. Image-guided surgery. Curr Probl Surg 2015;52:476–520.
14. Selesnick SH, Kacker A. Image-guided surgical navigation in otology and neuro-tology. Am J Otol 1999;20:688–93 [discussion: 93-7].
15. Ecke U, Luebben B, Maurer J, et al. Comparison of different computer-aided sur-gery systems in skull base surgery. Skull Base 2003;13:43–50.
16. Labadie RF, Majdani O, Fitzpatrick JM. Image-guided technique in neurotology. Otolaryngol Clin North Am 2007;40:611–624, x.
17. Kral F, Puschban EJ, Riechelmann H, et al. Comparison of optical and electro-magnetic tracking for navigated lateral skull base surgery. Int J Med Robot 2013;9:247–52.
18. Jödicke A, Ottenhausen M, Lenarz T. Clinical use of navigation in lateral skull base surgery: results of a multispecialty national survey among skull base sur-geons in Germany. J Neurol Surg B, Skull base 2018;79:545–53.
19. Wirtz CR. Intraoperative navigation, with focus on the skull base. HNO 2016;64: 635–40.
20. Zanoletti E, Mazzoni A, Martini A, et al. Surgery of the lateral skull base: a 50-year endeavour. Acta Otorhinolaryngol Ital 2019;39:S1–146.
21. Horsley V, Clarke RH. The structure and functions of the cerebellum examined by a new method. Brain 1908;31:45–124.
22. Caldemeyer KS, Sandrasegaran K, Shinaver CN, et al. Temporal bone: compar-ison of isotropic helical CT and conventional direct axial and coronal CT. AJR Am J Roentgenol 1999;172:1675–82.
23. Jäger L, Bonell H, Liebl M, et al. CT of the normal temporal bone: comparison of multi- and single-detector row CT. Radiology 2005;235:133–41.

24. Dalrymple NC, Prasad SR, El-Merhi FM, et al. Price of Isotropy in Multidetector CT. Radiographics 2007;27:49–62.
25. Ozgen B, Cunnane ME, Caruso PA, et al. Comparison of 45° oblique reformats with axial reformats in CT evaluation of the vestibular aqueduct. AJNR Am J Neuroradiol 2008;29:30–4.
26. Lane JI, Lindell EP, Witte RJ, et al. Middle and inner ear: improved depiction with multiplanar reconstruction of volumetric CT data. Radiographics 2006;26:115–24.
27. Hsieh J. Computed tomography principles, design, artifacts, and recent advances. Bellingham (WA): SPIE; 2015.
28. Rafferty MA, Siewerdsen JH, Chan Y, et al. Intraoperative cone-beam CT for guidance of temporal bone surgery. Otolaryngol Head Neck Surg 2006;134:801–8.
29. Bartling SH, Leinung M, Graute J, et al. Increase of accuracy in intraoperative navigation through high-resolution flat-panel volume computed tomography: experimental comparison with multislice computed tomography-based navigation. Otol Neurotol 2007;28:129–34.
30. Siewerdsen JH. Cone-Beam CT with a flat-panel detector: from image science to image-guided surgery. Nucl Instrum Methods Phys Res A 2011;648:S241–50.
31. Gupta R, Cheung AC, Bartling SH, et al. Flat-panel volume CT: fundamental principles, technology, and applications. Radiographics 2008;28:2009–22.
32. Majdani O, Thews K, Bartling S, et al. Temporal bone imaging: comparison of flat panel volume CT and multisection CT. AJNR Am J Neuroradiol 2009;30:1419.
33. Sparacia G, Iaia A. Diagnostic performance of reformatted isotropic thin-section helical CT images in the detection of superior semicircular canal dehiscence. Neuroradiol J 2017;30:216–21.
34. Rathgeb C, Anschuetz L, Schneider D, et al. Accuracy and feasibility of a dedicated image guidance solution for endoscopic lateral skull base surgery. Eur Arch Otorhinolaryngol 2018;275:905–11.
35. Juliano AF. Cross sectional imaging of the ear and temporal bone. Head Neck Pathol 2018;12:302–20.
36. Pillai P, Sammet S, Ammirati M. Application accuracy of computed tomography-based, image-guided navigation of temporal bone. Neurosurgery 2008;63:326–32 [discussion: 32-3].
37. Komune N, Matsushima K, Matsuo S, et al. The accuracy of an electromagnetic navigation system in lateral skull base approaches. Laryngoscope 2017;127:450–9.
38. Juliano AF, Ginat DT, Moonis G. Imaging review of the temporal bone: part I. Anatomy and inflammatory and neoplastic processes. Radiology 2013;269:17–33.
39. Baráth K, Huber AM, Stämpfli P, et al. Neuroradiology of cholesteatomas. AJNR Am J Neuroradiol 2011;32:221–9.
40. Corrales CE, Blevins NH. Imaging for evaluation of cholesteatoma: current concepts and future directions. Curr Opin Otolaryngol Head Neck Surg 2013;21:461–7.
41. Feigl GC, Hiergeist W, Fellner C, et al. Magnetic resonance imaging diffusion tensor tractography: evaluation of anatomic accuracy of different fiber tracking software packages. World Neurosurg 2014;81:144–50.
42. Barone DG, Lawrie TA, Hart MG. Image guided surgery for the resection of brain tumours. Cochrane Database Syst Rev 2014;2014:Cd009685.
43. Embleton KV, Haroon HA, Morris DM, et al. Distortion correction for diffusion-weighted MRI tractography and fMRI in the temporal lobes. Hum Brain Mapp 2010;31:1570–87.

44. Fitzpatrick JM, West JB. The distribution of target registration error in rigid-body point-based registration. IEEE Trans Med Imaging 2001;20:917–27.

45. West JB, Fitzpatrick JM, Toms SA, et al. Fiducial point placement and the accuracy of point-based, rigid body registration. Neurosurgery 2001;48:810–6 [discussion: 16-7].

46. West JB, Maurer CR. Designing optically tracked instruments for image-guided surgery. IEEE Trans Med Imaging 2004;23:533–45.

47. Calvin R. Maurer Jr, Jennifer J, et al. Michael Fitzpatrick. Estimation of accuracy in localizing externally attached markers in multimodal volume head images. Proc. SPIE 1898, Medical Imaging 1993: Image Processing.

48. Maurer CR Jr, Fitzpatrick JM, Wang MY, et al. Registration of head volume images using implantable fiducial markers. IIEEE Trans Med Imaging 1997;16:447–62.

49. Elfring R, de la Fuente M, Radermacher K. Assessment of optical localizer accuracy for computer aided surgery systems. Comput Aided Surg 2010;15:1–12.

50. Grauvogel TD, Soteriou E, Metzger MC, et al. Influence of different registration modalities on navigation accuracy in ear, nose, and throat surgery depending on the surgical field. Laryngoscope 2010;120:881–8.

51. Widmann G, Stoffner R, Sieb M, et al. Target registration and target positioning errors in computer-assisted neurosurgery: proposal for a standardized reporting of error assessment. Int J Med Robot 2009;5:355–65.

52. Kral F, Riechelmann H, Freysinger W. Navigated surgery at the lateral skull base and registration and preoperative imagery: experimental results. Arch Otolaryngol Head Neck Surg 2011;137:144–50.

53. Henderson JM, Smith KR, Bucholz RD. An accurate and ergonomic method of registration for image-guided neurosurgery. Comput Med Imaging Graph 1994; 18:273–7.

54. Kristin J, Burggraf M, Mucha D, et al. Automatic registration for navigation at the anterior and lateral skull base. Ann Otol Rhinol Laryngol 2019;128:894–902.

55. Grauvogel TD, Engelskirchen P, Semper-Hogg W, et al. Navigation accuracy after automatic- and hybrid-surface registration in sinus and skull base surgery. PloS one 2017;12:e0180975.

56. Wiltfang J, Rupprecht S, Ganslandt O, et al. Intraoperative image-guided surgery of the lateral and anterior skull base in patients with tumors or trauma. Skull base 2003;13:21–9.

57. Wei B, Sun G, Hu Q, et al. The safety and accuracy of surgical navigation technology in the treatment of lesions involving the skull base. J Craniofac Surg 2017; 28:1431–4.

58. Schneider D, Hermann J, Gerber KA, et al. Noninvasive registration strategies and advanced image guidance technology for submillimeter surgical navigation accuracy in the lateral skull base. Otol Neurotol 2018;39:1326–35.

59. Caversaccio F. Computer assistance for intraoperative navigation in ENT surgery. Minimally invasive therapy & allied technologies. Minim Invasive Ther Allied Technol 2003;12:36–51.

60. Franz AM, Haidegger T, Birkfellner W, et al. Electromagnetic tracking in medicine–a review of technology, validation, and applications. IEEE Trans Med Imaging 2014;33:1702–25.

61. Ecke U, Maurer J, Boor S, et al. Common errors of intraoperative navigation in lateral skull base surgery. HNO 2003;51:386–93.

62. Marchioni D, Alicandri-Ciufelli M, Rubini A, et al. Endoscopic transcanal corridors to the lateral skull base: Initial experiences. Laryngoscope 2015;125(Suppl 5): S1–13.

63. Marchioni D, Carner M, Rubini A, et al. The fully endoscopic acoustic neuroma surgery. Otolaryngol Clin North Am 2016;49:1227–36.
64. Pillai P, Sammet S, Ammirati M. Image-guided, endoscopic-assisted drilling and exposure of the whole length of the internal auditory canal and its fundus with preservation of the integrity of the labyrinth using a retrosigmoid approach: a laboratory investigation. Neurosurgery 2009;65:53–9 [discussion: 59].
65. Master A, Hamiter M, Cosetti M. Defining the limits of endoscopic access to internal auditory canal. J Int Adv Otol 2016;12:298–302.
66. Kempfle J, Kozin ED, Remenschneider AK, et al. Endoscopic Transcanal retrocochlear approach to the internal auditory canal with cochlear preservation: pilot cadaveric study. Otolaryngol Head Neck Surg 2016;154:920–3.
67. Trakimas DR, Kempfle JS, Reinshagen KL, et al. Transcanal endoscopic infracochlear vestibular neurectomy: a pilot cadaveric study. Am J Otolaryngol 2018;39: 731–6.
68. Kempfle JS, Fiorillo B, Kanumuri VV, et al. Quantitative imaging analysis of transcanal endoscopic Infracochlear approach to the internal auditory canal. Am J Otolaryngol 2017;38:518–20.
69. Liming BJ, Westbrook B, Bakken H, et al. Cadaveric study of an endoscopic keyhole middle fossa craniotomy approach to the superior semicircular canal. Otol Neurotol 2016;37:533–8.
70. Wick CC, Arnaoutakis D, Barnett SL, et al. Endoscopic transcanal transpromontorial approach for vestibular schwannoma resection: a case series. Otol Neurotol 2017;38:e490–4.
71. Creighton F Jr, Barber SR, Ward BK, et al. Underwater endoscopic repair of superior canal dehiscence. Otol Neurotol 2020;41:560.
72. Plontke SK, Kösling S, Schilde S, et al. The infracochlear approach for diagnostic petrous apicotomy. HNO 2019;67:791–5.
73. Barber SR, Wong K, Kanumuri V, et al. Augmented reality, surgical navigation, and 3D Printing for transcanal endoscopic approach to the petrous apex. OTO Open 2018;2. 2473974x18804492.
74. Zhou C, Anschuetz L, Weder S, et al. Surface matching for high-accuracy registration of the lateral skull base. Int J Comput Assist Radiol Surg 2016;11: 2097–103.
75. Roberts DS, Parikh P, Kashat L, et al. Augmented visualization surgical microscope assisted microvascular decompression for hemifacial spasm. Otol Neurotol 2020. https://doi.org/10.1097/MAO.0000000000002717.
76. Marroquin R, Lalande A, Hussain R, et al. Augmented reality of the middle ear combining otoendoscopy and temporal bone computed tomography. Otol Neurotol 2018;39:931–9.

Endoscopic-Assisted Drug Delivery for Inner Ear Regeneration

Judith S. Kempfle, MD

KEYWORDS

- Endoscopic ear surgery • Inner ear regeneration • Stem cell • Hair cell
- Spiral ganglion neuron • Drug delivery • Synaptopathy

KEY POINTS

- Endoscopic approaches for future drug delivery offer a minimally invasive approach to the inner ear that could be used in offices.
- Endogenous regeneration of inner ear cells after damage relies on drugs to stimulate remaining cells in the inner ear. One possible route of application includes transtympanic delivery.
- Indirect drug application onto the round window membrane may be feasible in patients with residual hearing and relies on diffusion of the drug into the inner ear.
- In patients without residual hearing, direct drug injection through the round window membrane or via cochleostomy could be performed with the endoscope to target supporting or glial cells and to stimulate regeneration.

INTRODUCTION

Hearing loss and deafness affect approximately 6% of the world's population, according to recent estimates of the World Health Organization.[1]

To date, sensorineural hearing loss is irreversible, because damaged sensory cells cannot regenerate.[2,3] Hearing rehabilitation attempts with hearing aids or cochlear implants can give back some degree of hearing, but often, especially in more severe cases, hearing quality remains below that of natural hearing. More recently, regenerative approaches targeting sensorineural hearing loss have gained significant interest, in particular, pharmacologic treatments, and, although most regeneration approaches still are highly experimental, first clinical trials hold promise. Novel therapies are geared toward specific subsets of inner ear cells and are focused on both exogenous and endogenous regeneration techniques.

Department of Otolaryngology, Massachusetts Eye and Ear Infirmary, Eaton-Peabody Laboratories, C360, 243 Charles Street, Boston, MA 02114, USA
E-mail address: Judith_Kempfle@MEEI.HARVARD.EDU

Otolaryngol Clin N Am 54 (2021) 189–200
https://doi.org/10.1016/j.otc.2020.09.022
0030-6665/21/© 2020 Elsevier Inc. All rights reserved.

Recent advances in endoscopic ear surgery have opened the door to minimally invasive delivery approaches to the middle and inner ear, which could be successfully used for inner ear regeneration treatments.[4]

BACKGROUND

When it comes to regeneration, a lot has been learned from lower vertebrates, such as fish, birds, and amphibians, which can replace sensory cells after damage and spontaneously throughout life. Mammals, however, have lost this capacity due to their more complex inner ear anatomy.[5,6] Endogenous regeneration relies on remaining nonsensory cells, such as supporting cells and inner ear glia, which harbor stem cell potential and survive in the inner ear long after damage of hair cells or neurons.[7,8] Activation of these cells can initiate proliferation and transdifferentiation, causing them to turn into hair cells or neurons.[9] Exogenous regeneration involves delivery of outside cells into the inner ear. Hair cells and neurons, generated from stem cells and progenitor cells in a dish, can be transplanted into the inner ear in an attempt to restore the auditory circuit and normal hearing.[10–12]

Lastly, gene therapy and synapse regeneration comprise newer areas within the field of hearing restoration. With the development of viral vectors and novel gene transduction methods, gene therapy has enabled successful gene alteration and phenotype modifications in hair cells and neurons in animal models.[13]

Loss of synapses between inner ear hair cells and neurons is termed, *synaptopathy or hidden hearing loss*, and novel neurotrophic therapies are under way, aiming at reconnecting both cells via drug-induced synapse regeneration.[14]

Delivery of cells, drugs, or viral vectors into the inner ear faces many challenges, but the endoscope may provide novel applications and delivery routes to aid in the quest for inner ear regeneration.

CURRENT STUDIES
Advances in Exogenous Inner Ear Regeneration

Exogenous regeneration of hair cells
The in vitro generation of hair cells from human or mouse embryonic stem cells (ESCs), induced pluripotent stem cells (iPSCs), or mesenchymal stem cells (MSCs) is initiated by stepwise differentiation of stem cells into progenitors with a more mature phenotype, which can be tracked by expression of various otic markers at each stage.[15–18] The most important key hair cell gene is ATOH1, a member of the family of basic helix-loop-helix transcription factors and necessary for hair cell fate.[19] Both generation and regeneration of a hair cell rely on transcriptional activation of Atoh1.[20] Other classical hair cell markers include MYO7A and OTOF. Low differentiation efficiency of stem cells in vitro has hindered groundbreaking success of this approach in favor of endogenous regeneration. Coculture of iPSCs with chicken utricle stroma cells yielded hair cell–like cells with an electrophysiologic profile close to mature hair cells, but differentiation efficiency was extremely low.[15]

Transplantation attempts of iPSC-derived hair cell like progenitors into a mouse model with nonfunctioning hair cells demonstrated surviving grafted hair cells in the organ of Corti, however, at extremely small numbers and too small to obtain any functional hearing improvement.[21,22]

Exogenous regeneration of spiral ganglion neurons
What has been a comparably difficult attempt in regard to hair cell regeneration has proved more successful for auditory neurons: neural progenitors and neuronal cells

derived from human or mouse ESCs, iPSCs, or MSCs have been transplanted into murine inner ears to replace damaged auditory neurons. Successful integration and differentiation into neurons depend on various factors, similar to hair cell generation: prior to transplantation, stepwise differentiation in vitro into neural progenitors, and subsequently neuron-like cells, increased chance of graft integration and successful reconnection to hair cells. Human ESC neural differentiation and synapse formation was enhanced by coculture with cochlear sensory epithelium.[16,23] Expression of PERIPHERIN, GATA3, TRKB, TRKC, and NGN1 in a small subset of the ESC-derived neurons suggested somewhat of a peripheral neuron phenotype. Although basic steps of neural differentiation can generate sufficient numbers of neural progenitors for transplantation, differentiation protocols have to be optimized to obtain a high yield of purely peripheral spiral ganglion neuron (SGNs).[11,24]

In vivo assays included transplantation of ESC-derived neural progenitors into the cochlea in gerbil and mouse models of auditory neuropathy.[25,26] Most often, these transplantation attempts targeted the modiolus at the base of the cochlea-replacing neuronal cell bodies directly at the site of damage in Rosenthal canal is an anatomically complex goal that has not yet been achieved. Successful transplantation in animals or humans would require (1) survival of the graft without rejection from the host environment, which generally means a concurrent prolonged course of immunosuppressant therapy; (2) integration of the graft into the host environment, which is dependent on neurotrophic cues from surrounding glial cells and sensory epithelium; and (3) proper neurite and axonal fiber outgrowth from the graft toward hair cells in the periphery and the brainstem centrally, to create functional synapse connections. This is a time-consuming process. Complete regeneration including survival, integration, and neural reconnection centrally and in periphery.[11,25] Alternative transplantation approaches involved direct round window injections or cochleostomies to deliver cells directly into the perilymph or endolymph; however, overall cell survival was low, and only few cells integrated in the area of the modiolus or Rosenthal canal.[26,27] Overall, modiolar transplantation demonstrated slightly higher cell survival, and functional improvements seen with auditory brainstem response testing hint at successful restoration of the auditory circuit, which suggests that this is a more promising approach.[25]

Advances in Endogenous Inner Ear Regeneration

Progenitors with stem cell capabilities are present in neonatal ears and still can spontaneously differentiate into hair cells and neurons in vitro, but in adulthood, these cells lose their plasticity and become dormant.[7,9]

In the neonatal mouse, such stem cells were found in the organ of Corti (supporting cells), the spiral ganglion and vestibular ganglion (glial cells), and the utricle (supporting cells). In vitro, these progenitors expand and can give rise to most cell types present within the inner ear, and will start to express classic stem cell genes, such as Sox2, Musashi, nestin, islet1, and Pax2. Upon differentiation, early progenitor markers are down-regulated and cells begin to express mature neural or sensory cell genes.[9,20]

Only the adult vestibular system retains some limited regenerative ability when expanded in vitro, based on few postmortem studies conducted on adult vestibular tissue.[8]

Endogenous hair cell regeneration

Endogenous regeneration may hold a possible key to hair cell renewal within the cochlea. It relies on stimulation of the remaining dormant cells with stem cell capabilities within the inner ear.

Recent studies have demonstrated that subsets of adult supporting cells in the murine inner ear have the capacity to proliferate and turn into hair cells after activation.[20,28–30] Supporting cells with stem cell characteristics can be reactivated from their dormant state via pharmacologic treatments or direct gene manipulation in order to regenerate new sensory cells.

The supporting cells with key roles in hair cell regeneration include the third row of Deiters cells and inner pillar and inner border cells as well as the greater epithelial ridge. These cells express Lgr5, a marker of the Wnt pathway, which plays an important role for proliferation and cell fate specification during inner ear development.[28] These cells function as hair cell precursors and can be stimulated with small molecule drugs that manipulate the Wnt and Notch signaling pathway.[28–30]

Endogenous regeneration of hair cells mainly occurs in 2 ways—by direct transdifferentiation and by asymmetric division (**Fig. 1**). Transdifferentiation involves direct differentiation of a supporting cell into a hair cell, usually by activation of hair cell specific genes. This is possible due to the relative similarity of these cells, because both originate from a common progenitor during development. Becaused proliferation does not occur in this process, the pool of remaining supporting cells is depleted, which may lead to its own challenges.[30,31]

Asymmetric division follows proliferation of supporting cells, which divide into a new hair cell in addition to a supporting cell, and replenish the pool of supporting cells at the same time (see **Fig. 1**).

Early phase I clinical trials focus on Notch inhibition for transdifferentiation of supporting cells into hair cells or a combined approach of Wnt and Notch manipulation for proliferation of supporting cells with asymmetric division into supporting cells and hair cells.[29,32]

Endogenous spiral ganglion neuron regeneration

Extensive work in the central and peripheral nervous system has shown that, similarly to the story of hair cells and supporting cells, neuronal and glial lineages are related developmentally through common progenitors.[33,34] Glia of the central nervous system can be forced into a neural phenotype upon overexpression of proneural genes, such as Ascl1 and Neurog1.[35–38] The author and others have found that a subset of cochlear glial cells may represent a dormant population of early stem cell–like cells that is responsive to reprogramming. These Plp-positive glial cells of the spiral ganglion are derived from neural crest and continue to express Plp postnatally in glial cells along the peripheral and central SGN axons as well as in satellite glial cells

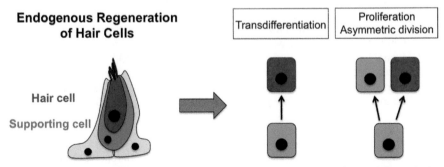

Fig. 1. Concept of endogenous hair cell regeneration. Comparison of transdifferentiation and asymmetric division. Hair cells are labeled in red; supporting cells are labeled in green.

surrounding SGN cell bodies.[39,40] In vitro and in vivo stimulation of these cells via direct delivery of proneural genes or drug treatments indicates that these glial cells can act to replenish lost auditory neurons in murine models of auditory neuropathy.[38,39,41,42]

Regeneration of Inner Ear Synapses for Treatment of Auditory Synaptopathy

Difficulty hearing in noise and tinnitus commonly are associated with hearing loss and may even be present in patients with normal thresholds in pure tone audiograms.[43] Recent work in animal models has characterized this hidden hearing loss as primary synaptopathy[44]: noise exposure resulted in a loss of synapses between hair cells and neurons, without loss of either cell type, which could be detected in auditory brainstem responses (**Fig. 2**).[44] In humans, cell bodies of hair cells and neurons persist for years after synaptic degradation,[45] which leaves an extended window for potential regeneration. Synapse regeneration in the ear relies on neurotrophic stimulation of neurons. Innate neurotrophins, namely neurotrophin-3 (NT3) and brain-derived neurotrophic factor (BDNF), are secreted in the inner ear throughout life and are crucial for neuronal survival and outgrowth. Neurons express tyrosine receptor kinases C and B, which act as receptors for NT3 and BDNF.[46,47]

Exogenous application of either neurotrophin or long-acting small molecule agonists in in vitro culture models clearly showed a positive effect on SGN survival and neurite outgrowth.[48–50] Overexpression of a neurotrophin gene or delivery of neurotrophin proteins to the inner ear in vivo similarly enhanced both neuron survival and axonal regrowth, in part with preserved electrophysiologic responsiveness of neurons.[51–55] Regenerative neurotrophic therapy with BDNF or NT3 or small molecule agonists not only presents a potential treatment of isolated synaptopathy but also may have a beneficial effect in patients with cochlear implants when performance is compromised by neurite retraction and additional neuronal damage.[56]

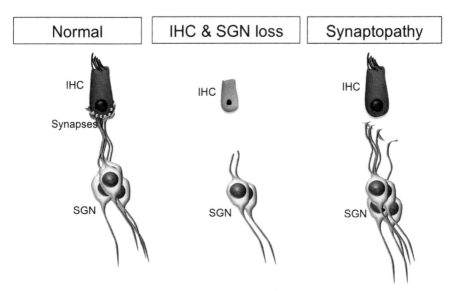

Fig. 2. Primary hair cell damage and primary or secondary neuron damage lead to loss of either cell type; synaptopathy is characterized by sole loss of synapses, whereas hair cells and neurons are maintained. IHC, inner hair cell.

Gene Therapy for Treatment of Hearing Loss

The advances in recombinant DNA techniques and viral vectors introduced the concept of single gene repair. Gene therapy aims at delivering specific genes into the inner ear for treatment of specific monogenetic diseases and potential regeneration.[13,57] Viruses, plasmids, nanoparticles, polymers, or lipid packages, to name a few, have been trialed as shuttle systems to gain access to the inner ear.[58–60] Various viral vectors with or without cell specificity successfully acted as vehicles for gene transfer, such as adenoviruses, adeno-associated viruses (AAVs), and lentiviruses.[61] Although adenoviruses are considered safe carriers and offer fast onset of gene expression, genes tend to be expressed only transiently because there is no integration into the host genome; but, on the flipside, they bear an increased risk of cell toxicity or immunogenic reaction.[13,61] AAVs offer another safe gene delivery vehicle, with longer-term gene expression (up to years) and reduced toxicity, but are limited in terms of packaging capacity and may therefore not be a suitable carrier for larger genes.[62] Lentiviruses or retroviruses are highly efficient in infecting a variety of cells in the inner ear and offer long-term gene expression and high packaging capacity but are considered much less commonly due to the high risk of toxicity and immune response.[61] Delivery of viruses carrying the Atoh1 gene into the inner ear in vitro and in vivo resulted in additional immature hair cells in nonsensory areas in the ear[63] and partially recovered hearing after gene therapy with Atoh1-AAV.[57,62]

First human clinical trials in a related sensory organ, the eye, have been successful in rescue of monogenetic defects, specifically retinitis pigmentosa and Leber congenital amaurosis, which resulted in partial vision restoration.[64] A phase I clinical trial is targeting supporting cell transdifferentiation via intracochlear viral delivery of ATOH1 in patients with sensorineural deafness, and several start-up companies have dedicated themselves to gene therapy approaches for treatment of hearing loss.[32,65,66]

Additional approaches are focusing on silencing and down-regulation of gene expression for treatment of hereditary diseases. Small interfering RNAi (siRNA) binds to complementary base sequences and, thereby, can interfere with transcription of genes. At the post-transcriptional level, microRNAs can inhibit messenger RNAs as a way to inhibit gene expression.[67] Transtympanic delivery of siRNA for single genes was successful in prevention of ototoxic damage, hair cell regeneration, and hearing recovery.[68,69]

Endoscopic Delivery Routes to the Inner Ear for Regeneration

Several possible routes for surgical access to the inner ear have been established in animal models and humans, many of which could be performed with an endoscope in the future.[70] Transtympanic delivery represents a relatively safe and indirect approach that keeps cochlear structures intact and could be chosen in cases of patients with residual hearing. Intratympanic injections of dexamethasone already are used commonly in cases of sudden sensorineural hearing loss and easily can be performed in a clinic.[71] Herein, the middle ear acts as a reservoir for a drug in solution, which can penetrate the round window membrane (RWM) and diffuse into the inner ear. This entails a sufficient fluid depot in contact with the RWM. Alternatively, a tympanomeatal flap could be raised endoscopically, and RWM could be visualized to allow RWM drug deposit (**Fig. 3**).

Larger molecules likely fail to cross the RWM in sufficient quantity or require prolonged application and a permeabilizing carrier to pass the RWM. Gel foam, alginate beads, poloxamer, and hyaluronic acid, among others just to name a few, have been used to increase permeability and contact time with the RWM.[72–74] In cases of direct

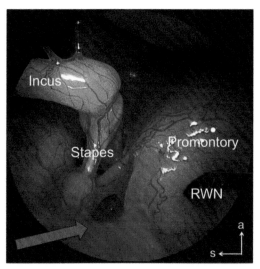

Fig. 3. Endoscopic view of the posterior inferior quadrant of a right middle ear (0° endoscope). Close proximity to the round window niche (RWN) makes this quadrant favorable for inner ear compound delivery (a, anterior; s, superior). Blue arrow demonstrates angle of injection.

delivery into the cochlea required, whether for cell transplantation or viral delivery, or in cases of larger-sized or negatively charged molecules, direct access through the RWM or via a cochleostomy could be performed under visualization with an endoscope. In certain select cases, endoscope-assisted canalostomies can be useful for viral delivery and in an attempt to preserve hearing. Direct intracochlear delivery likely results in highest treatment efficiency, with high drug or cell concentrations, and a high chance of reaching targets within the endolymph and the modiolus, but, as of now, this treatment modality is limited in its clinical applicability to deafened ears.[61]

In addition to the surgical approach itself, consideration should be given to the duration and degree of hearing loss. Cochlear fluid turnover suggests that drugs are eliminated from the cochlea within hours to days[75]: in cases of long-standing or extensive damage or loss of hair cells and neurons, stimulation of remaining endogenous cells may be insufficient to provide regeneration to a meaningful hearing threshold, or surviving neurons will require prolonged treatment over a significant amount of time for neurite regrowth.[76,77]

Multiple endoscopic procedures may be required to provide repeat treatments, or sustained delivery may be required. In this regard, first attempts with neurotrophin filled or prefilled or preloaded cochlear implants and osmotic pumps are under way to allow extended treatment for SGN regeneration and survival.[56,73,78] Current experimental approaches in animal models include a variety of viral vectors and bone-binding small molecules, all of which could be applied via a transcanal endoscopic procedure.[48,79] In rare cases of cochlea sparing, direct access to the auditory nerve that may be needed, a minimally invasive, endoscopic approach to the internal auditory canal via a subcochlear tunnel may be feasible.[80]

SUMMARY

Recent advances in auditory research have translated the concept of inner ear regeneration from bench to bedside. Currently, THE first gene therapy trials and small molecule trials are under way in humans, leading to the belief that the concept of inner ear regeneration, and with it, biological hearing restoration, may become reality in a lifetime. Endoscopic ear surgery offers a valuable tool for minimally invasive delivery of regenerative therapies to the inner ear.

DISCLOSURE

Consultant, Boston Pharmaceuticals.

REFERENCES

1. Organization WH. Deafness and hearing loss. WHO. 2020. Available at: https://www.who.int/health-topics/hearing-loss - tab=tab_2. Accessed August 05, 2020.
2. Lenoir M, Daudet N, Humbert G, et al. Morphological and molecular changes in the inner hair cell region of the rat cochlea after amikacin treatment. J Neurocytol 1999;28(10–11):925–37.
3. Raphael Y. Cochlear pathology, sensory cell death and regeneration. Br Med Bull 2002;63:25–38.
4. Kanzaki S. Gene delivery into the inner ear and its clinical implications for hearing and balance. Molecules 2018;23(10):2507.
5. Mammoto T, Ingber DE. Mechanical control of tissue and organ development. Development 2010;137(9):1407–20.
6. Warchol ME. Sensory regeneration in the vertebrate inner ear: differences at the levels of cells and species. Hear Res 2011;273(1–2):72–9.
7. Oshima K, Heller S. Sound from silence. Nat Med 2005;11(3):249–50.
8. Senn P, Mina A, Volkenstein S, et al. Progenitor cells from the adult human inner ear. Anatomical Rec 2020;303(3):461–70.
9. Martinez-Monedero R, Yi E, Oshima K, et al. Differentiation of inner ear stem cells to functional sensory neurons. Dev Neurobiol 2008;68(5):669–84.
10. Tang PC, Hashino E, Nelson RF. Progress in modeling and targeting inner ear disorders with pluripotent stem cells. Stem Cell Reports 2020;14(6):996–1008.
11. Shi F, Corrales CE, Liberman MC, et al. BMP4 induction of sensory neurons from human embryonic stem cells and reinnervation of sensory epithelium. Eur J Neurosci 2007;26(11):3016–23.
12. Rivolta MN, Li H, Heller S. Generation of inner ear cell types from embryonic stem cells. Methods Mol Biol 2006;330:71–92.
13. Shibata SB, West MB, Du X, et al. Gene therapy for hair cell regeneration: review and new data. Hear Res 2020;394:107981.
14. Liberman MC. Hidden hearing loss. Sci Am 2015;313(2):48–53.
15. Oshima K, Shin K, Diensthuber M, et al. Mechanosensitive hair cell-like cells from embryonic and induced pluripotent stem cells. Cell 2010;141(4):704–16.
16. Shi F, Edge AS. Prospects for replacement of auditory neurons by stem cells. Hear Res 2013;297:106–12.
17. Koehler KR, Nie J, Longworth-Mills E, et al. Generation of inner ear organoids containing functional hair cells from human pluripotent stem cells. Nat Biotechnol 2017;35(6):583–9.
18. Ronaghi M, Nasr M, Ealy M, et al. Inner ear hair cell-like cells from human embryonic stem cells. Stem Cells Dev 2014;23(11):1275–84.
19. Bermingham NA, Hassan BA, Price SD, et al. Math1: an essential gene for the generation of inner ear hair cells. Science 1999;284(5421):1837–41.
20. Kempfle JS, Turban JL, Edge AS. Sox2 in the differentiation of cochlear progenitor cells. Sci Rep 2016;6:23293.

21. Chen J, Guan L, Zhu H, et al. Transplantation of mouse-induced pluripotent stem cells into the cochlea for the treatment of sensorineural hearing loss. Acta Otolaryngol 2017;137(11):1136–42.

22. Chen J, Hong F, Zhang C, et al. Differentiation and transplantation of human induced pluripotent stem cell-derived otic epithelial progenitors in mouse cochlea. Stem Cell Res Ther 2018;9(1):230.

23. Hyakumura T, McDougall S, Finch S, et al. Organotypic cocultures of human pluripotent stem cell derived-neurons with mammalian inner ear hair cells and cochlear nucleus slices. Stem Cells Int 2019;2019:8419493.

24. Barboza LC Jr, Lezirovitz K, Zanatta DB, et al. Transplantation and survival of mouse inner ear progenitor/stem cells in the organ of Corti after cochleostomy of hearing-impaired guinea pigs: preliminary results. Braz J Med Biol Res 2016;49(4):e5064.

25. Chen W, Jongkamonwiwat N, Abbas L, et al. Restoration of auditory evoked responses by human ES-cell-derived otic progenitors. Nature 2012;490(7419):278–82.

26. Lang H, Schulte BA, Goddard JC, et al. Transplantation of mouse embryonic stem cells into the cochlea of an auditory-neuropathy animal model: effects of timing after injury. J Assoc Res Otolaryngol 2008;9(2):225–40.

27. Xu YP, Shan XD, Liu YY, et al. Olfactory epithelium neural stem cell implantation restores noise-induced hearing loss in rats. Neurosci Lett 2016;616:19–25.

28. Shi F, Kempfle JS, Edge AS. Wnt-responsive Lgr5-expressing stem cells are hair cell progenitors in the cochlea. J Neurosci 2012;32(28):9639–48.

29. McLean WJ, Yin X, Lu L, et al. Clonal expansion of Lgr5-positive cells from mammalian cochlea and high-purity generation of sensory hair cells. Cell Rep 2017;18(8):1917–29.

30. Mizutari K, Fujioka M, Hosoya M, et al. Notch inhibition induces cochlear hair cell regeneration and recovery of hearing after acoustic trauma. Neuron 2013;78(2):403.

31. Stone JS, Cotanche DA. Hair cell regeneration in the avian auditory epithelium. Int J Dev Biol 2007;51(6–7):633–47.

32. ClinicalTrials.gov. FX-322 in adults with stable sensorineural hearing loss. 2019. Available at: https://clinicaltrials.gov/ct2/show/NCT04120116. Accessed March 08, 2020.

33. Delaunay D, Heydon K, Cumano A, et al. Early neuronal and glial fate restriction of embryonic neural stem cells. J Neurosci 2008;28(10):2551–62.

34. Doetsch F. The glial identity of neural stem cells. Nat Neurosci 2003;6(11):1127–34.

35. Davis AA, Temple S. A self-renewing multipotential stem cell in embryonic rat cerebral cortex. Nature 1994;372(6503):263–6.

36. Ramachandran R, Fausett BV, Goldman D. Ascl1a regulates Muller glia dedifferentiation and retinal regeneration through a Lin-28-dependent, let-7 microRNA signalling pathway. Nat Cell Biol 2010;12(11):1101–7.

37. Wu SX, Goebbels S, Nakamura K, et al. Pyramidal neurons of upper cortical layers generated by NEX-positive progenitor cells in the subventricular zone. Proc Natl Acad Sci U S A 2005;102(47):17172–7.

38. Nishimura K, Weichert RM, Liu W, et al. Generation of induced neurons by direct reprogramming in the mammalian cochlea. Neuroscience 2014;275:125–35.

39. Kempfle JS, Luu NC, Petrillo M, et al. Lin28 reprograms inner ear glia to a neuronal fate. Stem Cells 2020. https://doi.org/10.1002/stem.3181.

40. Harlow DE, Saul KE, Culp CM, et al. Expression of proteolipid protein gene in spinal cord stem cells and early oligodendrocyte progenitor cells is dispensable for normal cell migration and myelination. J Neurosci 2014;34(4):1333–43.

41. Meas SJ, Zhang CL, Dabdoub A. Reprogramming glia into neurons in the peripheral auditory system as a solution for sensorineural hearing loss: lessons from the central nervous system. Front Mol Neurosci 2018;11:77.

42. Lang H, Xing Y, Brown LN, et al. Neural stem/progenitor cell properties of glial cells in the adult mouse auditory nerve. Sci Rep 2015;5:13383.

43. Liberman MC, Epstein MJ, Cleveland SS, et al. Toward a differential diagnosis of hidden hearing loss in humans. PloS One 2016;11(9):e0162726.

44. Kujawa SG, Liberman MC. Adding insult to injury: cochlear nerve degeneration after "temporary" noise-induced hearing loss. J Neurosci 2009;29(45):14077–85.

45. Viana LM, O'Malley JT, Burgess BJ, et al. Cochlear neuropathy in human presbycusis: confocal analysis of hidden hearing loss in post-mortem tissue. Hear Res 2015;327:78–88.

46. Green SH, Bailey E, Wang Q, et al. The Trk A, B, C's of neurotrophins in the cochlea. Anatomical Rec 2012;295(11):1877–95.

47. Ernfors P, Lee KF, Kucera J, et al. Lack of neurotrophin-3 leads to deficiencies in the peripheral nervous system and loss of limb proprioceptive afferents. Cell 1994;77(4):503–12.

48. Kempfle JS, Nguyen K, Hamadani C, et al. Bisphosphonate-linked TrkB agonist: cochlea-targeted delivery of a neurotrophic agent as a strategy for the treatment of hearing loss. Bioconjug Chem 2018;29(4):1240–50.

49. Yu Q, Chang Q, Liu X, et al. Protection of spiral ganglion neurons from degeneration using small-molecule TrkB receptor agonists. J Neurosci 2013;33(32):13042–52.

50. Richardson RT, O'Leary S, Wise A, et al. A single dose of neurotrophin-3 to the cochlea surrounds spiral ganglion neurons and provides trophic support. Hear Res 2005;204(1–2):37–47.

51. McGuinness SL, Shepherd RK. Exogenous BDNF rescues rat spiral ganglion neurons in vivo. Otol Neurotol 2005;26(5):1064–72.

52. Wan G, Gomez-Casati ME, Gigliello AR, et al. Neurotrophin-3 regulates ribbon synapse density in the cochlea and induces synapse regeneration after acoustic trauma. Elife 2014;3:e03564.

53. Suzuki J, Corfas G, Liberman MC. Round-window delivery of neurotrophin 3 regenerates cochlear synapses after acoustic overexposure. Sci Rep 2016;6:24907.

54. Sly DJ, Campbell L, Uschakov A, et al. Applying neurotrophins to the round window rescues auditory function and reduces inner hair cell synaptopathy after noise-induced hearing loss. Otol Neurotol 2016;37(9):1223–30.

55. Leake PA, Akil O, Lang H. Neurotrophin gene therapy to promote survival of spiral ganglion neurons after deafness. Hear Res 2020;394:107955.

56. Atkinson PJ, Wise AK, Flynn BO, et al. Neurotrophin gene therapy for sustained neural preservation after deafness. PLoS One 2012;7(12):e52338.

57. Izumikawa M, Minoda R, Kawamoto K, et al. Auditory hair cell replacement and hearing improvement by Atoh1 gene therapy in deaf mammals. Nat Med 2005;11(3):271–6.

58. Plontke SK, Salt AN. Local drug delivery to the inner ear: principles, practice, and future challenges. Hear Res 2018;368:1–2.

59. Salt AN, Hartsock JJ, Piu F, et al. Dexamethasone and dexamethasone phosphate entry into perilymph compared for middle ear applications in guinea pigs. Audiol Neurootol 2018;23(4):245–57.
60. Lajud SA, Nagda DA, Qiao P, et al. A novel chitosan-hydrogel-based nanoparticle delivery system for local inner ear application. Otol Neurotol 2015;36(2):341–7.
61. Fukui H, Raphael Y. Gene therapy for the inner ear. Hear Res 2013;297:99–105.
62. Akil O, Lustig L. AAV-mediated gene delivery to the inner ear. Methods Mol Biol 2019;1950:271–82.
63. Zheng JL, Gao WQ. Overexpression of Math1 induces robust production of extra hair cells in postnatal rat inner ears. Nat Neurosci 2000;3(6):580–6.
64. Tan MH, Smith AJ, Pawlyk B, et al. Gene therapy for retinitis pigmentosa and Leber congenital amaurosis caused by defects in AIPL1: effective rescue of mouse models of partial and complete Aipl1 deficiency using AAV2/2 and AAV2/8 vectors. Hum Mol Genet 2009;18(12):2099–114.
65. ClinicalTrials.gov. Safety, Tolerability and Efficacy for CGF166 in Patients With Unilateral or Bilateral Severe-to-profound Hearing Loss. 2014. Available at: https://clinicaltrials.gov/ct2/show/NCT02132130. Accessed March 08, 2020.
66. Akouos. 2020. Available at: https://akouos.com/. Accessed March 08, 2020.
67. Ambros V. The functions of animal microRNAs. Nature 2004;431(7006):350–5.
68. Mukherjea D, Jajoo S, Kaur T, et al. Transtympanic administration of short interfering (si)RNA for the NOX3 isoform of NADPH oxidase protects against cisplatin-induced hearing loss in the rat. Antioxid Redox Signal 2010;13(5):589–98.
69. Du X, Cai Q, West MB, et al. Regeneration of cochlear hair cells and hearing recovery through hes1 modulation with sirna nanoparticles in adult guinea pigs. Mol Ther 2018;26(5):1313–26.
70. Swan EE, Mescher MJ, Sewell WF, et al. Inner ear drug delivery for auditory applications. Adv Drug Deliv Rev 2008;60(15):1583–99.
71. Rauch SD, Halpin CF, Antonelli PJ, et al. Oral vs intratympanic corticosteroid therapy for idiopathic sudden sensorineural hearing loss: a randomized trial. JAMA 2011;305(20):2071–9.
72. Lambert PR, Carey J, Mikulec AA, et al. Intratympanic Sustained-exposure dexamethasone thermosensitive gel for symptoms of meniere's disease: randomized phase 2b safety and efficacy trial. Otol Neurotol 2016;37(10):1669–76.
73. Salt AN, Plontke SK. Principles of local drug delivery to the inner ear. Audiol Neurootol 2009;14(6):350–60.
74. Shibata SB, Cortez SR, Wiler JA, et al. Hyaluronic acid enhances gene delivery into the cochlea. Hum Gene Ther 2012;23(3):302–10.
75. Salt AN, Hartsock JJ, Gill RM, et al. Perilymph pharmacokinetics of locally-applied gentamicin in the guinea pig. Hear Res 2016;342:101–11.
76. Gillespie LN, Clark GM, Bartlett PF, et al. BDNF-induced survival of auditory neurons in vivo: cessation of treatment leads to accelerated loss of survival effects. J Neurosci Res 2003;71(6):785–90.
77. Gillespie LN, Zanin MP, Shepherd RK. Cell-based neurotrophin treatment supports long-term auditory neuron survival in the deaf guinea pig. J Control Release 2015;198:26–34.
78. Landry TG, Fallon JB, Wise AK, et al. Chronic neurotrophin delivery promotes ectopic neurite growth from the spiral ganglion of deafened cochleae without compromising the spatial selectivity of cochlear implants. J Comp Neurol 2013;521(12):2818–32.

79. Wise AK, Tu T, Atkinson PJ, et al. The effect of deafness duration on neurotrophin gene therapy for spiral ganglion neuron protection. Hear Res 2011;278(1–2): 69–76.
80. Kempfle J, Kozin ED, Remenschneider AK, et al. Endoscopic transcanal retrocochlear approach to the internal auditory canal with cochlear preservation: pilot cadaveric study. Otolaryngol Head Neck Surg 2016;154(5):920–3.

Pearls and Pitfalls in Endoscopic Ear Surgery

Sagit Stern Shavit, MD, Rahul K. Sharma, BS, Alexander Chern, MD,
Justin S. Golub, MD, MS*

KEYWORDS

- Pearls • Pitfalls • Surgical tips • Endoscopic ear surgery

KEY POINTS

- Using websites, formal endoscopic courses, and developing a mentor-protégé relationship with an experienced surgeon are useful tools while getting started with endoscopic ear surgery.
- Initially start with simple procedures such as myringotomy, tympanostomy tube insertion, endoscopic inspection of the middle ear, and raising a tympanomeatal flap.
- Dedicated tools such as suction round knife and up-curved and down-curved suctions are valuable for endoscopic ear surgery.
- Strategies to avoid and manage bleeding, prevent fogging, and familiarization with simple equipment troubleshooting are important to assure feasible, safe, and frustration-free endoscopic ear surgery.

INTRODUCTION

Within the past decade, we have seen a rapid increase in the popularity of endoscopic ear surgery (EES). The endoscope provides numerous visualization benefits for the surgeon, including a wider field of view, enlarged and detailed sight of the target, and high-intensity illumination of the middle ear. In addition, angled optics allow the surgeon to see and dissect around corners. Hidden recesses not seen by traditional microscopic ear surgery are revealed. These advantages help the surgeon overcome many of the visualization limitations of the traditional microscopic approach, reducing the need for a postauricular approach and extensive bone removal. Nevertheless, EES also has disadvantages, including lack of depth perception from the 2-dimensional (2D) view and the one-handed nature of surgery.

In this article, the authors discuss useful pearls and pitfalls of EES. Some of our recommendations may repeat those of other chapters, which is by design. The goal is for

Department of Otolaryngology—Head and Neck Surgery, Columbia University Vagelos College of Physicians and Surgeons, NewYork-Presbyterian/Columbia University Irving Medical Center, 180 Fort Washington Avenue, HP8, New York, NY 10032, USA
* Corresponding author.
E-mail address: justin.golub@columbia.edu
Twitter: @jsgolub (J.S.G.)

Otolaryngol Clin N Am 54 (2021) 201–209
https://doi.org/10.1016/j.otc.2020.09.016
0030-6665/21/© 2020 Elsevier Inc. All rights reserved.
oto.theclinics.com

the reader to understand common obstacles faced when learning EES along with their solutions. This includes how to get started, how to become familiar with common instruments and equipment, and how to gradually incorporate EES into the surgeon's existing practice. The authors also provide technical tips and ergonomic strategies that will help the learner become a more versatile and adaptive endoscopic ear surgeon.

GETTING STARTED

Microscopic surgery has generally been considered the gold-standard technique for accessing the middle ear, in part because there have been no compelling alternatives.[1] Because of its well-established role, most training programs emphasize or exclusively teach a microscopic approach to middle ear surgery. Therefore, most otolaryngology residents typically have little or no exposure to EES. Becoming a good endoscopic ear surgeon requires some initiative, self-directed training, patience, and a time commitment.

One of the major challenges of learning EES is simply knowing how to get started. Similar to all surgical training, utilization of online media such as videos and websites, as well review articles and textbooks are wise to consult before operating with the endoscope.[2] Two starting places are the websites of the International Working Group on Endoscopic Ear Surgery (www.iwgees.org) and several high-quality channels on YouTube (youtube.com). Online endoscopic videos are surprisingly high quality because the video feed, when maintained in high-definition (HD) resolution, mirrors precisely what the surgeon saw in the operating room (the same can never be said for microscopic videos). Formal courses throughout the United States and the world exist to teach and foster the use of EES in the modern otolaryngology practice. Although it is always wise to observe an experienced endoscopic ear surgeon in the operating room, seeing is quite different from doing. Therefore, utilization of a formal course focused on endoscopic technique can offer a more immersive, standardized, and rigorous approach. Courses generally involve cadaveric dissections on frozen specimens, which allow trainees to fully experiment with the endoscope and develop an understanding of the physical feel, novel angles and perspectives, and specific operative techniques. It is best to have this preliminary hands-on exposure outside the time-sensitive operative environment.

After completing a course, it is ideal to identify and keep in touch with a trained and experienced endoscopic ear surgeon. She or he can help answer the numerous individualized questions that will undoubtedly arise. This will also help uncover key nuances and pearls that might not be fully expressed in a teaching course. Geography permitting, observing actual procedures is helpful. However, observing recorded videos created by the mentor can also be high yield. Just as in residency and fellowship training, the mentor-protégé relationship will provide teaching, support, and guidance as a surgeon begin to practice endoscopic surgeries.

INCORPORATING ENDOSCOPIC EAR SURGERY INTO PRACTICE

Once a sufficient amount of preliminary preparation has been completed, it is appropriate to begin integrating the endoscope into practice. Initially, simple procedures or brief endoscopic inspections can be used to develop the hand-eye coordination required to progress to more advanced endoscopic procedures. Examples include myringotomy and tympanostomy tube insertion, endoscopic inspection of the middle ear during conventional microscopic surgery, myringoplasty, raising a tympanomeatal flap, and eventually simple tympanoplasties for small posteroinferior central tympanic membrane perforations. Given the high volume of tympanostomy tubes in common otolaryngologic practice, the authors highly recommend endoscopic tube placement as a way to get started even though there is little intrinsic benefit to performing the surgery with an endoscope as opposed to a microscope.

To avoid inappropriately challenging cases, which can be not only discouraging but potentially unsafe, the learner also begins performing EES under optimal conditions. For example, EES is far easier when the ear canal is wide. Thus, it is recommended to initially avoid procedures on patients with small ear canals, such as the very young or syndromic children with congenitally stenotic ear canals. Patients with large shoulders may restrict the movement and positioning of the surgeon, making it harder to operate. Similarly, most right-handed surgeons find it easier to begin with left ears, where a shoulder will not be pressed up against the right-sided dissecting hand. Moist, inflamed, or granulated ear canals can also make the surgical field drastically more difficult to navigate because of bleeding. Operating in an optimal environment will allow the surgeon to focus on the surgical technique and skills that will ultimately enable him or her to perform surgery in more difficult conditions.

Moreover, the authors suggest that the microscope be draped for all cases as one begins to incorporate EES into his or her practice. This will allow the surgeon to confirm EES views with the microscopic view and, more importantly, to easily abort endoscopy and approach with a more familiar two-handed microscopic surgery if necessary. Once the surgeon becomes more comfortable with endoscopic skills, he or she can refrain from draping the microscope.

To emphasize what has been alluded to previously, learning EES takes a great deal of patience, commitment, and practice. It is important to not give up too quickly because ease and comfort will happen; it simply takes time. Initially, longer operating times are expected and should be built into your schedule.

One important pearl is that when performing a tympanoplasty, one of the hardest steps with an endoscope is raising the tympanomeatal flap. Unfortunately, this is also one of the first steps of the procedure. When starting out with EES, the surgeon should consider performing this step with a microscope and then switching to the endoscope once the middle ear is reached. This can prevent the learner from getting immediately frustrated and discouraged. With time and experience, otolaryngologists can become efficient with using the endoscope and reap all the benefits of using a totally transcanal endoscopic approach to the middle ear from start to finish.

HELPFUL INSTRUMENTS

A small number of specialized instruments can increase the efficiency of the endoscopic ear surgeon, particularly when learning. The suction round knife is particularly helpful to decrease the difficulty in raising a tympanomeatal flap. Because of the one-handed nature of endoscopic surgery, a regular suction cannot be used simultaneously with a regular round knife. As familiar otolaryngologists well know, the skin of the ear canal is quite vascularized and it is common to encounter bleeding at first. Without a suction or specialized technique, the field can fill with blood within a second, obscuring dissection. The suction round knife combines both suctioning and dissecting, allows the surgeon to raise a tympanomeatal flap smoothly and continuously with good visibility of the surgical field (ie, not one obscured by blood). When a suction round knife is not available, a small gauze patty soaked in epinephrine can be used in concert with a traditional round knife. This technique is discussed further below.

Up-curved and down-curved suctions can also be helpful to reach around corners and under structures that can be seen with the endoscope, especially angled ones, but cannot be reached with straight instruments. Curved suctions are available in a variety of bends. To start, the authors recommend the minimally curved types, which will be easier to use.

As the surgeon's skills develop and case complexity increases, he or she may choose to purchase a dedicated endoscopic instrument set that includes a variety of angular dissectors as well as a diverse range of curved suctions. Examples include the Panetti endoscopic instrument set by Spiggle & Theis, Endo-Ear endoscopic instruments by Grace Medical, and other instruments and trays from manufacturers such as Karl Starz, Fentex Medical, and the like.

SETUP AND EQUIPMENT

The endoscope itself comes in variety of widths and lengths. When starting, the "sinus" endoscope, which is 4 mm $\times$ 18 cm, can be used for adults with large ear canals. The most commonly used "otologic" endoscope is 3 mm $\times$ 14 cm. Thinner endoscopes tend to enable better visualization at the expense of inferior optics.[3] Scopes shorter than 14 cm are not recommended because it will increase collisions between the surgeon's two hands.

The operating microscope requires a wide viewing portal for adequate illumination and visualization of the surgical field. Thus, additional exposure (ie, by drilling bone obscuring the view of the target) is often needed. In contrast, use of an endoscope allows the light source and optical element to bypass obstructions. Angled scopes facilitate this phenomenon by allowing views around corners and into recesses never seen with microscopy. Rigid endoscopes come with angles ranging from 0° to 70°. To begin, we recommend using the 0° exclusively. Eventually, the 30° can be added and finally, once advanced, the 45°. Larger angles increase the risk of inadvertently colliding into critical structures that are not in view (ie, the head of the stapes) and should only be used by more advanced endoscopic ear surgeons.

The 30° is helpful for visualizing peripheral anatomy, for example, the inferior hypotympanum, the epitympanum, or around a tortuous ear canal when raising a flap. The 45° endoscope is ideal for visualizing the mastoid antrum and the anterior epitympanum. Seventy-degree endoscopes are seldom used.

When using hotter light sources (eg, halogen or xenon) while operating, it is recommended that a light source intensity is turned as low as possible (usually under 50%) to avoid overheating.[4] Fiber-optic light sources were originally designed to illuminate large body cavities such as the abdomen. At approximately 1 mL in volume, the ear canal is significantly smaller in size and requires very little light to illuminate. Because of its small size, it also will heat up more quickly. Several studies have documented elevated temperatures in the middle ear due to heat transmission from the fiber-optic light source to the endoscope tip.[4] Heating can occur from distances up to 8 mm and was shown to cause thermal damage in vitro and in mice model studies.[5–7] Frequent repositioning of the endoscope, irrigation, and suction is recommended to facilitate adequate tissue cooling and prevent thermal injury. Overheating is less of a concern with newer, cooler light sources, such as LEDs.

The visualization elements of the endoscope consist of the light source, light cable, endoscope, camera, camera processing unit, and the video display. The surgeon should be familiar with common troubleshooting strategies when visualization is not adequate or simply nonfunctional. When faced with a poor image, one should first check and optimize the components. For image blurring, this includes first wiping the tip of the endoscope with moist saline followed by a defogging solution. If not improved, the back lens of the endoscope as well as the lens of the camera should also be wiped. All connections should be checked, including endoscope-camera, light cable-endoscope, and light cable-processing unit. Finally, the endoscopy tower (confirm power on, correct input) can be checked as well. Intermittent images (sudden change in color or flickers where the image turns off) can be due to a frayed camera cable. These checks are no different from what is employed in endoscopic sinus surgery.

The authors also recommend shutting off all operating room lights except for a single spot light for anesthesia and the surgical technician, which will reduce glare on the display and improve perceived contrast.

The use of HD digital cameras with compatible HD monitors, now fairly ubiquitous, is recommended. Three-chip cameras and HD digital cameras produce excellent quality images and feature automatic controls for color, exposure, white balance, and digital contrast enhancement. HD digital monitors as well as data management and documentation capabilities are considered standard equipment for the endoscope; they also exhibit better image quality when paired with the endoscope than with the microscope. High-quality images or videos may prove useful especially for teaching and sharing with the families. Newer 4K system scan provide even greater resolution.

TEACHING

Teaching otology using a microscope can be difficult due to the different views between the primary binocular lenses, the 2D side-optic, and the image displayed on the screen. The quality of the display is always inferior compared with the primary surgical view because it is stripped of 3D and brightness. Moreover, the area of interest may be entirely off-screen or out of focus during the surgery. Thus, the learner can easily have an inadequate view of the surgery and a suboptimal educational experience with microscopic ear surgery. In contrast, EES may provide greater educational benefits relative to microscopic ear surgery because the surgeon and observers all share the same view on a screen. This common view also allows the teacher to directly point out anatomic areas of interest and instruct the trainee on where to dissect. This also removes the need to switch positions so the teacher can first appreciate the optimal view (ie, via the primary binocular lens) before telling the trainee how to proceed with the surgery. Several studies have suggested that EES provides greater educational value than microscopic ear surgery.[8,9] In addition, otolaryngology resident physicians are often already adept with the endoscope prior to starting EES as a result of their experience with functional endoscopic sinus surgery.

ERGONOMICS

From an ergonomic perspective, EES is often considered to be superior to microscopic ear surgery. However, there is a paucity of literature comparing the ergonomics of endoscopic and microscopic ear surgery.[10]

The main ergonomic advantage of EES is the fact that it is a "heads-up" procedure, whereas microscopic surgery is a "heads-down" procedure. EES thus likely puts less strain on the neck and back compared with microscopic ear surgery.

Ergonomic recommendations for the endoscopic ear surgeon are aimed toward naturalizing neck and back position. It is recommended to set the monitor directly in front of the surgeon (**Fig. 1**). The monitor should be at or slightly below the surgeon's eye level. With such a position, the surgeon does need to turn his or her neck upwards, left, or right to properly view the monitor. The optimal monitor distance will depend on monitor size, image clarity, and surgeon preference. However, it is common for the distance to be between approximately 50 and 180 cm (20–65 inches).

Because of the seated nature of EES, using a specialized chair with both back support and arm support can delay fatigability and aches associated with prolonged sitting. Arm support should be adjusted to keep shoulders in a relaxed, neutral anatomic position to help resist the tendency of upward shoulder migration. The armrest height of the chair should be adjusted to allow for a 90- to 120-degree elbow joint angle when shoulders are relaxed (**Fig. 2**). Recognizing muscle fatigue and allowing for adequate break times is important to prevent long-term complications of chronic muscle strain.

THE SURGICAL PROCEDURE

Ultimately, the operative course is determined by both the pathology and the unique anatomy of each individual patient. However, following a few simple guidelines during EES can optimize workflow and improve the efficiency of operations.

One of the first steps is meticulously trimming hair from the ear canal. Ear canal hairs collect and retain blood droplets. Inadequate trimming will result in frequent soaking of endoscope tip with blood, which deteriorates image quality. Trimming can be performed using Bellucci scissors held parallel to the ear canal. Alternatively, small iris or Stevens scissors can also be used for larger, more lateral hairs.

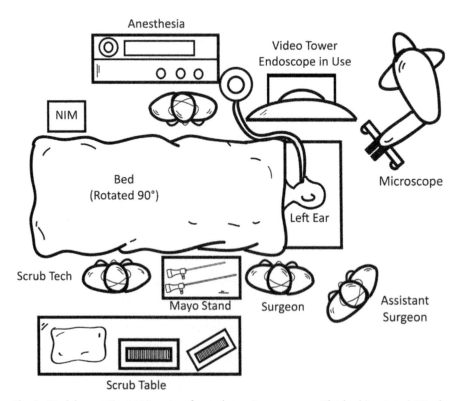

Fig. 1. Model operating room setup for endoscopic ear surgery. The bed is rotated 90°, the surgeon and assistant are seated in front of the ear, and the monitor is positioned directly across from the surgeon. This setup allows easy switching between endoscope and microscope. Alternative setups with 180° bed rotation are also possible. NIM, nerve integrity monitor.

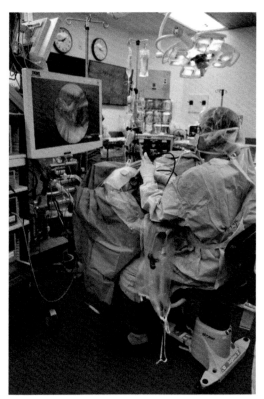

Fig. 2. Recommended ergonomic posture for EES. The surgeon is sitting with his/her back perpendicular to the ground. His/her arms are using the arm rest, allowing the shoulders to be relaxed. The screen is positioned directly in front of the surgeon, allowing him/her to keep a "heads up" neutral position.

Bleeding can be a major impediment to the success of EES, as hemostasis in the narrow space of the ear canal can be difficult, especially when the dissection instrument does not contain a built-in suction port. It is important to have multiple strategies to manage bleeding. Having the anesthesiologist lower the blood pressure and raise the head of the bed to reduce blood flow to the head and neck region can reduce bleeding. Opting for total intravenous anesthesia (TIVA) (eg, remifentanil and propofol), as opposed to use of inhalation agents, for general anesthesia is another strategy that may prevent excess bleeding. TIVA has been shown to be associated with less bleeding in endoscopic sinus surgery.[11]

Cottonoids, neuro-pledgets, or cotton balls soaked in 1:1000 epinephrine and applied topically can help achieve hemostasis. When using these topical agents, it is important to wait long enough for them to take effect before suctioning and working on the area again; working in another region can be done in the meantime. Absorbable hemostatic agents consisting of oxidized regenerated cellulose, such as Surgicel (Johnson & Johnson) or FloSeal (Baxter), are another alternative. Finally, frequent warm saline irrigation can help clear the field and also allow a moment to strategize for the next step.

Instruments containing integrated suctions can also be helpful for managing bleeding. A specially designed suction round knife is particularly helpful when raising the tympanomeatal flap. When a suction round knife is not available, a small (usually hand-cut) gauze patty or cotton ball soaked in 1:1000 epinephrine can be used. The patty is placed directly next to the dissecting round knife, which absorbs blood and buys more time before the field is obscured by bleeding. The patty itself can also be used to raise the flap, with the round knife applying advancing pressure from behind. The moment before entering the middle ear is often one of the most bloody. It is helpful to have a patty acting as a sink for blood, while a small pick or round knife is used to puncture the mucosa under the annulus and enter the middle ear. Once the middle ear space is opened, visualization usually improves.

Fogging or misting of the endoscope tip is another common problem faced during EES. This can blur and obscure the view. The use of a commercial anti-fog solution is recommended. However, these antifog solutions (which typically consist of alcohol, surfactants, glycerin, and water) have been shown to be ototoxic in guinea pig models.[12] Therefore, judicious use is advised. Wet gauze can also be used to wipe blood from the endoscope tip before rubbing it on the antifog sponge.

The one-handed nature of the endoscope is one of the most challenging aspects of EES. This is especially true with the management and positioning of ossicular prosthesis. One strategy to overcome this difficulty while positioning an ossicular prosthesis (eg, a PORP, TORP, or stapes prothesis) is to place small amount of Gelfoam on both sides of the stapes and lay the prosthesis on the Gelfoam. Using one hand, the prosthesis can be elevated onto the stapes head.

It is also important to think of the endoscope as a surgical tool used to achieve an optimal surgical outcome, as opposed to a goal in itself. Understanding when not to use the endoscope is just as important as using the endoscope. This is especially true in the management of antral and attic cholesteatoma. When learning the endoscopic approach, it is tempting to spend considerable time chasing the cholesteatoma and avoiding a mastoidectomy. However, failing to convert to a mastoidectomy earlier in the procedure when necessary can be a pitfall of EES. Consider designating a specific time frame for the cholesteatoma resection before converting to mastoidectomy.

SUMMARY

Understanding the challenges of EES and the solutions is crucial in developing the skills necessary to be successful with the technique. With sufficient knowledge, training, experience, and a few select tools, EES can be used by any otolaryngologist and incorporated into his or her practice. In addition, understanding the unique advantages of both the microscope and endoscope can facilitate development of a tailored approach to specific clinical situations. This will allow an otolaryngologist to become more efficient and versatile in addressing the pathology he or she intends to treat.

DISCLOSURES

Sagit Stern-Shavit: none. Rahul K. Sharma: none. Alexander Chern: none. Justin S. Golub: travel expenses for industry-sponsored meetings (Cochlear, Advanced Bionics, Oticon Medical), consulting fees or honoraria (Oticon Medical, Auditory Insight, Optinose, Abbott, Decibel Therapeutics), department received unrestricted educational grants (Storz, Stryker, Acclarent, 3NT, Decibel Therapeutics).

REFERENCES

1. Presutti L, Gioacchini FM, Alicandri-Ciufelli M, et al. Results of endoscopic middle ear surgery for cholesteatoma treatment: a systematic review. Acta Otorhinolaryngol Ital 2014;34(3):153–7.

2. Shariff U, Seretis C, Lee D, et al. The role of multimedia in surgical skills training and assessment. Surgeon 2016;14(3):150–63.
3. Neel GS, Kau RL, Bansberg SF, et al. Comparison of 3 mm versus 4 mm rigid endoscope in diagnostic nasal endoscopy. World J Otorhinolaryngol Head Neck Surg 2017;3(1):32–6.
4. Mitchell S, Coulson C. Endoscopic ear surgery: a hot topic? J Laryngol Otol 2017; 131(2):117–22.
5. Tomazic PV, Hammer GP, Gerstenberger C, et al. Heat development at nasal endoscopes' tips: danger of tissue damage? A laboratory study. Laryngoscope 2012;122(8):1670–3.
6. Kozin ED, Lehmann A, Carter M, et al. Thermal effects of endoscopy in a human temporal bone model: implications for endoscopic ear surgery. Laryngoscope 2014;124(8):E332–9.
7. Kozin E, Lee D. Staying safe during endoscopic ear surgery. ENT Audiol News 2016;25(2):3–6.
8. Anschuetz L, Huwendiek S, Stricker D, et al. Assessment of middle ear anatomy teaching methodologies using microscopy versus endoscopy: a randomized comparative study. Anat Sci Educ 2019;12(5):507–17.
9. Anschuetz L, Stricker D, Yacoub A, et al. Acquisition of basic ear surgery skills: a randomized comparison between endoscopic and microscopic techniques. BMC Med Educ 2019;19(1):357.
10. Shavit SS, Golub JS, Lustig LR. The risks of being otologist, an ergonomic and Occupational Hazard review. Otol Neurotol 2020;41(9):1182–9.
11. Wormald PJ, van Renen G, Perks J, et al. The effect of the total intravenous anesthesia compared with inhalational anesthesia on the surgical field during endoscopic sinus surgery. Am J Rhinol 2005;19(5):514–20.
12. Nomura K, Oshima H, Yamauchi D, et al. Ototoxic effect of Ultrastop antifog solution applied to the guinea pig middle ear. Otolaryngol Head Neck Surg 2014; 151(5):840–4.

The Role for Microsurgery of the Ear

Sujana S. Chandrasekhar, MD[a,b,c,]*, Sandra Ho, MD[d], John W. House, MD[e]

KEYWORDS

• Microsurgery • Otology • Ear surgery • Otoendoscopy

KEY POINTS

• Microscope-assisted middle ear and mastoid surgery remains the mainstay of currently accepted techniques.
• Endoscope-assisted middle ear surgery offers some advantages and some disadvantages when compare to the microscope.
• Understanding the history of ear microsurgery will help otologic surgeons mold the future of endoscopic ear surgery.

HISTORY OF MICROSURGERY OF THE EAR

In 1921, 100 years ago, the microscope was used for the first time in ear surgery by Swedish otologist Carl-Olof Nylén, when he transformed an ordinary laboratory microscope into an operating microscope.[1] The following year, this monocular microscope was replaced by a binocular microscope developed by Gunnar Holmgren. Because of its limited field of vision, very short focal distance, poor light quality, and instability, however, this microscope initially seldom was used, and many different models were developed. In 1951, the Littmann and Zeiss companies introduced a model that was easy to use and with which focal distance could be maintained while changing magnification. This allowed for the development of tympanoplasties and stapes surgery.

Anatomic examination of the ear began in the Western world only during the seventeenth century, and magnification was added to those studies at the end of the eighteenth century.[2] The clinical specialty of otology began in the mid-nineteenth century in Europe and progressed explosively in German-speaking countries at the end of that

[a] ENT & Allergy Associates, LLP, 18 East 48th Street, 2nd Floor, New York, NY 10017, USA; [b] Zucker School of Medicine; [c] Icahn School of Medicine; [d] TJH Medical Services, P.C., 89-06 135th Street, Suite 7D, Jamaica, NY 11418, USA; [e] House Ear Institute, Geffen-UCLA Medical Center, 2100 West Third Street, Los Angeles, CA 90210, USA
* Corresponding author. ENT & Allergy Associates, LLP, 18 East 48th Street, 2nd Floor, New York, NY 10017.
E-mail address: ssc@nyotology.com
Twitter: @DrSujanaENT (S.S.C.)

Otolaryngol Clin N Am 54 (2021) 211–219
https://doi.org/10.1016/j.otc.2020.09.025
0030-6665/21/© 2020 Elsevier Inc. All rights reserved.
oto.theclinics.com

century. Since 1860, loupe magnification was employed for ear surgery but only in rare cases.[3] As the Zeiss products brought microsurgery to the mainstream, in the 1960s, novel techniques, instruments and even suture materials were developed, to support not only ear surgery but also ophthalmology, plastic and reconstructive surgery, and neurosurgery.

Since the 1950s, the quality of surgical microscopes has of course improved. No longer does the lens have to be physically changed out reach the correct focal length for, say, otology versus laryngology procedures; the microscope can do this. The viewer now has a binocular piece. The closed-circuit image is clear and parfocal, enabling all in the room to see, learn, and participate. Exoscopes now are available, offering 3-dimensional microscopic views on screens for what has been termed, *heads-up microsurgery*.

HISTORY OF ENDOSCOPIC SURGERY IN OTOLARYNGOLOGY

Otolaryngologists have been comfortable with endoscopic surgical techniques since the mid-1980s. After some early attempts, endoscopes were introduced into paranasal sinus surgery with (Harold H.) Hopkins rods in the 1960s. Professor Walter's landmark book on diagnostic endoscopy of the nose was published in 1978. Given the frequent failures of Caldwell-Luc surgery, the morbidity of frontal sinus osteoplasty, and bleeding and visualization difficulties of performing headlight intranasal ethmoidectomy, there was a strong rationale for trying to improve surgical techniques for chronic sinusitis, and thus endoscopic sinus surgery was adopted, initially as an adjunct and subsequently as a stand-alone technique, called functional endoscopic sinus surgery (FESS).[4]

Dennis Poe and colleagues introduced the concept of endoscope-assisted ear surgery in 1995.[5] They presented results of 32 otologic and neurotologic operations, performed since 1993, that incorporated endoscope-guided dissection as a principal part of the procedure to reduce incision size, exposure width, and operative time or to access areas otherwise inaccessible. Initially, narrow sinus endoscopes were used; over time, more appropriately sized (length and diameter) ear endoscopes and then endoscopic ear instruments were developed, as interest has grown in this technique. The number of publications on use of endoscopes in ear surgery increased from 6 in 1990 to an accumulated total of 451 in 2018.[6] There was a clear shift away from diagnostic endoscopy, to endoscope-assisted surgery, and then, similar to the FESS evolution, to transcanal EES (TEES). That same article contained results of a survey further showing the increased awareness of the value of the endoscope and its increased use in clinical otologic practice.

ADVANTAGES AND DISADVANTAGES OF THE TWO APPROACHES

Rates of adoption of EES are seen that mirror but are not as complete as those for FESS 30 years ago. It might be wondered, Why is that? One problem is that some otologic surgeons do not perceive a problem with MES. With excellent outcomes and patient satisfaction, they may feel that adding endoscopes is not worth the time and energy or financial cost. Some still are on the upslope of the learning curve, either still using an endoscope-assisted technique or finding that endoscope-only cases take much longer as they learn to use the new instruments. Some are unwilling to work with the single-handed technique of EES for cases that could as easily be done with 2 hands under a microscope. Concerns regarding risk with concentrated light in the middle ear have been raised. A cadaver temporal bone study found that endoscopes maximally powered by xenon or light-emitting diode light sources resulted in a rapid temperature elevation up to 46°C within 0.5 mm to 1 mm from the tip of the endoscope within 30 seconds to 124 seconds and that elevated temperatures occurred up to 8 mm from the endoscope tip.[7] The temperature decreased rapidly within 20 seconds to 88 seconds of turning off the light source or applying suction. In vivo damage has not been reported. Caution should be taken, therefore, to ensure that the surgical support staff does not turn the light source up to the levels commonly used for endoscopic sinus surgery.

What are the potential advantages of TEES or EES, then? The list includes avoidance of a postauricular scar, allowing the entire operating room staff to see just as well as the surgeon, being able to see past a narrow ear canal to the anterior tympanic membrane, and being able to see around corners in the middle ear, hypotympanum, epitympanum, and protympanum; these are discussed fully in the other articles in this issue. Additionally, in low-resource settings, the cost of an operating microscope may be prohibitive whereas endoscopic ear instruments may be affordable; however, where the microscope already exists, it may be costly to bring in endoscopes and the necessary video tower.

In the authors' opinion, MES is not exclusively done postauricularly. There are many transcanal MES (TMES) procedures that are appropriate for the patient and the pathology. Because there often is a small postauricular incision made to obtain a fascia graft, making that slightly longer is not a significant morbidity. With gentle manipulation of the tissue, pain appears to be a minimal if any postoperative concern even with a postauricular approach. Avoiding even the small postauricular scar by using artificial materials, the authors believe, adds unnecessary cost and risk to a straightforward operation with ample local tissue available for repair. When performing middle ear and tympanic membrane surgery transcanal with a microscope, the authors find that the ability to use instruments in both hands allows for precise and efficient dissection. Any small amount of bleeding does not necessitate replacement of the dissecting instrument in the dominant hand with a suction. Using endoscopy to repair a small anterior perforation could be helpful; the authors often see larger perforations that extend anteriorly and may not be amenable to TEES.

The visibility around corners and the beautiful illustration of anatomy seen in cadaver EES dissections not always is seen in the living patient with inflammation and bleeding. This can be frustrating and result in conversion of a case to MES.

MASTOIDECTOMY

Three instrumental periods are recognizable in the history of mastoidectomy: the trepan period, the chisel and gouge period, and the electrical drill period.[8] Mastoidectomy, first performed in 1736 by Petit using trephination, then was codified using chisels and gouges by Schwartze in 1873 and then, at the end of the nineteenth century, Macewen introduced the electrical dental drill to ear surgery but it only gained popularity in the 1950s as microscopes and improvements in suction-irrigation were developed. The current ability to see clearly around corners with otoendoscopes appears to offer a nice advantage to the prior use of micromirrors. This may result in fewer mastoidectomies performed, particularly for cholesteatomas in the epitympanum. A study of 78 patients with attic cholesteatoma showed that TEES cases were done with better exposure, in less time, and with less postoperative pain than were the microscopic cases. No difference was seen for vertigo or air-bone gap (ABG) closure, and long-term outcome may have been better after TEES.[9] Perhaps EES is heralding a fourth phase wherein the indications for mastoidectomy become more limited.

THE LEARNING CURVE IN ENDOSCOPIC EAR SURGERY

The learning curve is familiar from other areas of otologic surgery. EES, however, provides new data that may be unexpected. A study of students, residents, and consultant surgeons showed that the younger people caught on to the endoscopic technique earlier and enjoyed it more.[10] A more traditional learning curve study looked at 20 type I tympanoplasty cases by an experienced microsurgeon in a teaching institution compared with the same surgeon's first 20 EES cases and the same surgeon's next 20 EES cases. Outcomes were either the same between groups or better in the second 20 EES cases; after an initial few slow EES cases, surgical times were the same between all groups. In the first EES group, 1 of 5 were converted to microscopic, whereas none of the second EES group was. The investigators concluded that maintenance of good outcomes and similar results can be maintained during a surgeon's transition to adopting endoscopic tympanoplasty and teaching it to residents.[11]

MYRINGOPLASTY AND TYMPANOPLASTY

Myringoplasty outcomes seem to be similar when comparing endoscopic and microscopic approaches, with the exception of more pain reported (from the postauricular incision) in the microscopic group in a study of 120 cases, and 3-dB better ABG gain in the microscopic group, which was statistically significant.[12] Pediatric myringoplasty can pose more of a challenge. particularly with anterior perforations in the setting of a narrow canal. A review of 22 children with tympanic membrane perforations showed that the anterior edge of the perforation could not be seen with a microscope alone but additional of the endoscope allowed the operation to proceed transcanal. The authors report 100% surgical success using this transcanal microscope-assisted endoscopic myringoplasty technique.[13] Another study looked at 73 patients undergoing type I tympanoplasty, retrospectively.[14] One-third underwent EES; two-thirds underwent postauricular microscopic tympanoplasty. Time of surgery was longer for the microscopic cases and there was a difference in pain on postoperative day 1, which was significant but does not appear to be clinically relevant. Otherwise, outcomes were the same between groups.

STAPES SURGERY

As endoscopic ear surgeons have become more comfortable, the use of endoscopes specifically for stapes surgery, first described in 1999, recently has gained popularity, with large case series published from other countries around the world. The United States has not been an early adopter. Those series report that otoendoscopes provide superior visibility and ease of use, while achieving similar outcomes as the microscope. The authors recently performed a systematic review and meta-analysis[15] comparing both techniques and found an increase in hearing outcomes in favor of endoscopy (2.6 dB), which was statistically significant but may be clinically trivial. There also was 15.2% greater incidence of dysgeusia in patients undergoing microscopy that was statistically significant. The heterogeneity of data must be taken into concern, however, and may negate these differences to at least some degree. The authors did not find differences in rates of vertigo or chorda tympani nerve manipulation or sacrifice between the groups.

Other systematic reviews comparing outcomes between endoscopic versus microscopic stapes surgery have shown mixed results. Nikolaos and colleagues[16] included 7 studies in their meta-analysis and found that there was no difference between the groups in postoperative ABG closures to less than 10 dB. They also found a 69%

lower chance of developing dysgeusia postoperatively and 98% lower chance of scutum drilling in the endoscopic group.[16] Koukkoullis and colleagues[17] reported on 6 studies and found no difference between groups in achieving an ABG of less than 10 dB. They found that chorda tympani nerve injury was more than 3 times more likely and dysgeusia more than 2 times more likely to happen with microscopic stapes surgery. They found no difference between tympanic membrane perforations or postoperative pain or dizziness between the groups.[17] Of the 5 articles comparing endoscopic to microscopic stapes surgery, Manna and colleagues[18] described significantly decreased postoperative pain and decreased rates of injury to the chorda tympani nerve in the endoscopy group compared with microscopy. They did not find any difference between the rates of postoperative dizziness, mean improvement in ABG, or operative times.[18] Pauna and colleagues[19] performed a qualitative analysis of 14 studies and found that, of the 5 comparative studies that were included, the prevalence of transient vertigo and chorda tympani nerve injury was significantly lower among endoscopy patients. They found no differences in prevalence of tympanic membrane perforation or facial nerve paralysis between the 2 groups.[19] Hall and colleagues[20] performed a systematic review looking at endoscopic stapes surgery only. They included 14 studies in their analysis and found that 95.3% and 76.6% of patients closed their ABGs to less than 20 dB and 10 dB, respectively. Chorda tympani nerve injury was found in 3.5% of the cases and dysgeusia in 5%. Of the 313 cases that were included in their review, they found 2 patients that had moderate sensorineural hearing loss postoperatively that occurred within a single series (0.6%), which is consistent with sensorineural hearing loss (SNHL) rates from stapes surgery in the literature (0.5%–1%).[20] They also found that perilymphatic fistula occurred on 4 occasions (1.3%), requiring subsequent conversion to microscope.

ERGONOMICS IN EAR SURGERY

Another reason given for conversion from microsurgery to endosurgery is improved ergonomics for the surgeon. Musculoskeletal (MSK) injuries are reported across otolaryngology procedures, worse with standing than sitting, but reported with both microsurgery and endoscopic procedures.[21] Maintaining 90° angles at the ankles, knees, and hips; shoulder and elbow support; and neck flexion of 25° or less results in the least amount of MSK injury in the long run.[22] For longer cases, even with using ergonomically sound positioning, it is prudent to push back every so often and even stand up to stretch out muscles and joints for 1 minute or 2 minutes. There are some anecdotal reports of surgeons using chair yoga techniques that can be done while maintaining sterility and without undue interference in terms of anesthetic time.

Some ear surgeons hunch over in order to operate through the microscope; others lean back without proper lower back or upper arm support, craning their necks. These are poor techniques. It is important that trainees are instructed in the proper positioning of the body, arms, and neck so that they can remain comfortable under the microscope in order to perform the delicate 2-handed microsurgery that is required. This aspect of education is, unfortunately, not commonly seen across surgical specialties.[23] **Fig. 1** shows examples of poor and good positioning for microsurgery.

Ergonomics issues can affect endoscopic ear surgeons as well. Some sinus surgeons report poor hand and scope size match; this problem is not of concern with smaller, lighter ear endoscopes. Keeping the nondominant hand that is holding the endoscope still as the other hand is operating can cause MSK strain, and elbow support is important. The monitor should be kept at the correct height so that the surgeon is not over-flexing or craning the neck in order to see. The term, *heads-up ear surgery*,

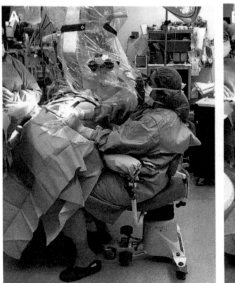
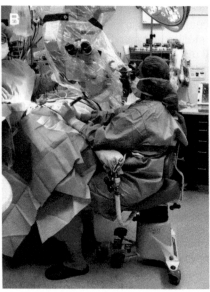

Fig. 1. (*A*) Poor microsurgical position of the surgeon. (*B*) Ergonomically sound positioning for ear microsurgery.

refers to using endoscopes or exoscopes to perform middle ear procedures; the correct position is head straight or slightly up as opposed to craning of the neck. **Figs. 2** and **3** show exoscope and endoscope surgeon positioning, respectively. In **Fig. 3**A, the screen is just above the full line of sight of the surgeon whereas in **Fig. 3**B, the screen has been moved down so that the surgeon's neck remains in neutral position. In both cases, the operating microscope is also in the room—visible in **Fig. 3**A and not in **Fig. 3**B.

Approaching the ear for transcanal or postauricular otomicroscopic or endoscopic procedures can be challenging in the obese patient. It remains to be studied whether using longer but appropriately narrow endoscopes in the ear provides MSK relief for the surgeon while affording adequate visualization and flexibility.

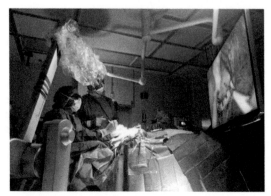

Fig. 2. Ergonomics of the surgeon during exoscope craniectomy procedure. (*Courtesy of* David Langer, MD Lenox Hill Hospital, NYC; with permission.)

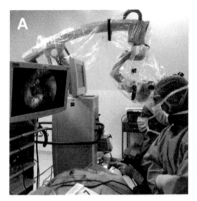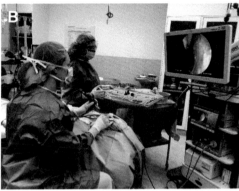

Fig. 3. (*A*) EES. The surgeon is seated squared to the patient; the assistant is standing; the microscope is draped and ready in the background. (*B*) EES. Note the placement of the monitor in the surgeon's full line of sight, avoiding neck strain, but slightly away so the surgeon is at an angle to the patient. ([*A*] *Courtesy of* Daniel Lee MD, Massachusetts Eye and Ear Infirmary, Boston, MA; with permission.)

DISCUSSION

Microsurgery of the ear remains the standard by which other approaches must be gauged. The importance of the ability to use both hands to operate, using suction while dissecting, using 2 microinstruments for dissection or placement of a prosthesis, and so forth, should not be minimized. Large classical series of chronic ear surgeries demonstrate excellent outcomes with MES for these conditions. Unlike the superiority of laser over microdrill in certain otosclerosis cases, it remains unclear whether EES affords any advantage over MES in this condition.

The authors encourage the otologic surgeon to retain comfortable familiarity with MES, while also developing comfort and skills in EES. Endoscope-assisted surgery is a reasonable way for the experienced MES surgeon to enter the EES world. No matter which technique is used, paying attention to ergonomics ensures physician comfort and improved patient outcomes for the case at hand and for the longevity of a surgeon's career. When doing MES, the surgeon should be aware of the limitations, particularly as they relate to a large anterior canal wall overhang or disease in the hypotympanum, sinus tympani, and epitympanum. When doing EES, the surgeon should be aware of the potential risk to middle ear structures if the light is too bright or held in 1 place for too long and that they may have trouble dissecting free disease correctly identified in previously hidden spaces and need to convert back to MES/endoscopic-assisted surgery techniques.

It is exhilarating to watch otologic surgery flourish and embrace new techniques. Surgeons, however, all took the oath, in whatever language they did so, of *primum non nocere*, or, *first, do no harm*. As surgical interventions are considered for patients, surgeons must pay heed to what is best for their hearing and healing outcome.

CLINICS CARE POINTS

- MES has been the mainstay of chronic ear and middle ear hearing restoration surgery for several decades.

- Endoscopes allow the surgeon and the team to see around corners that previously were relatively hidden and allow the entire operating room personnel to see what the surgeon is seeing.
- Proper ergonomic positioning is critical for all ear surgeons, no matter which approach is used.
- Two-handed surgical techniques used with MES have to be modified to single-handed techniques for EES, and the surgeon should prepare for a learning curve to adapt.
- The surgeon must be cognizant of potential trauma from the endoscope itself or from the concentrated light intensity on the middle ear structures.
- Mastoidectomy is done with microscopes; however, in epitympanic cholesteatomas, EES may facilitate in complete transcanal removal and avoidance of some percentage of mastoidectomies.
- Remaining facile with all techniques allows surgeons to offer the correct operation for the disease and the patient.

DISCLOSURE

The authors have nothing to disclose.

REFERENCES

1. Mudry A. The history of the microscope for use in ear surgery. Am J Otol 2000; 21(6):877–86.
2. Pappas DG. Otology through the ages. Otolaryngol Head Neck Surg 1996; 114(2):173–96.
3. Haeseker B. Microchirurgie, de 'kleine' chirurgische revolutie uit de medische geschiedenis van de afgelopen eeuw. [[Microsurgery, a 'small' surgical revolution in the medical history of the 20th century]]. Ned Tijdschr Geneeskd 1999;143(16): 858–64.
4. Tajudeen BA, Kennedy DW. Thirty years of endoscopic sinus surgery: what have we learned? World J Otorhinolaryngol Head Neck Surg 2017;3(2):115–21.
5. Bollrill ID, Poe DS. Endoscopic ear surgery, ANS papers. The Am J Otology 1995;158–63.
6. Kapadiya M, Tarabichi M. An overview of endoscopic ear surgery in 2018. Laryngoscope Investig Otolaryngol 2019;4(3):365–73.
7. Kozin ED, Lehmann A, Carter M, et al. Thermal effects of endoscopy in a human temporal bone model: implications for endoscopic ear surgery. Laryngoscope 2014;124(8):E332–9.
8. Mudry A. History of instruments used for mastoidectomy. J Laryngol Otol 2009; 123(6):583–9.
9. Das A, Mitra S, Ghosh D, et al. Endoscopic versus microscopic management of attic cholesteatoma: a randomized controlled trial. Laryngoscope 2019;130(10): 2461–6.
10. Anschuetz L, Stricker D, Yacoub A, et al. Acquisition of basic ear surgery skills: a randomized comparison between endoscopic and microscopic techniques. BMC Med Educ 2019;19(1):357.
11. Li B, Asche S, Yang R, et al. Outcomes of adopting endoscopic tympanoplasty in an academic teaching hospital. Ann Otol Rhinol Laryngol 2019;128(6):548–55.

12. Jyothi AC, Shrikrishna BH, Kulkarni NH, et al. Endoscopic myringoplasty versus microscopic myringoplasty in tubotympanic CSOM: A comparative study of 120 cases. Indian J Otolaryngol Head Neck Surg 2017;69(3):357–62.
13. Migirov L, Wolf M. Transcanal microscope-assisted endoscopic myringoplasty in children. BMC Pediatr 2015;15:32.
14. Choi N, Noh Y, Park W, et al. Comparison of endoscopic tympanoplasty to microscopic tympanoplasty. Clin Exp Otorhinolaryngol 2017;10(1):44–9.
15. Ho S, Patel P, Ballard D, et al, in press.
16. Nikolaos T, Aikaterini T, Dimitrios D, et al. Does endoscopic stapedotomy increase hearing restoration rates comparing to microscopic? A systematic review and meta-analysis. Eur Arch Otorhinolaryngol 2018;275(12):2905–13.
17. Koukkoullis A, Tóth I, Gede N, et al. Endoscopic versus microscopic stapes surgery outcomes: a meta-analysis and systematic review. Laryngoscope 2019;130(8):2019–27.
18. Manna S, Kaul VF, Gray ML, et al. Endoscopic versus microscopic middle ear surgery: a meta-analysis of outcomes following tympanoplasty and stapes surgery. Otol Neurotol 2019 Sep;40(8):983–93.
19. Pauna HF, Pereira RC, Monsanto RC, et al. A comparison between endoscopic and microscopic approaches for stapes surgery: a systematic review. J Laryngol Otol 2020;134(5):398–403.
20. Hall AC, Mandavia R, Selvadurai D. Total endoscopic stapes surgery: Systematic review and pooled analysis of audiological outcomes. Laryngoscope 2019;130(5):1282–6.
21. Vaisbuch Y, Aaron KA, Moore JM, et al. Ergonomic hazards in otolaryngology. Laryngoscope 2019;129(2):370–6.
22. Available at: https://surgery.duke.edu/news/duke-surgery-introduces-ergonomics-program-improve-surgeon-health#:%7E:text=Peer%2DBased%20Ergonomics%20Training,on%20correct%20postures%20during%20surgery. Accessed October 17, 2020.
23. Epstein S, Tran BN, Capone AC, et al. The current state of surgical ergonomics education in U.S. surgical training. Ann Surg 2019;269(4):778–84.

Future of Endoscopic Ear Surgery

Joao Flavio Nogueira, MD[a],*, Raquel de Sousa Lobo Ferreira Querido, MD[b],
Janaina Gonçalves da Silva Leite, MD, MS[c], Ticiana Cabral da Costa, MD[d]

KEYWORDS

- Endoscopic ear surgery • Transcanal endoscopic ear surgery • Ear surgery
- Minimally invasive ear surgery • Otoendoscopy

INTRODUCTION

Endoscopic ear surgery (EES) has gained popularity in recent years, becoming standard practice in otology centers around the world as an adjunct to conventional microscopic surgery and as a sole tool for limited disease.

Reports on EES started to appear in the literature in 1990 thanks to the work of Thomassin and colleagues,[1,2] Tarabich and colleagues,[3] and Poe and colleagues.[4] Thomassin used the endoscope as an adjuvant tool to work on the epitympanic recess and posterior sinus. Later, McKennan[5] described the technique of endoscopic "second look," establishing the effectiveness of the endoscope in detecting residual or recurrent disease. Magnan and colleagues[6] used the endoscope in the cerebellopontine angle and they were the first to use the expression "looking around the corner," now widely cited by endoscopic ear surgeons as one of the advantages of the endoscope over the microscope. In 1997, Tarabichi[3] was the first to describe a fully endoscopic technique for removal of middle ear cholesteatoma.

In 2004 we started seeing a gradual introduction of transcanal endoscopic techniques to treat middle ear diseases. Endoscopes were primarily used for the visualization of hidden areas, such as the posterior epitympanum during classic microscopic tympanoplasties.[7] Gradually, it was also used during operations, such as myringoplasty, tympanoplasty, ossiculoplasty, and cholesteatoma resection, to replace the microscope as the main tool in middle ear surgery.[8,9]

Now we like the term "transcanal endoscopic ear surgery" (TEES) to describe fully endoscopic minimally invasive procedures. Such surgeries offers several benefits when compared with conventional binocular retroauricular microscopic

[a] Medicine Faculty, State University of Ceará, Dr. Silas Munguba Av., 1700, Fortaleza 60741-000, Brazil; [b] Columbia University, Department of Otolaryngology–Head and Neck Surgery, P & S 11-452, 630 W. 168th Street, New York, NY 10032, USA; [c] Federal University of Ceará, Costa Mendes St., 1608, Fortaleza 60416-200, Brazil; [d] Cepto – Otos, Carolina Sucupira St., 1151, Fortaleza 60140-120, Brazil
* Corresponding author.
E-mail address: joaoflavioce@hotmail.com

Otolaryngol Clin N Am 54 (2021) 221–231
https://doi.org/10.1016/j.otc.2020.09.023
0030-6665/21/© 2020 Elsevier Inc. All rights reserved.

approaches, including a wide visualization of the surgical field,[10] enhanced optics with higher amplification, ocular access to hidden areas of the middle ear, avoidance of unnecessary incisions and soft tissue dissections, and a decreased operative time and less postoperative morbidity. However, the main disadvantage of EES is that the surgery has to be performed with one single hand, which is certainly restrictive for an ear surgeon who has been trained operating with two hands under otologic microscopic views for years and this certainly requires a learning period and perseverance.

Endoscopic instrumentation, techniques, and knowledge have improved during the last few years, and we believe that, in the future, endoscopic surgical techniques will gain even more importance in otologic surgery.

ENDOSCOPIC EAR SURGERY EQUIPMENT

Fundamental tools needed for endoscopic middle ear surgery incorporates[11] a light source, rigid endoscopes (0° and 30°, and in some cases 45°),[12] and an HD3-CCD camera and video screen.[13] Choices of different lights at different prices are easily accessible, such as halogen, light-emanating diode (LED), and xenon lights. There is no conclusive information advocating any of the sources of light and presently the choice depends on the surgeon's inclinations and accessibility.[14] It is important to mention that any of these light sources should never be at fully 100% capability. The middle ear cavity is small and to have a great view the surgeon needs no more than 40% of light power. This also reduces the probability of thermal injuries in middle ear structures.

Endoscopic camera systems are accessible through an assortment of sellers. The fundamental necessity for a camera system is a 3-CCD camera. The 3-CCD cameras allow for high-definition and clear video picture quality by depending on individual CCDs for red, green, and blue light. Single CCD cameras tend to "red out" and become saturated when used in a small area that contains bleeding. Currently, otologic and sinus surgery light sources are indistinguishable and are commonly accessible in otolaryngology operating theaters. Although not essential, nowadays there are 3-CCD high-definition (1080p) and 4K cameras. These produce a high-quality image (**Figs. 1–3**).

The diameters for the rigid endoscopes used in ear surgery are usually 2.7, 3, and 4 mm. If the outer canal is wide enough, EES or TEES is completed using a 4-mm

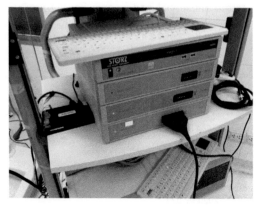

Fig. 1. 3-CCD HD camera.

3mm diameter x 14cm length

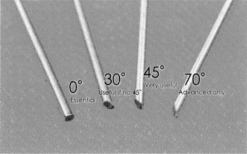

Fig. 2. Examples of the most used endoscopes in current EES.

diameter scope. TEES endoscopic shaft lengths are ordinarily 11, 14, and 18 cm in length. There is no evidence to conclude that there is an ideal endoscopic measurement and the choice depends on the surgeon's inclination, accessibility, and patient anatomy.[14]

HOLDER

Endoscope/camera holders have been designed to facilitate and allow two-handed EES. An ideal endoscope holder should be easy to set up, easily controlled, provide

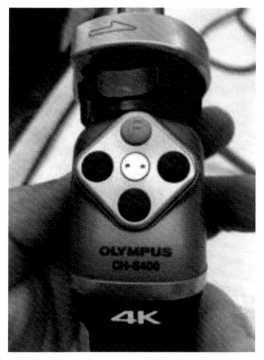

Fig. 3. Example of a 4K camera.

a variety of angled views, and allow the surgeon to operate with two hands, thus facilitating tympanomeatal flap elevation, delicate dissections of diseases from the ossicular chain, and allowing constant suctioning when needed for a blood-free operative site.[15]

Although endoscope holders have been designed to facilitate two-handed procedures, there are still some certain technical difficulties: (1) because of the narrowness of the external ear canal, in addition to the endoscope, there must be sufficient room for two surgical instruments; (2) during hemorrhage, the manipulation of the endoscope in and out of the operative field may be time consuming; (3) if the patient moves abruptly during the operation, an endoscope placed in the fixed position could cause injury to the outer and/or middle ear canal; and (4) because of the heat generated and thermal trauma risk of the stationary endoscope in the middle ear certain questions are raised regarding its long-term safety (**Fig. 4**).[16]

THREE-DIMENSIONAL ENDOSCOPIC EAR SURGERY

EES started to gain popularity with the release of high-definition camera systems with image quality a thousand times more detailed than with a standard camera. Considering the microscopic size of middle ear structures and the presence of important neurovascular structures in a small space the use of low-definition systems could negatively affect the performance and outcomes of EES. Since the studies by Presutti[7] and Marchioni and colleagues[9,17,18] who used the new high-definition system to study the endoscopic anatomy of the attic and retrotympanum, EES started to become a widely accepted technique for the management of middle ear disease.

Despite these technical improvements, the lack of depth perception provided by the two-dimensional (2D) vision and the need to operate with only one hand are the most cited limitation in EES. Even though an experienced endoscopic surgeon could overcome the loss of the sense of depth using other visual cues and anatomic knowledge,

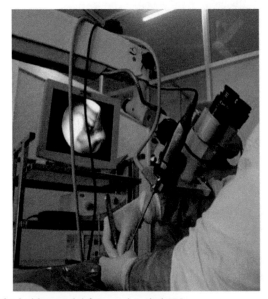

Fig. 4. Example of a holder model for two-handed EES.

a system that provides a three-dimensional (3D) image could be beneficial for beginners and more experienced surgeons.

The use of a 3D high-definition system has already been reported in some experimental studies in the laparoscopic and gynecologic fields.[19,20] However, the diameter (more than 4 mm) of the endoscope limited their use in ear surgery because the diameter of the external auditory canal is an important limiting factor.

With the release of a 4-mm high-definition 3D endoscope, this technology is now suitable for use in ear surgery (**Figs. 5** and **6**).

In their study, Bernardeschi and colleagues[21] used 4-mm 0° and 30° angled 3D endoscopes. These endoscopes incorporated the HD camera with a resolution of 1920 × 1080 pixels with two integrated video chips. The frame rate was 50/60 Hz, working length was 175 mm, and weight was 295 g. The light source was a POWER LED 300 cold light source. It was possible to change from 3D to 2D high-resolution images with the click of a button, which is an attractive feature for those surgeons who are not comfortable with 3D vision.[21]

However this new system showed some limitations: (1) no diameters less than 4 mm are available, and this could be an issue when dealing with a narrow external auditory canal or in pediatric cases; (2) only two angled endoscopes (0° and 30°) are currently available; and (3) the 3D endoscope has digital zoom capability compared with the 2D system, which has optical zoom, and this could induce some loss of resolution when zooming with the 3D system.

THREE-DIMENSIONAL EXOSCOPES

The microscope has long been considered the best tool for microsurgical visualization.[22] However, it is limited by positioning at extreme angles, and otolaryngologists are often forced into awkward positions with little freedom of motion for extended periods of time, which can explain the high prevalence of neck and back pain with long-term detrimental effects.[23]

A new surgical visualization system called the 3D exoscope system is a viable alternative to surgical microscopes for otologic and neurotologic surgery.[24,25] The 3D exoscope is meant to be exterior to the body surface like a microscope and to have dual image sensors for 3D visualization. The images obtained from the 3D exoscope are visualized on a monitor, and a surgeon observes 3D stereoscopic images wearing 3D glasses (**Figs. 7** and **8**).

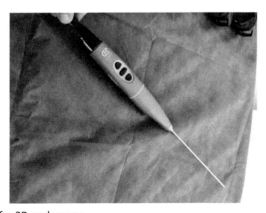

Fig. 5. Example of a 3D endoscope.

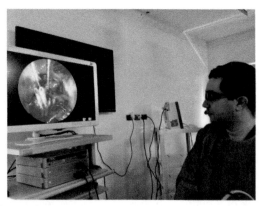

Fig. 6. Example of 3D endoscope.

An exoscope allows for excellent visualization at extreme angles because the surgeons are able to independently position themselves and they no longer depend on the eyepiece but operate using the monitors. Better ergonomics also extends to the assistant and the entire surgical team, which also allows better instrument exchange and communication between team members (including residents, anesthesiologists, and nurses), allowing an active participation in procedures and education and thus increasing patient's safety.[26]

The main drawbacks of exoscopes are: (1) limited depth perception, which is overcome using newer monitors, such as 3D or 3D 4K monitors; (2) low lighting, especially when visualizing through narrow surgical fields; and (3) lower image quality when compared with the microscope, which can be improved with continued device development.

4K TECHNOLOGY AND NARROW-BAND IMAGING IN OTOLOGY

Some of the greatest advantages of using an endoscope includes the higher magnification and wide angled views, allowing the surgeon to access and remove disease from delicate areas in a safer manner.

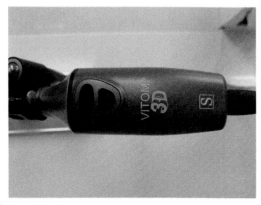

Fig. 7. Example of 3D exoscope.

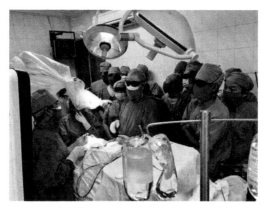

Fig. 8. Exoscope in action during live surgery.

Advances in optical technology have led to the development of high-definition visualization, such as 4K technology, which increases the magnification even further. The increased resolution improves image sharpness and provides a much more detailed view of all anatomic and pathologic structures (when compared with standard systems currently in use), which is particularly important when working around delicate and critical structures, improving the safety and efficacy of the surgical procedure.

Narrow band imaging (NBI), which has been implemented in oncologic surgery in all fields,[27] uses a filter that allows different wavelengths of narrow band light (415 and 540 nm wavelengths), in a sequential red-green-blue illumination, to pick up hypervascularity,[27] which could indicate areas of dysplasia. Recently there has been interest in using this technology in noncancer cases.[28]

In otologic surgery there is a difference in how structures and disease in the middle ear appear under the narrow band filter compared with ordinary white light. Because of the avascular nature of tympanosclerosis and cholesteatoma, they appear whiter than usual on NBI, whereas hypervascular structures, such as granulation tissue, are highlighted by the filter.[28]

The association of 4K magnification with NBI technology could improve the identification and dissection of middle ear pathology, such as cholesteatoma during middle ear surgery. The 4K magnification would allow a better visualization of the sinus tympani, facial recess, and stapes foot plate while dissecting the disease. However, NBI not only allows assessment of the extent of disease, but also ensures small residual disease is not left behind at the time of operation.

Further studies using the same NBI technology combined with 4K resolution and rigid scope are necessary to validate this extremely interesting potential.

NEURONAVIGATION

Advances in microsurgical techniques have led to an expansion of minimally invasive otologic/neurotologic procedures. Simultaneously, the complexity and proximity of critical anatomic structures, particularly on the skull base, sometimes requires the intraoperative use of navigation techniques.

Surgical approaches through the temporal bone require some form of temporal bone drilling to create an adequate access toward the surgical target. Skull base surgeons use anatomic landmarks as means of orientation during temporal bone drilling, to optimize access creation while minimizing bone removal and evading critical structures, such as the facial nerve and sigmoid sinus. However, these landmarks are subject to high interindividual variability[29] and is eroded by tumor, inflammation, or previous surgery.

To reduce the risks during the procedure, surgical navigation systems have been increasingly used in otologic surgery.[30,31] These image-guidance systems are developed to help surgeons to identify critical anatomic landmarks intraoperatively; however, it cannot substitute a thorough knowledge of the surgical anatomy. Initially developed for neurosurgical procedures, these systems use computerized tracking devices to monitor the position of the endoscopes or instruments relative to the patient's anatomic landmarks. The system displays the location of the tip of a tracked drill, and other instruments, in real-time, on a navigation map of the patient's preoperative anatomy image (computed tomography or MRI).[32,33]

However, the cost and lack of portability make the current image-guidance systems unavailable in many institutions and hard to transport to different hospitals.[32,34]

In their study, Nogueira and colleagues[35] used a third-generation camera and a predefined black and white pattern for optical tracking. The camera was attached in a holder at a distance from 60 cm to 100 cm from the patient's marker, and it was linked to an up-to-date laptop through a standard firewire port. This port provides a power supply and a fast hub for information exchange, because the orientation functions needed to be performed repeatedly at real-time rates.[35]

The laptop-based image-guidance system achieved an accuracy rate of 1.16 mm, showing its effectiveness and possible use in real patients (**Figs. 9 and 10**).

NEW SURGICAL APPROACHES

In recent years, technical improvements and growing expertise in the handling of the endoscope allowed introducing an exclusive endoscopic approach to the middle ear, lateral skull base, middle cranial fossa, and posterior fossa/cerebellopontine angle pathologies.

Although the endoscope has been commonly used in transcanal middle ear surgeries, which have proved to be highly successful, EES has also proven to be a feasible option in the approach of cochlear schwannoma involving internal auditory canal.

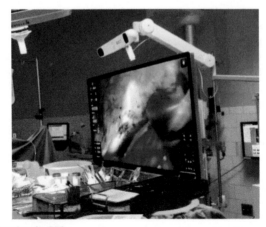

Fig. 9. Neuronavigation in EES.

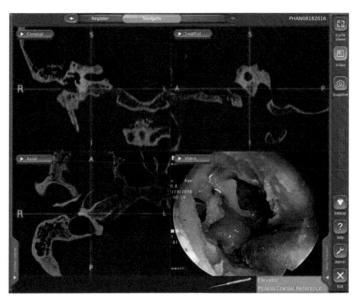

Fig. 10. Neuronavigation in EES.

There are no proven indications against the advisability of EES. Any otologic surgery that is conducted with a microscope can also use an endoscope. Therefore, these are some of the current indications for EES.

1. External ear: Cholesteatoma, exostosis repair, canalplasty, debridement, and biopsy.
2. Middle ear: Myringotomy, myringoplasty, medial graft tympanoplasty, lateral graft tympanoplasty, the retraction of the tympanic membrane, acquired cholesteatoma, congenital cholesteatoma, neoplasms of middle ear (eg, glomus tympanicum), ossiculoplasty, and stapes surgery.
3. Inner ear/skullbase: Intracochlear schwannoma, small symptomatic neoplasms of internal auditory canal fundus of facial nerve, petrous apex cyst, and the repair of perilymph fistulas (congenital or traumatic).
4. Middle cranial fossa: The repair of superior canal dehiscence.
5. Posterior fossa/cerebellopontine angle: Establishing enduring schwannoma in internal auditory canal fundus, and localization and sealing of externalized air cells during the decompression of internal auditory canal to reduce the risk of cerebrospinal fluid leaks.

DISCLOSURE

The Authors have nothing to disclose.

REFERENCES

1. Thomassin JM, Duchon-Doris JM, Emram B, et al. Endoscopic ear surgery. Initial evaluation. Ann Otolaryngol Chir Cervicofa 1990;107:564–70.
2. Thomassin JM, Korchia D, Doris JM. Endoscopic-guided otosurgery in the prevention of residual cholesteatomas. Laryngoscope 1993;103:939–43.

3. Tarabichi M. Endoscopic management of acquired cholesteatoma. Am J Otol 1997;18:544–9.
4. Poe D, Rebeiz E, Pankratov M, et al. Transtympanic endoscopy of the middle ear. Laryngoscope 1992;102:993–6.
5. McKennan KX. Endoscopic "second look" mastoidoscopy to rule out residual epitympanic/mastoid cholesteatoma. Laryngoscope 1993;103:810–4.
6. Magnan J, Chays A, Lepetre C, et al. Surgical perspectives of endoscopy of the cerebellopontine angle. Am J Otol 1994;15:366–70.
7. Presutti L, Marchioni D, Mattioli F, et al. Endoscopic management of acquired cholesteatoma: our experience. J Otolaryngol Head Neck Surg 2008;37(4): 481–7.
8. Tarabichi M. Endoscopic management of limited attic cholesteatoma. Laryngoscope 2004;114(7):1157–62.
9. Marchioni D, Alicandri-Ciufelli M, Molteni G, et al. Endoscopic tympanoplasty in patients with attic retraction pockets. Laryngoscope 2010;120(9):1847–55.
10. Marchioni D, Alicandri-Ciufelli M, Piccinini A, et al. Inferior retrotympanum revisited: an endoscopic anatomic study. Laryngoscope 2010;120(9):1880–6.
11. Kozin ED, Gulati S, Kaplan AB, et al. Systematic review of outcomes following observational and operative endoscopic middle ear surgery. Laryngoscope 2015;125(5):1205–14.
12. Bottrill I, Perrault D, Poe D. In vitro and in vivo determination of the thermal effect of middle ear endoscopy. Laryngoscope 1994;106:213–6.
13. Kozin ED, Lehmann A, Carter M, et al. Thermal effects of endoscopy in a human temporal bone model: implications for endoscopic ear surgery. Laryngoscope 2014;124(8):E332–9.
14. Kozin ED, Daniel JL. Basic principles of endoscopic ear surgery. Oper Tech Otolaryngol Head Neck Surg 2017;28:2–10.
15. Khan MM, Parab SR. Endoscopic cartilage tympanoplasty: a two-handed technique using an endoscope holder. Laryngoscope 2016;126:1893–8.
16. Ito T, Kubota T, Takagi A, et al. Safety of heat generated by endoscope light sources in simulated transcanal endoscopic ear surgery. Auris Nasus Larynx 2016; 43:501–6.
17. Marchioni D, Mattioli F, Alicandri-Ciufelli M, et al. Endoscopic approach to tensor fold in patients with attic cholesteatoma. Acta Otolaryngol (Stockh) 2009;129: 946–54.
18. Marchioni D, Mattioli F, Alicandri-Ciufelli M, et al. Transcanal endoscopic approach to the sinus tympani: a clinical report. Otol Neurotol Otol Neurotol 2009;30:758–65.
19. Storz P, Buess GF, Kunert W, et al. 3D HD versus 2D HD: surgical task efficiency in standardised phantom tasks. Surg Endosc 2012;26:1454–60.
20. Spille J, Wenners A, von Hehn U, et al. 2D versus 3D in laparoscopic surgery by beginners and experts: a randomized controlled trial on a Pelvitrainer in objectively graded surgical steps. J Surg Educ 2017. https://doi.org/10.1016/j.jsurg. 2017.01.011.
21. Bernardeschi D, Lahlou G, Seta D, et al. 3D endoscopic ear surgery: a clinical pilot study. Eur Arch Otorhinolaryngol 2017. https://doi.org/10.1007/s00405-017-4839-6.
22. Uluc K, Kujoth GC, Baskaya MK. Operating microscopes: past, present, and future. Neurosurg Focus 2009;27:E4.
23. Carlucci C, Fasanella L, Ricci Maccarini A. Exolaryngoscopy: a new technique for laryngeal surgery. Acta Otorhinolaryngol Ital 2012;32:326–8.

24. Rossini Z, Cardia A, Milani D, et al. VITOM 3D: preliminary experience in cranial surgery. World Neurosurg 2017;107:663–8.
25. Sack J, Steinberg JA, Rennert RC, et al. Initial experience using a high-definition 3-dimensional exoscope system for microneurosurgery. Oper Neurosurg 2018; 14:395–401.
26. Mamelak AN, Drazin D, Shirzadi A, et al. Infratentorial supracerebellar resection of a pineal tumor using a high definition video exoscope (VITOM). J Clin Neurosci 2012;19:306–9.
27. Ochsner M, Klein A. The utility of narrow band imaging in the treatment of laryngeal papillomatosis in awake patients. J Voice 2015;29(3):349–51.
28. Plaat B, Zwakenberg MA, Zwol JGV, et al. Narrow-band imaging in transoral laser surgery for early glottic can-cer in relation to clinical outcome. Head Neck 2017; 39(7):1343–8.
29. Gharabaghi A, Rosahl SK, Feigl GC, et al. Image-guided lateral suboccipital approach: part 1-individualized landmarks for surgical planning. Neurosurgery 2008;62:18–22.
30. Miller RS, Hashisaki GT, Kesser BW. Image-guided localization of the internal auditory canal via the middle cranial fossa approach. Otolaryngol Head Neck Surg 2006;134:778–82.
31. Woerdeman PA, Willems PW, Noordmans HJ, et al. Auditory feedback during frameless image-guided surgery in a phantom model and initial clinical experience. J Neurosurg 2009;110:257–62.
32. Stamm AC, Pignatari S, Sebusiani S, et al. Image-guided endoscopic sinus and skull base surgery. Rev Bras Otorinolaringol 2002;68:502–9.
33. Metson R, Cosenza M, Gliklish RE, et al. The role of image-guidance systems for head and neck surgery. Arch Otolaryngol Head Neck Surg 1999;125:1100–4.
34. Chu ST. Endoscopic sinus surgery under navigation system: analysis report of 79 cases. J Chin Med Assoc 2006;69:529–33.
35. Nogueira JF Jr, Stamm AC, Lyra M. Novel compact laptop-based image-guidance system: preliminary study. Laryngoscope 2009;119:576–9.

Special Article Series: Intentionally Shaping the Future of Otolaryngology

Editor

JENNIFER A. VILLWOCK

OTOLARYNGOLOGIC CLINICS OF NORTH AMERICA

www.oto.theclinics.com

Consulting Editor
SUJANA S. CHANDRASEKHAR

February 2021 • Volume 54 • Number 1

Special Foreword

Tackling Gender and Racial Discrimination in Otolaryngology, Head (and Neck) On

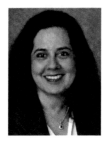

Sujana S. Chandrasekhar, MD, FACS, FAAOHNS
Consulting Editor

This issue of *Otolaryngologic Clinics of North America* features the third installment in our Special Article Series: Intentionally Shaping the Future of Otolaryngology, Guest Edited by Dr Jennifer A. Villwock. The first 2 articles of the series highlighted the importance of leadership in our field. The second 2 articles focused on the current state of the Otolaryngology workforce and the importance of devoting attention to diversity and inclusion in our field in order to improve the care that we deliver to a diverse population. The current 2 articles delve deeper into the structural barriers against the entry and progression of women and racial minorities in medicine and surgery in the United States.

In the United States and Canada, underrepresentation of women in medicine and surgery is no longer an issue in medical schools. Half of matriculating students are women. However, this parity disappears quickly as one ascends the hierarchy, with less than 20% of Department Chairs or Deans of Medical Schools being women. **Figs. 1** and **2** from the American Association of Medical Colleges (AAMC) and the Association of Faculties of Medicine of Canada demonstrate the problem.[1,2]

However, black, Hispanic, and American Indian/Alaskan Native (AIAN) students remain underrepresented among medical school matriculants compared with the US population. This underrepresentation has not changed significantly since the institution of the Liaison Committee of Medical Education diversity accreditation guidelines in 2009. A study by Lett and colleagues[3] looked at the data using a representation quotient (RQ), defined as the ratio of proportion of a particular subgroup among the total population of applicants or matriculants relative to the corresponding estimated proportion of that subgroup in the US population. An RQ greater than 1 indicates that a subgroup is overrepresented among medical school applicants, matriculants, or

Otolaryngol Clin N Am 54 (2021) xxiii–xxvii
https://doi.org/10.1016/j.otc.2020.10.003
0030-6665/21/© 2020 Published by Elsevier Inc.

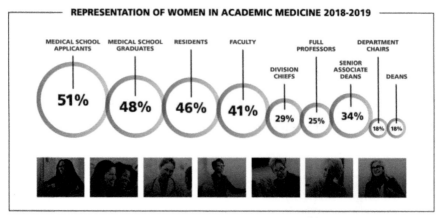

Fig. 1. Representation of Women in Academic Medicine, US, 2018-2019. (*From* Lautenberger DM, Dandar VM. The state of women in academic medicine 2018-2019: exploring pathways to equity. Association of American Medical Colleges, AAMC 2020. Available at: https://store.aamc.org/downloadable/download/sample/sample_id/330/. Accessed November 4, 2020.)

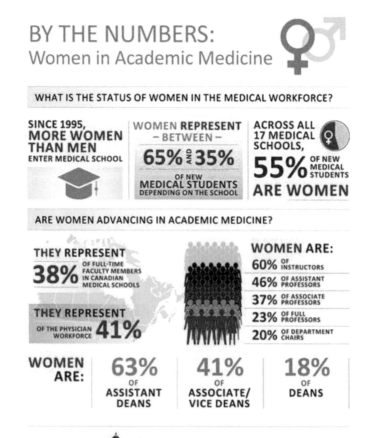

Fig. 2. Women in Academic Medicine, Canada. (*From* the Association of Faculties of Medicine of Canada. Available at: http://www.afmc.ca/. Accessed November 4, 2020.)

enrollees relative to the US population; an RQ less than 1 indicates a subgroup is underrepresented. The magnitude of the RQ is also interpretable. An RQ of 0.50 indicates that the representation for that subgroup is 50% of that subgroup's representation in the total US population, and an RQ of 1.75 indicates that the representation of that subgroup is 75% greater than its representation in the US population. **Fig. 3** shows the overrepresentation of Asians and the severe underrepresentation of underrepresented minorities (URM) in medical school classes in the United States.

The problem continues beyond medical education and is exemplified in the data regarding URM physicians in academic leadership. A December 2016 report by the AAMC shows this in graphical form in **Fig. 4**.[4] Note the abysmal percentages for assistant, associate, and full professor status: maximally 10%, 8%, and 5.9% in Clinical Departments, respectively. These percentages are even worse in Basic Science Departments: 7%, 6.5%, and 4%. These data are deeply troubling and

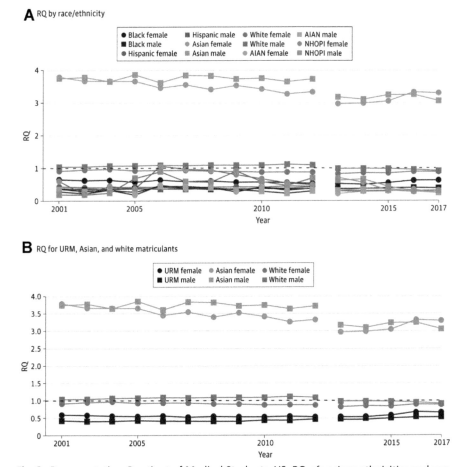

Fig. 3. Representation Quotient of Medical Students, US. RQ of various ethnicities and genders in US medical schools. NHOPI, Native Hawaiian or Other Pacific Islander. (*From* Lett LA, Murdock HM, Orji WU, Aysola J, Sebro R. Trends in racial/ethnic representation among US medical students. JAMA Netw Open. 2019;2(9):e1910490.)

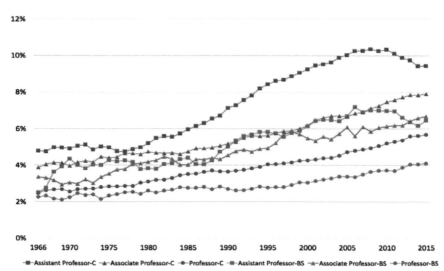

Fig. 4. US medical school URM faculty diversity trends by rank and department type, 1966 to 2015. US medical school URM faculty diversity trends by rank and department type, 1966 to 2015. BS, basic science department; C, clinical department. (*From* Xierali IM, Fair MA, Nivet MA. Faculty diversity in US medical schools: progress and gaps coexist. analysis in brief. Association of American Medical Colleges, 16:16 (2016). Available at: https://www.aamc.org/system/files/reports/1/december2016facultydiversityinu.s.medicalschoolsprogressandgaps.pdf. Accessed November 4, 2020.)

cannot be "explained away" by "pipeline problems" or other excuses. Furthermore, it is critical for patients and prospective students to see themselves represented in a meaningful way in our health care establishment. This may be the best way to immediately demonstrate a meaningful commitment to culturally competent care and optimizing outcomes for diverse patients. In turn, these commitments facilitate the active participation and open dialogue that are critical to informing and improving health outcomes. Without adequate diversity and representation, we are losing out as a society.

Drs Lindsay Sobin, Scott Harrison, and Barry Kriegsman and Drs Michelle Liu and Candace Flagg have provided thoughtful, sobering information that we must know about the current conditions for women and persons of color in the House of Medicine. There is a clear need for the development and evaluation of more robust policies and programs to create a physician workforce that is demographically representative of the US population. We need meaningful discussion and training around inherent biases so that they may be tamed, and so that racist and sexist behavior is completely unacceptable in our profession.

Sujana S. Chandrasekhar, MD, FACS, FAAOHNS
Consulting Editor
Otolaryngologic Clinics of North America
Past President
American Academy of Otolaryngology–
Head and Neck Surgery
Secretary-Treasurer
American Otological Society
Partner, ENT & Allergy Associates LLP
18 East 48th Street, 2nd Floor
New York, NY 10017, USA

Clinical Professor
Department of Otolaryngology–
Head and Neck Surgery
Zucker School of Medicine at Hofstra-Northwell
Hempstead, NY, USA

Clinical Associate Professor
Department of Otolaryngology–
Head and Neck Surgery
Icahn School of Medicine at Mount Sinai
New York, NY, USA

E-mail address:
ssc@nyotology.com

Website:
http://www.ears.nyc

REFERENCES

1. Available at: https://store.aamc.org/the-state-of-women-in-academic-medicine-2018-2019-exploring-pathways-to-equity.html?utm_source=twitter&utm_medium=aamctoday&utm_content=53bd0014-e00e-4b73-bc93-9e89345ff1f6. Accessed November 4, 2020.
2. Available at: http://www.afmc.ca/. Accessed November 4, 2020.
3. Lett LA, Murdock HM, WU Orji, et al. Trends in racial/ethnic representation among US medical students. JAMA Netw Open 2019;2(9):e1910490.
4. Available at: https://www.aamc.org/system/files/reports/1/december2016 facultydiversityinu.s.medicalschoolsprogressandgaps.pdf. Accessed November 4, 2020.

Special Preface
False Dichotomies

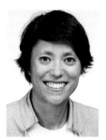

Jennifer A. Villwock, MD, FAAOA
Editor

There will be no shortage of things for which the year 2020 will be remembered. Among these events are the losses of numerous pioneers, including NASA mathematician Katherine Johnson, Congressman John Lewis, and Supreme Court Justice Ruth Bader Ginsburg. I feature their words in this preface not only to honor their lives and legacies but also because they ring true.

The late legendary civil right leader Congressman John Lewis wrote in *Across That Bridge: A Vision for Change and Future of America* that "it is only through examining history that you become aware of where you stand within the continuum of change." It is for this reason that this issue's special articles begin with the review article by Dr Lindsay Sobin and colleagues, "Women and Minorities in Surgery: A Historical Perspective," of the known contributions of women and minorities in surgery and otolaryngology. Recognizing the efforts of these pioneering trailblazers reminds us of our history and the subsequent progress of our profession. In our remembrances, we must also send our thanks to those whose names were never associated with their enduring contributions.

As noted by Margot Lee Shetterly in the book, *Hidden Figures: The American Dream and the Untold Story of the Black Women Mathematicians Who Helped Win the Space Race*, "[t]he work of most women…was anonymous. Even a woman who had worked closely with an engineer on the content of a research report was rarely rewarded by seeing her name alongside his on the final publication. Why would the computers have the same desire for recognition that they did? Many engineers figured. There were women, after all."

Drs Flagg and Liu's article, "The Work Is Just Beginning: Racism in Medicine," reflecting on their lived experiences as Black otolaryngologists is a poignant reminder that we are writing our history now. As late Justice Ruth Bader Ginsburg said, "We should not be held back from pursuing our full talents, from contributing what we could contribute to the society, because we fit into a certain mold—because we belong to a

Otolaryngol Clin N Am 54 (2021) xxix–xxx
https://doi.org/10.1016/j.otc.2020.10.004
0030-6665/21/© 2020 Published by Elsevier Inc.

group that historically has been the object of discrimination." There is clearly room for improvement.

Once, at the end of a grand rounds talk, I was fielding questions. Two people raised their hands at the same time. One was an attending physician who was young and a woman. The other was an older, white man. Making the decision about whose raised hand to recognize first was a reflex. Who do you think I called on? We must also recognize the false dichotomies that prevent progress. Calling on the man first did not make me a "bad" person. But it did highlight cultural programming I need to work on. I personally apologized to the woman, and we had a nice chat. Rather than trying to forget and quickly move on from this event, I continue to carry this story with me. I do so as a reminder of my own fallibility and how to respond with kindness, grace, and a friendly challenge to do better in the future.

Doing better takes courage. We must listen and hold space for stories we may find uncomfortable. We must recognize that it is not the responsibility of the oppressed or disenfranchised to educate us. We must explore our own culturally ingrained biases and be accountable for the impact of our actions, regardless of our intentions.

It seems fitting to end this preface as I began, by borrowing the words of Representative John Lewis. As with any ideal we strive toward, "Freedom is not a state; it is an act. It is not some enchanted garden perched high on a distant plateau where we can finally sit down and rest. Freedom is the continuous action we all must take, and each generation must do its part to create an even more fair, more just society."

Jennifer A. Villwock, MD, FAAOA
Department of Otolaryngology, Head
and Neck Surgery
University of Kansas Medical Center
3901 Rainbow Boulevard, MS 3010
Kansas City, KS 66160, USA

E-mail address:
jvillwock@kumc.edu

Women and Minorities in Otolaryngology

A Historical Perspective and Analysis of Current Representation

Barry Kriegsman, BS[a], Scott Harrison, PhD[b], Lindsay Sobin, MD[c],*

KEYWORDS

- Women • Minorities • Otolaryngology • History • Representation

KEY POINTS

- Visionary women and minority otolaryngologists–head and neck surgeons made significant contributions to the field throughout the twentieth century. However, the true volume, depth, and importance of these contributions is likely unknown given the long tradition of women and minorities not receiving just credit for their work in science and medicine.
- Women and racial minorities, particularly African Americans, remain underrepresented in otolaryngology.
- Mentorship opportunities during undergraduate medical education may help increase the presence of women and minorities in otolaryngology.

INTRODUCTION

Women and minorities have long been underrepresented in medicine as a whole and, in particular, in the surgical subspecialties, such as otolaryngology–head and neck surgery. Additionally, early female practitioners have largely been excluded from the historical narrative. This is explained by the Matilda effect, a well-documented phenomenon in which accomplishments by women are overshadowed by their male counterparts.[1] Because of the efforts of some pioneering surgeons who paved the way for today's women and minority otolaryngologists, gender and minority disparities have decreased and there is increased emphasis on the importance of equity, diversity, and inclusion. Here, we shine a light on some of these inspirational individuals' contributions to otolaryngology and the implications for otolaryngology's future.

[a] University of Massachusetts Medical School, 55 Lake Avenue North, Worcester, MA 01655, USA; [b] Boston Architectural College, Boston, 320 Newbury Street, Boston, MA 02115, USA; [c] Department of Otolaryngology, University of Massachusetts Medical School, 55 Lake Avenue North, Worcester, MA 01655, USA
* Corresponding author.
E-mail address: Lindsay.Sobin@umassmemorial.org

Otolaryngol Clin N Am 54 (2021) 233–238
https://doi.org/10.1016/j.otc.2020.09.017
0030-6665/21/© 2020 Elsevier Inc. All rights reserved.

HISTORICAL PERSPECTIVE

Until the late nineteenth century, women were barred from applying to most US medical school programs because of the gendered notion that women were unsuited for the profession of medicine. Arguments, such as those of Harvard Medical School professor, Edward Clark, who warned that "higher education in women produces monstrous brains and puny bodies," were used to justify women's exclusion from medicine.[2] The efforts of some enterprising individuals (**Table 1**), such as Elizabeth Blackwell, who became the first woman to receive a medical degree in the United States and who later founded the New York Infirmary for Women and Children, led to increasing numbers of women entering the medical profession in the late nineteenth century.[3]

One of the first women to specialize in otolaryngology was Dr Alice Bryant. She graduated from the Women's Medical College of New York in 1890 and then practiced at the New England Hospital for Women and Children and at the New England Deaconess Hospital. Dr Bryant was well known for being a talented clinician and an innovator, inventing various surgical tools, such as the tonsil tenaculum, tonsil snare cannula, bone-gripping forceps, and nasal polyp hook.[4,5] She was also a humanitarian, instituting flexible hours for the convenience of her patients in response to the changing times and demands of the working poor. A highly productive member of the scientific community, she authored more than 75 articles ranging from suppurative ear disease to adenoid infections.[6,7] In June 1914, Dr Bryant was one of the first two women to be admitted to the American College of Surgeons.

Dr Margaret Butler and Dr Emily Van Loon demonstrated decisive leadership at the Women's Medical College of Pennsylvania. Dr Butler, a graduate of the Women's Medical College of Pennsylvania in 1894, became a Clinical Professor of Laryngology

Table 1
Summary of highlighted individuals' contributions to medicine and otolaryngology

Name	Significant Contributions
Dr Elizabeth Blackwell	Founded the New York Infirmary for Women and Children
Dr Alice Bryant	Invented several surgical tools including the tonsil tenaculum, tonsil snare cannula, bone-gripping forceps, and nasal polyp hook
Dr Margaret Butler	Invented the Butler tonsil snare and nasal septum splint
Dr Emily Van Loon	Established methods of removing foreign bodies by bronchoscopy
Dr Lucja Frey	Described auriculotemporal nerve syndrome
Dr Margaret Dix	Described the maneuver used to diagnose benign paroxysmal positional vertigo
Dr Eleanor Bennett	Established the otolaryngology residency program at the University of Wisconsin after becoming the first female chairperson at any major US medical school
Dr Rebecca Lee Crumpler	First African American woman to earn a medical degree in the United States
Dr Harry Barnes	First African American board-certified otolaryngologist
Dr Dana Thompson	Public advocate for diversity and inclusion in otolaryngology after being one of the first African American female residents in otolaryngology

and Chief of the Nose and Throat Department of her alma mater in 1906. In addition to spending long hours in the operating room performing procedures, Dr Butler invented multiple otolaryngologic instruments, including the Butler tonsil snare and a nasal septum splint designed for use after submucosal resections.[8] Following in Dr Butler's footsteps, Dr Van Loon became the Chief of Otolaryngology at the Women's Medical College of Pennsylvania. Most notably, Dr Van Loon, along with Dr Chevalier Jackson, developed the bronchoscope and established methods of bronchoscopic removal of foreign bodies.[4]

A Polish-Jewish physician named Dr Lucja Frey was one of the first female academic neurologists in Europe. A couple decades after receiving her medical degree from the University of Lviv in 1923, Dr Frey and 136,000 others of Jewish nationality were escorted to live in the Ghetto Lemberg.[9] Before her tragic death at the hands of the Nazis, Dr Frey made many contributions to the medical literature, including the publication of auriculotemporal nerve syndrome.[10] This postoperative otolaryngologic phenomenon of gustatory sweating, widely known as Frey syndrome, is particularly pertinent to surgical resections of the parotid gland.[11]

Dr Margaret Dix was a British neuro-otologist who published landmark papers on vertigo and how to differentiate between its causes. She is just one example of how national and global upheavals shaped the lives of women practicing in otolaryngology. A graduate of the Royal Free Hospital of Medicine in 1937, Dr Dix's career as a surgeon was cut short after a World War II air raid disfigured her face and lodged fragments of glass in her eyes.[12] Despite this, she accomplished groundbreaking research on auditory, vestibular, and neurologic conditions at the National Hospital in London, publishing more than 100 articles. Notably, along with Dr Charles Hallpike, Dr Dix described the eponymous Dix-Hallpike maneuver to diagnose benign paroxysmal positional vertigo.[13,14]

Dr Eleanor Bennett was a highly successful female otolaryngologist of the mid-twentieth century. After graduating from medical school at the University of Nebraska, Omaha in 1942, she proceeded to become the first female chairperson in any major US medical school, serving as the Professor and Chair of Otolaryngology at the University of Wisconsin, Madison in 1963. Dr Bennett was also the first woman admitted to the American Laryngological, Rhinological, and Otological (Triological) Society. Her commitment to educating future generations of physicians was exemplified by her establishment of the otolaryngology residency program at the University of Wisconsin.[4,8]

In 1864, Dr Rebecca Lee Crumpler became the first African American woman to earn a medical degree in the United States, graduating from the New England Female Medical College in Boston, Massachusetts.[15] For more than a century thereafter, no African American women practiced in otolaryngology–head and neck surgery. This time lapse may be caused, in part, by the aftermath of the Flexner Report. Although it has been credited with modernizing and standardizing medical education, the Flexner Report also resulted in the closure of many medical schools that admitted women and minorities.[16] In 1927, Dr Harry Barnes became the first African American board-certified otolaryngologist and it was not until the late-twentieth century that African American women, such as Dr Dana Thompson, entered the field.[17] After graduating from the University of Missouri, Kansas City School of Medicine, Dr Thompson attended the Mayo Medical School where she completed her otolaryngology residency in 1996. At that time, she was one of the first female otolaryngology residents and one of the first African American otolaryngology residents.[18] Dr Thompson is a renowned pediatric otolaryngologist, authoring more than 50 publications in the field, and is currently the Division Head in Otorhinolaryngology at the Lurie Children's

Hospital of Chicago. Beyond her academic leadership, she has continued to advocate for changes in otolaryngology to help advance diversity and inclusion.

CURRENT REPRESENTATION

Over the past 40 years, the number of women entering otolaryngology has steadily increased. In 2017, approximately 17.1% of active otolaryngologists were women, as compared with less than 1% in 1980.[4,19] The percentage of women actively practicing in other specialties is variable, ranging from 5.3% of orthopedic surgeons to 63.3% of pediatricians.[19] Among the surgical fields, otolaryngology has a lower percentage of women than obstetrics and gynecology (57.0%) or general surgery (20.6%) but a higher percentage than plastic (16.0%), vascular (13.1%), or neurologic surgery (8.4%).[19] In terms of rank within academic positions, the sex disparity is even more pronounced. In 2019, only 85 of the 531 otolaryngology professors were women (16.0%) and only 3 of the 87 otolaryngology department chairs were women (3.4%).[20,21]

Current trends in residency programs suggest that these figures for female otolaryngologists will gradually increase over the next few decades. In 2019, 36.2% of otolaryngology residents were female, up from 30.8% a decade prior.[22,23] According to Lopez and colleagues,[23] over the decade spanning 2008 to 2018, a significantly higher proportion of women made up the otolaryngology residency workforce in the second half of the decade than in the first half. Yet surprisingly, the number of female otolaryngology applicants has not significantly changed over this decade.[23] Furthermore, in 2016, there was a significantly smaller proportion of female otolaryngology applicants (33.3%) than female medical school graduates (47.4%), a difference that was not observed in any other demographic group.[24] The fact that more women are now entering otolaryngology training despite a stagnation in the number of female applicants suggests that residency programs may have an increased awareness of the gender gap in medicine and that additional mentorship opportunities during medical school may be helpful in furthering the representation of women in the field.

Racial minorities remain underrepresented in otolaryngology at the resident and faculty level. From 2013 to 2018, there were significantly more minorities in the otolaryngology resident workforce than in the 5 years prior; however, this was largely a reflection of the overall increase in otolaryngology residents during that time.[23] Furthermore, not all minority groups have experienced the same trends; the number of Asian and Hispanic otolaryngology residents has increased in the last decade, whereas the number of African American otolaryngology residents has decreased since 2010.[23,24] In 2016, only 2.1% of otolaryngology residents were African American, the lowest percentage of any surgical subspecialty.[24]

To improve diversity within the workforce, efforts must be made to understand the perceptual and structural barriers that surgeons of color face. A recent study by Ulloa and colleagues[25] revealed that for African American and Latino surgeons, early identification of mentors who could help mediate a sense of belonging in surgical culture is incredibly important. The degree of racial diversity among otolaryngology faculty seems similar to that among residents; in 2018, the percentage of active female otolaryngologists who were African American was only 4.3%, lower than that in orthopedic (4.7%), plastic (5.0%), or general surgery (8.0%).[26] Regarding academic positions, underrepresented minority faculty have historically been promoted at lower rates when compared with white faculty.[27] In 2019, only 21.1% of otolaryngology professors and 19.5% of otolaryngology department chairs were from self-reported racial minority groups.[28]

There are multiple ways in which we can work to address these disparities and increase diversity and inclusion in otolaryngology. As examples, leadership and professional development opportunities are widely available through conferences and national organizations. At the institutional level, most medical schools have formed diversity committees and may use resources, such as those provided by the American College of Surgeons, to establish cultural competency, recognize implicit bias, and create diverse surgical teams. Additionally, trainee mentorship efforts during medical school and residency can foster an increased sense of belonging in the surgical community. However, with all of these approaches, we must be cognizant of the minority tax, that is, the additional effort taken on by minority leaders to help address the systemic issues preventing greater representation.

SUMMARY

Women and minority otolaryngologists have made substantial and lasting contributions to our field. Their perseverance in the face of bias, racism, and discrimination has inspired generations of women and minorities thereafter to pursue what has historically been a white male–predominant surgical subspecialty. Here, we bring to the foreground the voices and life narratives of individuals whose contributions are not well recognized. Today, there continues to be a need for greater diversity within otolaryngology–head and neck surgery; the growing numbers of women and underrepresented minorities over the past decade suggests that we are approaching a critical time in defining how these disparities will evolve in the twenty-first century. The underrepresentation of racial minorities in otolaryngology, particularly African Americans, requires attention to improve diversity within the field. Mentorship opportunities during undergraduate medical education may be particularly helpful on this front. Eliminating overt exclusionary practices is not sufficient. To facilitate the next generation of greatness in otolaryngology, the culture must evolve toward celebrating diversity and inclusion.

DISCLOSURE

The authors have nothing to disclose.

REFERENCES

1. Knobloch-Westerwick S, Glynn CJ, Huge M. The Matilda Effect in Science Communication: an experiment on gender bias in publication quality perceptions and collaboration interest. Sci Commun 2013;35(5):603–25.
2. Jefferson L, Bloor K, Maynard A. Women in medicine: historical perspectives and recent trends. Br Med Bull 2015;114(1):5–15.
3. Wynn R. Saints and sinners: women and the practice of medicine throughout the ages. JAMA 2000;283(5):668–9.
4. Konstantinidou S, Adams M. Women in otorhinolaryngology: a historical perspective. J Laryngol Otol 2018;132(8):670–2.
5. Stanley A. Mothers and daughters of invention: notes for a revised history of technology. NJ (New Brunswick): Rutgers University Press; 1995.
6. Bryant AG. The importance of early recognition of suppurative ear disease. Medical Record (1866-1922): W. Wood; New York. 1905. vol. 67(19).
7. Bryant AG. Streptococcic infections of the pharyngeal adenoid tissue in adults. JAMA 1908 ;L(24):1963-6.

8. Friedman R, Fang CH, Zubair M, et al. Women's role in otolaryngologic medicine. Bull Am Coll Surg 2016;101(12):40–5.

9. Grzybowski A, Sak J. Lucja Frey (1889-1942). J Neurol 2016;263(11):2358–9.

10. Moltrecht M, Michel O. The woman behind Frey's syndrome: the tragic life of Lucja Frey. Laryngoscope 2004;114(12):2205–9.

11. Motz KM, Kim YJ. Auriculotemporal syndrome (Frey syndrome). Otolaryngol Clin North Am 2016;49(2):501–9.

12. Royal College of Surgeons of England. Margaret Ruth Dix. London: RCS ENG; Plarr's lives of the Fellows 2015.

13. Dix MR, Hallpike CS. The pathology, symptomatology and diagnosis of certain common disorders of the vestibular system. Ann Otol Rhinol Laryngol 1952; 61(4):987–1016.

14. Dix MR, Hallpike CS. The pathology symptomatology and diagnosis of certain common disorders of the vestibular system. Proc R Soc Med 1952;45(6):341–54.

15. Crumpler RL. US National Library of Medicine changing the face of medicine. Bethesda (MD): USA.gov; 2003.

16. Sullivan LW, Suez Mittman I. The state of diversity in the health professions a century after Flexner. Seattle (WA): Blackpast.org; Acad Med 2010;85(2):246–53.

17. Mahoney E. William Henry Barnes (1887-1945) 2017.

18. Quinn R. Dana Thompson, MD, addresses bias and diversity in otolaryngology. ENTtoday 2018;13(6):1–3.

19. AAMC. Active Physicians by Sex and Specialty, 2017. Table 1.3. Number and Percentage of Active Physicians by Sex and Specialty, 2017.

20. AAMC. 2019 U.S. Medical School Faculty. Table 13: Sex, Rank, and Department.

21. AAMC. 2019 U.S. medical school faculty. Supplemental Table C: Department Chairs by Department, Sex, and Race/Ethnicity.

22. AAMC. Report on residents. Table B3: Number of Active Residents, by Type of Medical School, GME Specialty, and Sex.

23. Lopez EM, Farzal Z, Ebert CS Jr, et al. Recent trends in female and racial/ethnic minority groups in U.S. otolaryngology residency programs. Laryngoscope 2020. https://doi.org/10.1002/lary.28603.

24. Ukatu CC, Welby Berra L, Wu Q, et al. The state of diversity based on race, ethnicity, and sex in otolaryngology in 2016. Laryngoscope 2019. https://doi.org/10.1002/lary.28447.

25. Ulloa JG, Viramontes O, Ryan G, et al. Perceptual and structural facilitators and barriers to becoming a surgeon: a qualitative study of African American and Latino surgeons. Acad Med 2018;93(9):1326–34.

26. AAMC. Diversity in medicine: facts and figures 2019. Table 12. Practice Specialty, Females by Race/Ethnicity, 2018.

27. Fang D, Moy E, Colburn L, et al. Racial and ethnic disparities in faculty promotion in academic medicine. JAMA 2000;284(9):1085–92.

28. AAMC. 2019 U.S. medical school faculty. Table 19: Sex, Race/Ethnicity, Rank, and Department.

The Work Is Just Beginning— Racism in Medicine

Candace A. Flagg, MD[a], Michelle F. Liu, MD, MPH[b],*

KEYWORDS

- Racism • Antiracism • Implicit bias • Diversity • Inclusion
- Cultural and structural competency • Underrepresented in medicine (URM)
- Sponsorship

KEY POINTS

- Diversity, equity, and inclusion efforts are nothing without first creating safe spaces for minority experiences to be shared. This fosters an environment where conversations begin, stay honest, and cultivate understanding.
- The growth rate of African American residents in otolaryngology programs has remained statistically insignificant since 1975, making it apparent that institutional change is lacking despite previous calls to action for diversity in medicine.
- An increasingly diverse medical workforce has two functions: more culturally competent providers who can sensitively care for minority patients and creation of academic medicine pipelines to support current and future URM physicians.
- Health care providers must ask themselves how to engage in personal and professional spaces as a deliberate antiracist; what are the more proactive steps to become culturally sensitive and advocate for minority colleagues or friends, and, even more so, protect minority patients?
- Sponsorship is the cornerstone of an Otolaryngology training program committed to diversity and inclusion, and a feature sought by URM who are acutely aware of their potential to experience racism and isolation during training.

INTRODUCTION

I remember standing in the kitchen a few days following my big news from The Match, still on and off of the phone with long-distance friends and family sharing how I'd officially been selected to become an otolaryngologist. It felt good to say. I was preparing a dinner recipe I had long wanted to try when suddenly my phone rang again. My friend shared with me "I heard that one of our classmates said, 'I didn't match because of a Black girl.'"

[a] Department of Otolaryngology–Head and Neck Surgery, San Antonio Uniformed Services Health Education Consortium, 3551 Roger Brooke Drive, Ft. Sam Houston, TX 78234, USA;
[b] Department of Otolaryngology–Head and Neck Surgery, Walter Reed Military Medical Center, 8901 Wisconsin Avenue, Bethesda, MD 20889, USA
* Corresponding author.
E-mail address: michelle.f.liu.mil@mail.mil

Otolaryngol Clin N Am 54 (2021) 239–245
https://doi.org/10.1016/j.otc.2020.09.018 oto.theclinics.com
0030-6665/21/Published by Elsevier Inc.

My stomach was instantly in knots. The back and forth of that conversation, as I tried desperately to figure out where this rumor came from, became more frustrating than helpful. I knew it had already worked through a grapevine more complicated than I could deal with. Just days later, there were more rumors that this classmate had filed a formal complaint.

BECOMING MINORITIZED

I grew up in a suburban town in Maryland, where now I consider myself fortunate to have attended school with plenty of other students and teachers that looked like me—Black. It wasn't until high school when I noticed always being one of the few Black students in my advanced classes. Then, in college, I was often the *only* Black person in the room at all. I realized then the comfort I had in earlier schooling was conditional. Although I missed the feeling of familiarity, I eventually grew unalarmed to strange looks I would receive, as though I was walking into the wrong class. "Maybe I just had something on my shirt," or "they weren't really staring at me, calm down, Candace." Deep down I knew the truth: I was seen as out of place.

By the time I attended medical school, though, I was a pro. I could let the looks brush off my shoulders, find meaningful friendships regardless of race, and stuck to the books like any good student would. Sure, I experienced microaggressions and implicit biases along the way, but I rarely spent energy on people or explanations I could tell would be a waste of time. "But, being articulate is a good thing," or "I only kid about Obama's birth certificate because we're rotating in Hawaii." People, always white, believed their compliments or jokes to be harmless. They were honestly surprised at my reactions because they were "not racist" and "taught not to see color." The dodgy excuses were endless, and I allowed a learned helplessness to stop me from saying anything more. It wasn't until my successful match into otolaryngology was dismissed as an unfair selection due to my race—a charity case—that I found both the words and the courage to confront what I had previously chosen to just let go.

Had I mistaken my entire interview season? I could remember being told by several attendings that I was competitive, and they'd even be happy to have me in their program. But now I sunk in my seat and let the whispers of those who didn't match, who had *never* been told "no" in their lives, linger. The feelings of confusion and anger were equally matched with, what I am now embarrassed to admit, immense anxiety and self-doubt. I was the *only* Black otolaryngology candidate in the military match at all during my application cycle... to think that I had felt unstoppable now felt shameful. It hurt to look in the mirror at someone who had been apologetically Black just to make it through medical school. No longer could I choose to ignore the subtle comments. The line was drawn.

CALLING OUT THE PROBLEM

The problem couldn't have been more obvious to me. Racism. Implicit bias. Microaggressions. Cultural incompetence. White privilege. The problem is my blackness can somehow be weaponized as cause for another's personal failure. Perceived as though I had traded in my "Black card" for academic success. The problem is privilege, whether conscious or subconscious, has taught the societal majority that they belong and are more deserving, even when it's simply not true. I was only one of nine applicants, with five others also successfully matching into otolaryngology, but singled out for the color of my skin.

For years, there has been a seemingly unattainable stereotype of the sorts of students that could match into otolaryngology: exceedingly high US Medical Licensing

Examination Step scores, acceptance into Alpha Omega Alpha, and multiple research activities and publications.[1] Although no combination of requirements has been proven to correlate to resident performance, otolaryngology still remains intimidatingly competitive . . . even for White colleagues. One can imagine how validating it felt to have made it into a residency program in the first place, but then to be labeled as undeserving left me wondering if it was possible to have truly "taken" a spot from someone else? I began pouring over the numbers, tables, and graphs that would prove two things: I *earned* my spot against the odds, and sadly, there's even less representation of minorities in otolaryngology than I imagined before this writing.

EXACTLY HOW MANY OTOLARYNGOLOGISTS LOOK LIKE ME?

In 2019, the Association of American Medical Colleges reported, "the growth of Black or African American [medical school] applicants, matriculants, and graduates lagged behind other groups."[2] Only 11.8% of medical school graduates from the 2018 to 2019 academic year (1 year ahead of my graduation) self-identified as Underrepresented in Medicine (URM; 6.2% Black or African American; 5.3% Hispanic, Latino, or of Spanish origin; 0.2% American Indian or Alaska Native; 0.1% Native Hawaiian or Other Pacific Islander).[3] Within the field of otolaryngology specifically, data from the 2019 to 2020 application cycle show that only 6.7% of applicants self-identified as URM (3.1% Black or African American; 3.6% Hispanic, Latino, or of Spanish origin; 0% American Indian or Alaska Native; 0% Native Hawaiian or Other Pacific Islander).[4]

Unfortunately, the annual growth rates of African American and American Indian otolaryngology residents have not been found statistically significant since 1975, according to Schwartz and colleagues[5] in 2013. Although Hispanic growth rates were statistically significant, they *still* did not match the overall US Hispanic population growth. In addition, an interesting survey study published in 2018 found that 37.5% of otolaryngology residency program directors admitted that there was matriculation of zero to one URM residents over a 15-year time period.[6] It's clear how the odds were not, and never have been, in my favor. To whomever might think my selection was based on race, give me a break. The pressure to prove myself and validate my existence in the otolaryngology community is an additional layer on top of an already hurtful narrative that URM candidates aren't deserving.

THE RIPPLE EFFECTS OF IMPLICIT BIAS

I don't share my story because it's unique. In fact, when venting to close friends and mentors, they *all* shared similar experiences—so-called 'lucky' to be Black. These stories of ours shine light on the bias and racism remaining deeply woven into our medical society.[7] I once thought of medicine as a field too academic, smart, and objective for these sorts of issues, but if anything, racial biases are only more difficult to address because they appear in dangerously subtle ways. Racially driven comments in academic settings are easy to miss or write off as nonproblematic, especially because they're coming from highly educated peers, co-residents, and teachers; these comments are coming from *doctors*. This begs a question that's been posed so many times before: what does this mean for our patients of color?

We have all heard of the health disparities existing in the US health care system, even after controlling for socioeconomic and insurance status.[8] We've also heard that Black patients are less likely to receive a narcotic prescription because their pain is often ignored,[9–12] or that Black mothers have an alarmingly higher maternal death rate than White mothers.[13–15] The same racial biases permeating self-proclaimed "diverse" medical schools, as in my experience, serve as the foundation from which health care providers learn what is acceptable treatment for patients based on the color of their skin. It's why I've seen Black patients get interrupted in the middle of sentences far more often than White patients, or why nurses and attendings can roll their eyes and say, "She's a complainer," when a Black woman asks questions during her weekly chemotherapy. For Black patients, sometimes the signs and symptoms don't determine the care they receive, and worse, their lives don't always seem to matter.

There are several reasons why race-concordant encounters between patients and their providers lead to better patient care: increased patient participation/satisfaction, more consistent visits, and strengthened trust in the health care system.[16] In my opinion, Black providers take more personal ownership of Black patients because too often it feels like no one else will. What our patients need, and what I need, is to know that medicine can be the safe space for equal treatment and respect I once thought it to be.

WHAT IS THE REAL NEXT STEP?

It's about time the medical community moves beyond lip service and gets serious about implicit bias and racism to address the ultimate impact they carry throughout the health care system. I can remember just *one* lecture during medical school on health disparities, and just *one* unsurprisingly uncomfortable reflective practice session on the topic of racism. We checked the boxes, went about our days, and remained right where we started. It's not surprising, then, that so many physicians remain culturally incompetent and/or insensitive. Existing literature on diversity suggests organizations start promoting diversity and inclusion as an institutional priority, or that some specialties, especially otolaryngology, should work to increase exposure throughout medical school curricula to enhance URM student recruitment.[5] Although these solutions are important measures to take, they don't address the underlying issue of bias.

No one will openly argue that diversity shouldn't be adopted as an organizational priority, but rather, it's within everyday conversations we realize shifting the culture begins with shifting individual mindsets. How can we do this? By mandating longitudinal curricula to (1) educate our health care providers on the topics of structural racism and implicit bias and (2) promote antiracist actions or behaviors. This sort of curriculum would not only advance cultural competency, but also over time lessen the awkward or uncomfortable posturing that ensues when discussing racial dynamics.

Hospital organizations should seek out URM candidates for leadership roles to bring more valuable opinions to the table, increase opportunities for sponsorship, and create new pipelines that will give longevity to URM leadership roles and representation. Individual residency programs or entire graduate medical education organizations institutions might also consider establishing a Diversity and Inclusion Council dedicated to incident resolution, outreach events within minority communities, and providing additional emotional support for URM residents and faculty. Having such a governing body would be bold, defining, and noticed; it would foster a greater sense of belonging for URM residents and relieve them of the "minority tax" (the assumed responsibility of minorities to solely create and sustain diversity efforts).[17]

The majority in society also needs to do more in their day-to-day lives, and not just in the workplace. Now is a *critical* moment to dedicate more time to learning and studying the history that shaped current societal inequities. Research unfamiliar terms (macroaggressions or microaggressions, implicit or unconscious bias, structural and cultural competency, antiracism, performative allyship, virtue signaling, and so forth), watch videos on these same terms, or read books delving into racial dynamics. Do not mistake a singular social media post, or a sympathetic text to your Black friend/colleague, as enough—it's not. These types of work are easy and temporary and often occur in moments when situations are so dire that it becomes "trendy" to speak up. People of color deserve more from White people, and progress is made only when our collective knowledge grows and allyship is consistent.

A HARD TRUTH TO FACE

The lesson I've learned is to stay engaged. Facing structural racism, microaggressions, and implicit bias laced within the fabric of the medical community will be far more frustrating at times than rewarding, but the work is worthwhile. Seemingly small, passive comments or actions are in fact the smouldering embers that allow biases to survive and thrive. Neither anyone else nor I can afford to avoid tough conversations anymore because enough is enough. To ignore opportunities to speak up is to ignore the ultimate impact biased opinions will have on the remainder of my education and training, and more importantly, on minority patients' health care. If my personal story does nothing else but rouse medical colleagues to question the state of racial dynamics in their institution or workplace, I'd consider that a win. There are similar stories that have come before this, and I'm sure there are more to come. If you're reading this and can relate, know that you're not alone. To everyone else, I ask you to move forward and become an ally first by keeping an open mind, knowing it is much less difficult than what your URM colleagues and friends battle against every day. Now is the time for all of us to choose to do better.
   –C.A.F.

THE WORK IS JUST BEGINNING—THE SPONSOR'S POINT OF VIEW

The truth is, meeting Dr. Flagg did more for me than she will ever know. Our brief conversation at a coffee shop to discuss her interest in otolaryngology was followed by several text messages and e-mails, and ultimately an invitation to her medical school graduation, which was virtual because of the coronavirus disease pandemic. The pride I had seeing her photo across the computer screen, one of eight African – American students in a class of 172, took me back to my own experience. Furthermore, when we met for the second time in person, she shared her distress concerning the discrediting rumors, and I empathized with her. Little did she know, that while I sat and listened, I was navigating my own experience of feeling isolated, devalued, and disheartened as a practicing otolaryngologist two decades her senior. Somehow, the timing was perfect; the opportunity to mentor and sponsor her reignited a spark that surgeons of all races experience when faced with the responsibility of fostering a bright, young clinician seeking guidance.

In a prospective study at Johns Hopkins University, financial assistance and faculty mentorship were provided to URM medical students during either a 3-month research clerkship or a 1-month clinical rotation, resulting in a favorable impact on their decision to apply for otolaryngology residency training. Furthermore, most students acquired at least 1 publication as a result of the rotation or clerkship; 46% of the URM students applied for otolaryngology residency, and 85% of those matched successfully.[18] Intentional and visible sponsorship for those URM has been demonstrated to be a characteristic of programs that attract students and uphold them as residents.

Although all sponsorship makes a difference in a residency experience, there is value in the presence of URM faculty to foster comfort, support, and feelings of belonging. Race alone is not the qualifier for a good sponsor. It is a teachable skill, and one that can be modeled. The intent to listen, to encourage, to share both vulnerability and curiosity, and to create psychological safety for all residents, URM in particular, is to take a step toward inclusivity. Not having a "blind eye" to the disparities in health care neither to the disproportionate faculty representation and selection of otolaryngology by URM students is another step. Finally, being bothered by the lack of increase in URM in otolaryngology should lead colleagues to support and collaborate, rather than question the qualifications of URM faculty and trainees, as both authors have unfortunately experienced firsthand. It's worth questioning why there are only 1% Black physicians specifically in otolaryngology nationwide and why similarly it is the medical specialty with the lowest representation of Black trainees,[19] disproportionate to the 12% of the national population constituted by African Americans. Our universal response should be one of intentional mentorship and sponsorship, which offers a double reward: inclusivity for both involved parties and the promise of better health care for all.

—M.L.F.

DISCLOSURE

The views expressed herein are those of the authors and do not reflect the official policy or position of Brooke Army Medical Center, Walter Reed National Military Medical Center, the US Army Medical Corps, the US Army Office of the Surgeon General, the Department of the Army, the Department of the Navy, the Department of Defense, the Defense Health Agency, or the US government. The authors have nothing to disclose.

REFERENCES

1. Bowe SN, Schmalbach CE, Laury AM. The state of the otolaryngology match: a review of applicant trends, "impossible" qualifications, and implications. Otolaryngol Head Neck Surg 2017;156(6):985–90.
2. AAMC. Diversity in medicine: facts and figures 2019. 2020. Available at: https://www.aamc.org/data-reports/workforce/report/diversity-medicine-facts-and-figures-2019. Accessed May 20, 2020.
3. AAMC. Figure 13. Percentage of U.S. medical school graduates by race/ethnicity (alone), academic year 2018-2019. 2019. Available at: https://www.aamc.org/data-reports/workforce/interactive-data/figure-13-percentage-us-medical-school-graduates-race/ethnicity-alone-academic-year-2018-2019. Accessed May 20, 2020.
4. AAMC. Table C-5. Residency applicants from U.S. MD-granting medical schools to ACGME-accredited programs by specialty and race/ethnicity, 2019-2020.
5. Schwartz JS, Young M, Velly AM, et al. The evolution of racial, ethnic, and gender diversity in US otolaryngology residency programs. Otolaryngol Head Neck Surg 2013;149(1):71–6.
6. Newsome H, Faucett EA, Chelius T, et al. Diversity in otolaryngology residency programs: a survey of otolaryngology program directors. Otolaryngol Head Neck Surg 2018;158(6):995–1001.
7. Evans MK, Rosenbaum L, Malina D, et al. Diagnosing and treating systemic racism. N Engl J Med 2020;383(3):274–6.
8. Smedley BD, Stith AY, Nelson AR. Unequal treatment: confronting racial and ethnic disparities. Washington, DC: The National Academies Press; 2003.
9. Narayan MC. Culture's effects on pain assessment and management. Am J Nurs 2010;110(4):38–47 [quiz: 48–9].
10. Anderson KO, Mendoza TR, Valero V, et al. Minority cancer patients and their providers: pain management attitudes and practice. Cancer 2000;88(8):1929–38.

11. Anderson KO, Green CR, Payne R. Racial and ethnic disparities in pain: causes and consequences of unequal care. J Pain 2009;10(12):1187–204.
12. Cintron A, Morrison RS. Pain and ethnicity in the United States: a systematic review. J Palliat Med 2006;9(6):1454–73.
13. Ozimek JA, Kilpatrick SJ. Maternal mortality in the twenty-first century. Obstet Gynecol Clin North Am 2018;45(2):175–86.
14. Howell EA, Egorova N, Balbierz A, et al. Black-white differences in severe maternal morbidity and site of care. Am J Obstet Gynecol 2016;214(1):122.e1-7.
15. Amankwaa LC, Records K, Kenner C, et al. African-American mothers' persistent excessive maternal death rates. Nurs Outlook 2018;66(3):316–8.
16. Cooper-Patrick L, Gallo JJ, Gonzales JJ, et al. Race, gender, and partnership in the patient-physician relationship. JAMA 1999;282(6):583–9.
17. Rodríguez JE, Campbell KM, Pololi LH. Addressing disparities in academic medicine: what of the minority tax? BMC Med Educ 2015;15(1):6.
18. Nellis JC, Eisele DW, Francis HW, et al. Impact of a mentored student clerkship on underrepresented minority diversity in otolaryngology–head and neck surgery. Laryngoscope 2016;126(12):2684–8.
19. Deville C, Hwang W-T, Burgos R, et al. Diversity in graduate medical education in the United States by race, ethnicity, and sex, 2012. JAMA Intern Med 2015;175(10):1706–8.

Moving?

Make sure your subscription moves with you!

To notify us of your new address, find your **Clinics Account Number** (located on your mailing label above your name), and contact customer service at:

Email: journalscustomerservice-usa@elsevier.com

800-654-2452 (subscribers in the U.S. & Canada)
314-447-8871 (subscribers outside of the U.S. & Canada)

Fax number: 314-447-8029

Elsevier Health Sciences Division
Subscription Customer Service
3251 Riverport Lane
Maryland Heights, MO 63043

*To ensure uninterrupted delivery of your subscription, please notify us at least 4 weeks in advance of move.

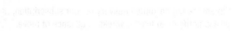

Printed and bound by CPI Group (UK) Ltd, Croydon, CR0 4YY

03/10/2024

01040405-0007